Statistics for Biology and Health

Series Editors

Mitchell Gail, Division of Cancer Epidemiology and Genetics, National Cancer Institute, Rockville, MD, USA

Jonathan M. Samet, Department of Epidemiology, School of Public Health, Johns Hopkins University, Baltimore, MD, USA

Statistics for Biology and Health (SBH) includes monographs and advanced textbooks on statistical topics relating to biostatistics, epidemiology, biology, and ecology.

More information about this series at http://www.springer.com/series/2848

Shahjahan Khan

Meta-Analysis

Methods for Health and Experimental Studies

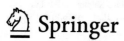 Springer

Shahjahan Khan
University of Southern Queensland
Toowoomba, QLD, Australia

ISSN 1431-8776   ISSN 2197-5671   (electronic)
Statistics for Biology and Health
ISBN 978-981-15-5034-8   ISBN 978-981-15-5032-4   (eBook)
https://doi.org/10.1007/978-981-15-5032-4

This Springer imprint is published by the registered company Springer Nature Singapore Pte Ltd.
The registered company address is: 152 Beach Road, #21-01/04 Gateway East, Singapore 189721, Singapore

This book is dedicated to my late parents Alhajj Moksudul Haque Khan and Zayeda Khatum. May their souls rest in heaven.

Shahjahan Khan

Preface

The main purpose of this book is to make meta-analysis easy for all researchers and users, especially for the students, health scientists, public health workers and nontechnical scholars who wish to perform meta-analysis and interpret the results for the first time. It simplifies all concepts, methods, computations and models related to meta-analysis through heuristic examples and illustrations using real-life data. It takes a step-by-step approach to performing meta-analyses using different statistical models for various effect size measures.

Evidence-based approach has been adopted in many areas of modern decision-making. It is more frequently used in all branches of the health sciences as well as in education, psychology and social sciences. The evidence-based decision-making primarily relies on the systematic reviews which often includes meta-analysis.

Meta-analysis is a very important component of many systematic reviews and is the best way to provide systematic review of quantitative data. It enables researchers to pool summary statistics/data of individual independent studies to synthesise the results for all the studies under investigation.

The idea of writing this book evolved from my efforts in preparing notes and making presentations in a series of workshops on statistical meta-analysis with applications in health sciences in Malaysia, Brunei, Japan and Bangladesh.

Effect Size

Meta-analyses are conducted on the summary data on various effect size measures that numerically evaluate the effectiveness of any intervention or treatment. In most studies, meta-analytic methods are used to estimate the unknown common population effect size. The effect size is the common name to a family of indices that measure the magnitude of a treatment or intervention effect. Depending on the type of study and the underlying outcome variables, there are various measures that can be used to determine the effect size for the intervention of interest.

If the underlying outcome variable is binary (or categorical with two arms), the effect size is measured by Relative Risk or Risk Ratio (RR) or Odds Ratio (OR) or simple proportion or difference of two proportions. If the outcome variable is continuous, the effect size is measured by Standardised Mean Difference (SMD) or Weighted Mean Difference (WMD). If the outcome of interest is the linear relationship between two quantitative variables, the correlation coefficient is the effect size measure.

Statistical Model

Every meta-analysis uses statistical models regardless of the effect size measure involved in the investigation. The oldest statistical model is the Fixed Effect (FE) model. This is applicable when effect size of interest is homogeneous across all studies, that is, there is no heterogeneity in the data, and variation among the observed effect size is only due to within studies random fluctuation attributable to chance causes. It also assumes that the random error (in the data) follows a normal distribution. To address the issue of heterogeneity, the Random Effects (REs) model is used. Under this model, the studies included in any investigations are considered to be a random sample from the population of all studies, and there is significant between-study variation along with the within-study variation. It assumes that both random error and treatment effect follow normal distribution. A more recent approach to tackle heterogeneity is the Inverse Variance Heterogeneity (IVhet) model that does not require any of the unrealistic assumptions of REs.

Meta-analysis is about estimating the common population effect size of all studies based on the observed data available from the selected primary studies. Normally point estimates (and standard deviations) of the common effect size observed from the individual studies are used to obtain the confidence intervals. The results produced by any meta-analysis are usually presented in a forest plot which is a scatterplot of 95% confidence intervals of the effect size of every individual studies, and that of the common effect size using the pooled/synthesised estimate.

In any specific investigation involving meta-analysis, the researcher requires to identify the type of outcome variable involved, decide appropriate effect size measure, select correct statistical model and then proceed to perform meta-analysis using preferred statistical software (e.g. MetaXL), and finally interpret the results produced by the meta-analytic methods.

Simplified Approach

This book simplifies meta-analytical methods by dedicating a chapter for each of the commonly used effect size measures such as RR, OR, SMD, WMD, etc. When any researcher identifies the effect size measure of interest, it is easy to go to the relevant chapter of the book to find all related concepts, methods and step-by-step guidance to perform meta-analysis.

The book uses a very easy to use free software as an add-on to MS Excel to demonstrate meta-analytical methods with real datasets. The MetaXL package is available for free download from Internet and comes with an Instruction Manual to guide the users to perform meta-analysis. For the benefit of the users, the book also provides Stata codes to perform meta-analysis on each of the popularly known effect size measures.

The Contents Covered

Chapter 1 introduces the systematic review as a general premise of synthesising independent studies within the framework of evidence-based decision-making. The second chapter discusses elementary concepts related to meta-analysis along with introducing some issues and statistical fundamentals. These two chapters form Part I of the book.

Part II of the book consists of three chapters on general introduction to the relevant concepts, definitions, illustrations and interpretation of effect size measures for binary outcomes of two arms studies. Chapter 3 introduces the relative risk or risk ratio and odds ratio. Chapter 4 covers meta-analysis of Relative Risk (RR) with illustrative examples including construction of forest plot using MetaXl under different statistical models and interpretation of results. Similar contents on odds ratio (OR) are provided in Chap. 5. Subgroup analysis and detection of publications bias (details in Chapter 2) using funnel plot and Doi plot are briefly introduced in these chapters. The one proportion problem is covered in Chap. 6, and the risk difference in Chap. 7.

The meta-analytic methods for continuous outcome variables are covered in Part III which includes Standardised Mean Difference (SMD) in Chap. 8, Weighted Mean Difference (WMD) in Chap. 9 and correlation coefficient in Chap. 10.

Part IV includes special topics in meta-analysis, namely, Meta-regression in Chap. 11, Publication bias in Chap. 12, and Dose-response meta-analysis in Chap. 13.

Words of Thanks

I am grateful to the School of Sciences; Faculty of Health, Engineering and Sciences; University of Southern Queensland, Australia for allowing me leave to prepare and finalise the manuscript of the book.

Finally, I must thank my late parents who cared and sacrificed so much to ensure my high quality education; dedicated wife Anarkali L Nahar for her patience and continuing support; and proud sons Imran, Adnun and Albab; daughters-in-law, Naafiya, Farhana and Anika, and lovely grandchildren Zara, Zayena, Aydin, Aarib and Esme for their inspiration.

Toowoomba, Australia

Shahjahan Khan

Acknowledgements

I am grateful to my co-contributor Prof. Suhail A. R. Doi, Qatar University, Qatar for his contribution and professional involvement throughout the period of preparing/finalising the proposal and writing the manuscript of the book. The great contribution of his students/colleagues, Dr. Luis Furuya-Kanamori (Chap. 12), Australian National University, Australia and Dr. Chang Xu, Department of population medicine, Qatar University (Chaps. 11 and 13) in preparing the final part of the book is highly acknowledged.

I sincerely thank Dr. Md. Mizanur Rahman, Department of Global Public Health Policy, Tokyo University, Japan, and Professor Muhammed Ashraf Memon, School of Medicine, University of Queensland, Australia for reading a number of chapters of the draft manuscript and providing detailed feedback to improve the contents and presentation of the book. Special thanks to Dr. Luis Furuya-Kanamori of Australian National University, Australia, and Dr. Md. Shafiur Rahman, Department of Global Public Health Policy, Tokyo University, Japan for helping with the Stata codes.

I am indebted to my research partner Dr. M. A. Memon, University of Queensland, Australia for inviting me to work on meta-analysis when he migrated to Australia from the UK in 2007 and introducing me to the area, and to my former Ph.D. student, Dr. Rossita M. Yunus, Institute of Mathematical Sciences, University of Malaya, Malaysia for providing computational support as a co-author in many of our high impact research publications.

My sincere gratitude to late Prof. M. Safiul Haq, University of Western Ontario, Canada and Emeritus Prof. A. K. Md. Ehsanes Saleh, Carleton University, Canada for teaching me research and inspiring me to achieve excellence in research.

I am indebted to Jahangirnagar University, Bangladesh and University of Western Ontario, Canada for providing me higher education in statistics, and Institute of Statistical Research and Training (ISRT), University of Dhaka, Bangladesh for enabling me to start my academic career.

Contents

Part I
Introduction to Systematic Review and Meta-Analysis

Chapter 1
Introduction to Systematic Review

In the era of evidence-based decision-making systematic reviews and meta-analyses are being widely used in many medical practices, public health departments, government programs, business offices, and academic disciplines including education and psychology. Obviously, not everyone involved in the evidence-based decision-making is evidence-informed, and aware of the various levels and/or quality of the evidence as well as the issues that directly impact on the validity and trustworthiness of the results. Research synthesis is an essential part of evidence-based decision-making.

1.1 Introduction to Evidence-Based Decision-Making

The world is increasingly moving towards evidence-based decision-making due to its proven ability to guide practitioners and policy makers to find out which interventions or methods or programs work effectively and which don't. It enables decision-making on programs, methods, interventions, treatments, practices, or policies based on the best available evidence in the form of historical record, experiential outcome, relevant data, contextual understanding and discipline knowledge. The main emphasis is to find out the method or procedure that has produced expected and reliable results and delivered the targeted outcome. The decision-makers use evidence to decide which method/intervention works the best to achieve the objectives, and avoid the ones that are ineffective. Thus the effectiveness of the evidence-based decisions directly depend on the quality of the evidence and it is crucial to be evidence-informed, that is, the decision-makers must be aware of the factors that impact on the quality of evidence along with any shortcomings in the process of gathering, processing and presenting evidence.

© Springer Nature Singapore Pte Ltd. 2020
S. Khan, *Meta-Analysis*, Statistics for Biology and Health,
https://doi.org/10.1007/978-981-15-5032-4_1

Although evidence-based decision-making originated and has been frequently used in medical procedures and health sciences, it is also used in a wide range of areas including agriculture, education, management, business, psychology, and social sciences. Obviously the validity of overall evidence, and hence the decisions based on them, are directly dependent on the quality of the underlying sources of evidence and the methodology employed to extract and process them. Hence the quality of evidence is crucial to any good evidence-based decision-making.

In an article (Breckon 2016) states that the policy-makers often pay lip-service to the idea of basing decisions on available evidence, but anyone who has ever tried to get evidence listened to and acted upon knows how hard it can be to achieve cut-through. What, then, are the best ways for getting research used by public decision-makers? It is hard to know when there are so many approaches to choose from. A recent review, conducted by the Evidence for Policy and Practice Information and Co-ordinating Centre (EPPI-Centre) at University College London, counted 150 different techniques in all. This article cited the recent work of (Langer et al. 2016) to summarise the grouping of the above techniques used to form evidences into six categories: Awareness, Agree, Access and communication, Interact, Skills, and Structure and process.

1.2   Gathering Research Data

Gathering of research data is a crucial first part of any systematic review, and research synthesis is the foundation of evidence-based decision-making. Evidence from different sources on a specific research question or topic of interest is gathered and analysed using systematic review methodologies. This is followed by the combination of quantitative study outcomes from independent studies to find an estimate of the synthesized outcome representing the unknown population parameter of interest—a process known as meta-analysis. The strict implementation, assessment and monitoring of the underlying selection and exclusion criteria, study protocol and quality assessment ensure that the results of the synthesis are reproducible.

Gathering and reviewing data systematically is called the systematic review whose first step is to identify studies that satisfy the predetermined inclusion criteria, and extract the relevant summary statistics from the selected studies adhering to agreed review procedures and protocols. Meta-analysis, on the other hand, is the quantitative part of the synthesis and enables us to arrive at a numerical summary of results (discussed in detail in other chapters).

The quality of the results produced through research synthesis depends on the quality of the studies and their design. If the selected studies are of high quality, then the results constitute the highest level of evidence. However, there are genuine issues related to such syntheses that directly impact on the quality of the final result. It is absolutely essential that policy-makers, and the producers and end users of such syntheses are aware of the weaknesses and strengths of the underlying processes and techniques so that they could assess the robustness of their results. This chapter introduces some basic concepts and methods in research synthesis and critically examines the strengths and weaknesses of the technique to provide insightful guidance to help professionals who are engaged in evidence-based decision-making.

Introduction of research synthesis in the process of the evidence-based decision-making is a milestone to avoid selection bias, achieve consistency and maintain high quality in assessing the studies with uniform standard. A number of rigorous systems with specific selection criteria have been introduced to improve the systematic reviews to achieve repeatability or reproducibility of studies. The statistical meta-analysis is the key to synthesise quantitative summary data from independent studies to estimate the common effect size (Khan et al. 2016).

1.3 Essentials of the Systematic Review

In a general term, the synthesis starts off with a systematic review which is a process of searching, gathering and investigating the literature on a specific topic to identify, select and analyse any evidence of interest. It is rigorous and comprehensive to make it transparent, minimise bias and enable future replicability. In the past, narrative reviews were used to assess evidence and was conducted by key leaders in the field on broad topics in some informal, unsystematic and subjective ways. Since the narrative reviews are conducted by individuals there is a very high chance of personal bias in the conclusion or evidence even if the authors are expert in the area. Narrative reviews are normally not objective in assessing the literature and evidence, and hence not replicable. The systematic review, on the other hand, is an attempt to objectively identify all the relevant literature with a view to selecting studies based on specific criteria, collect the documents, review their contents and critically analyse them to assess the underlying evidence. This kind of review is objective and free from personal bias or preferences. Khan et al. (2003) describes five different steps in performing a systematic review to ensure its objectivity.

1.3.1 Steps in Systematic Reviews

Systematic reviews must be comprehensive, exhaustive and meet the expectation of reproducibility. To ensure these key characteristics, the following five steps have been suggested: (1) Framing the research or study questions for the intended review, (2) identifying all relevant work in the published and unpublished literature, (3) assessing the quality of studies, (4) extracting and summarizing the evidence, and (5) interpreting the findings.

There are studies, including (Yannascoli et al. 2013), that provide comprehensive summary of the steps in conducting good quality systematic reviews. In spite of some differences in the details, the key steps in any systematic review literature are about the same. Readers may find a recent study by Memon et al. (2020) useful.

Any systematic review should start with good planning and agreed strategies to implement the plan focused to addressing the research question. The research team requires agreement on the list of tasks and the strartegies to handle any foreseeable problems to be addressed. The team should decide on an agreed list of what to be done, who will do what, how the tasks will be distributed/managed, and under what timeframe they will work. The distribution of the tasks to the members of the team and any back-up arrangements should also be a part of the planning. The successful implementation of the planning would require regular monitoring, assessment and review of the progress and adjustment in any areas of the review.

To implement any systematic review, formation of a research team comprising of experts from all relevant areas covering the study topic is the first step.

(a) **Reasons for the study**

The research team must clearly specify and agree on the reasons for the study as these are the driving force for any systematic reviews. The team must be fully aware and convinced of the reasons behind the proposed review and why the study is important. If the reasons behind any systematic review are not convincing and strong and the potential outcomes are not important it may not be worth spending time and resources. The stronger the reasons for the review, the firmer will be the commitment of the members of the research team and better will be the quality of the outcome. It is essential to keep in mind that the expected contribution of the review to the existing literature and how to minimize, if not eliminate any review bias to make it reproducible.

(b) **Research question**

One of the very first and key issues the research team must address is the formulation of the research question. This requires initial literature review to check if the research question to be investigated has already been addressed by others, and if there are enough accessible materials to answer the research question. Once determined, research question is the key driver of the review. All the planning considerations and activities will be centred around the research question. The review team must critically discuss the appropriateness of the research question, its importance and validity, and how to address it with the available literature relevant to the problem.

(c) **Inclusion and exclusion criteria**

Strict inclusion and exclusion criteria to be laid down at the outset of gathering research data to determine which identified studies to be included in the review are essential to avoid personal or selection bias in selecting studies identified by literature search. The specific conditions and protocols to select studies or articles in the proposed review should be explicitly stated before searching databases. There are many considerations that could potentially impact on the inclusion/exclusion criteria but the most relevant ones (e.g., study period, study type/design, RCTs, language, outcome measures) must be clearly stated and implemented throughout the searching process of the review.

1.4   Literature Search—Strategies, Terms, and Databases

Extensive and comprehensive search of all literature relevant to the research question are undertaken to identify and collect all materials pertaining to the review. Search should be inclusive of all published and unpublished studies in any language and from any country. Before embarking on the search, the team must prepare a search strategy, list the relevant databases and appropriate search engines, create access account to databases (e.g. PubMed, Cochrane, EMBASE, Medline, ISI etc. for health/medical studies), if needed. Study time period should be specified for the search to reflect that only the studies conducted within the relevant period are considered for the review. During the search all different combinations of the key/technical words, phrases and terms as well as their all possible combinations related to the topic of interest must be included using all available search engines. The search should be extended to all major languages to make sure that the publications in non-English languages are fully covered. It is important to record the search date to note the cut-off date up to which the review entries are included from a particular database.

(a)   **Reviewing the search outcomes—independent search**

At least two members of the review team should conduct independent searches in all relevant databases and resources taking into account both electronic and paper version of the materials, and then reconcile the information gathered independently by members of the team from the identified studies. If needed, a third reviewer may be engaged to reach agreement on the selection of any disputed studies. Any limitations or weaknesses of the search should be documented and included in the review report.

At the first stage, the selection of studies is based on the checking the title/heading of the articles by the independent reviewers. The studies selected at the first stage are then critically analysed and checked based on the abstract to decide next stage of selection. The full-text review is then conducted on the studies selected in the second stage. Thus the identified studies could be excluded in several stages (title, abstract, full-text) based on the selection and exclusion criteria.

The list of references or bibliographies of the items selected by full-text checking should be reviewed to identify any additional studies on the topic of interest. The same search, review, and checking processes and stages should be applied to any studies identified during this reference search stage to decide on their inclusion/exclusion. Use of platforms such as Rayyan (rayyan.qcri.org) and Endnote should be considered when selecting studies for inclusion/exclusion.

(b)   Collection of studies and extraction of data

Once the members of the team who are responsible to conduct the search independently identify the articles/studies to be included in the systematic review all related documents, and records including full-text article, must be collected and listed for review and record. A well-documented summary of key information on each study may help conduct the review in a systematic and orderly way. The analytical and critical review of these documents would lead to the review report and ultimate evidence to address the research question.

Data extraction from the included study documents is the next step. Data on the items of interest should be independently collected on a spreadsheet in a predetermined format. The format should allow sufficient flexibility to accommodate variation as different author may report the data in different format or scale or unit. It may be a good idea to pilot the data extraction sheet with a subset of the studies to make sure that the format is robust enough to deal with the diversities, if any. Data extraction should be conducted by at least two independent reviewers. The data from independent studies should be compared item by item, and agreement should be reached on the final figures before embarking on the analyses of the data. In case of any dispute/disagreement a third reviewer or an expert in the field should be called to make the final choice.

For the better management of resources all relevant documents from the selected studies may be saved in a separate folder with a back-up copy in a separate device. Referencing softwares such as EndNote are invaluable to keep track of all documents and make referencing easy and handy. In case of any missing or confusing data, the authors of the relevant articles should be contacted for clarification or requesting the missing information.

1.4.1   Reporting a Flow-Chart for Study Selection

Here is an example of reporting flowchart of selecting studies for the systematic review of D1 versus D2 gastrectomy for gastric adenocarcinoma (cf. Memon et al. 2011). In this study the initial search resulted in 29 records, but finally only 6 of them satisfied the inclusion critera and were included in the meta-analysis (Fig. 1.1).

If any other team of researchers were doing the same systematic review and meta-analysis independently they should be reporting exactly the same flowchart up till date of the search. This is because every systematic review must be reproducible.

1.5   Levels of Evidence

Not every type of study provides the same level of evidence. The level of evidence in any systematic review depends on the design of the primary studies. Often the

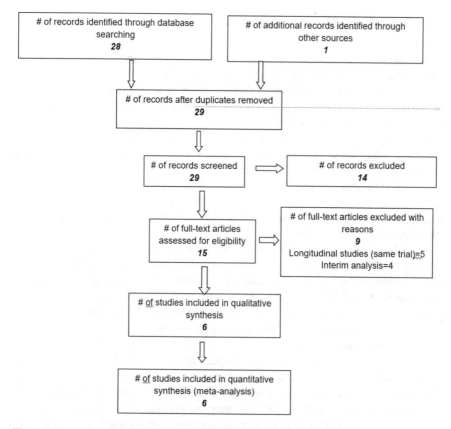

Fig. 1.1 Flow chart providing information through the different phases of study selection

research question of the investigation determines the choice of study design. The primary studies provide the original data and analysis for the research synthesis. An example of a primary literature source is a peer-reviewed research article. Other primary sources include preprints, theses, reports and conference proceedings.

The level of evidence from primary sources are broadly categorised based on the study design as follows (highest to lowest):

(a) Experimental: Randomised or non-randomised controlled trials
(b) Quasi-experimental studies (such as before-and-after study, interrupted time series)
(c) Observational analytic studies (e.g. cohort study, case-control study).

More detailed rating (highest to lowest) of level of evidence for quantitative questions in the healthcare studies is found in (Melnyk and Fineout-Overholt 2011).

1.6   Assessing Quality of Studies

The quality of the selected studies that meet inclusion criteria in the systematic review directly impact on the quality of evidence produced by the review.

By quality we mean the internal validity of the studies. *Internal validity* is the extent to which the analytic study is free from systematic errors and any difference between interventions is therefore only due to the intervention of interest. The internal validity is threatened by the methodological errors and varieties of biases such as selection, information and confounding biases. Depending on the type of study, scholars/experts have suggested different tools to improve study quality. There are more than a hundred such tools, and sometimes classified by study design. In addition, checklists exist to ensure the reporting protocol for the systematic reviews. The most popular and frequently used tools for assessing quality of primary studies are summarised in the next section.

The Meta-analysis Of Observational Studies in Epidemiology (MOOSE) group (Moher et al. 2000) proposed a checklist containing specifications for reporting of meta-analyses of observational studies. On the other hand the Preferred Reporting Items for Systematic review and Meta-Analysis Protocols (Moher et al. 2009) was published in 2015 aiming to facilitate the development and reporting of systematic review protocols that can be adopted for randomised controlled trials.

There are several measures of study quality in the literature. One old measure to assess the quality of studies to be included in meta-analysis that are based on the randomised controlled trials is the Jadad score (Jadad et al. 1996). This score is also known as the Oxford Quality Scoring System which ranges from zero to five, zero being the lowest quality and five being the highest achievable quality based on reporting of randomization, blinding, and withdrawals reported during the study period.

In qualitative syntheses, researchers stop at the systematic review stage and the information from independent studies selected by systematic search addresses the findings without conducting meta-analysis. However, in quantitative syntheses, numerical data from the selected studies are pooled through meta-analysis. In both cases the synthesis must be based on all the trials/studies, both published and unpublished, selected via a comprehensive literature search. A general perception is that the quality of meta-analysis is of the highest level if the study is based on independent randomised controlled trials (RCTs).

1.6.1   Tools for Assessing Study Quality

To make sure that the evidence is of high quality various tools have been suggested to assess the quality of the study. Researchers have been continuously trying to come up with safeguards against biases and design flaws of the individual studies. These safeguards comprise the tools against which studies are assessed. A brief summary of some key tools are discussed below.

QUOROM   The Quality of Reporting of Meta-analyses (QUOROM) addresses standards for improving the quality of reporting of meta-analyses of clinical randomised controlled trials (RCTs) was proposed by Moher et al. (1999). The QUOROM document consists of statements, a checklist, and a flow diagram. The checklist describes the preferred way to present the abstract, introduction, methods, results, and discussion sections of a report of a meta-analysis. The flow diagram provides information about both the numbers of RCTs identified, included and excluded, and the reasons for exclusion of trials.

CONSORT   Consolidated Standards of Reporting Trials encompasses various initiatives developed by the CONSORT Group (Moher et al. 2012) to deal with the problems arising from inadequate reporting of randomized controlled trials (RCT). The CONSORT Statement consists of a minimum set of recommendations for reporting randomized trials. It offers a standard way for authors to prepare reports of trial findings, facilitating their complete and transparent reporting, and aiding their critical appraisal and interpretation.

PRISMA   Preferred Reporting Items for Systematic Reviews and Meta-Analyses (PRISMA) is an evidence-based minimum set of items for reporting in systematic reviews and meta-analyses (Moher et al. 2009). PRISMA team focuses on the reporting of reviews evaluating randomized trials, but can also be used as a basis for reporting systematic reviews of other types of research, particularly evaluations of interventions.

PRISMA-P   Preferred Reporting Items for Systematic Review and Meta-Analysis Protocols (Moher et al. 2015) aiming to facilitate the development and reporting of systematic review protocols.

MOOSE   The Meta-analysis Of Observational Studies in Epidemiology (MOOSE) group (Stroup et al. 2000) proposed a checklist containing specifications for reporting of meta-analyses of observational studies in epidemiology, including background, search strategy, methods, results, discussion, and conclusion. Use of the checklist should improve the usefulness of meta-analyses for authors, reviewers, editors, readers, and decision makers.

ROBINS-I   Risk Of Bias In Non-randomised Studies of Interventions (ROBINS-I) proposed by Sterne et al. (2016) is a new tool for evaluating risk of bias in estimates of the comparative effectiveness (harm or benefit) of interventions from studies that did not use randomisation to allocate units (individuals or clusters of individuals) to comparison groups. The tool is particularly useful to those undertaking systematic reviews that include non-randomised studies.

The main aim of all these processes and protocols is to make the systematic review as objective as possible by removing potential bias from all possible sources to ensure high level of evidence. Needless to say that the success of these protocols depends on the strict adherence to the criteria throughout the systematic review.

1.7   Concluding Remarks

It is inevitable that more and more decision-makers and organisations will be using systematic reviews and meta-analyses as the practice of evidence-based decision-making continues to grow wider. It is essential that everyone involved in the evidence-based decision-making be evidence-informed so that they could evaluate the studies for inclusion and their quality so that any recommendations by any systematic review can be viewed in the context of their overall study quality. The research team must be well-skilled to decide on what should and should not be included strictly following the agreed procedure and criteria as well as meeting the underlying assumptions and satisfying the technical requirements. In case of disagreement/dispute, expert opinion, past experience and discipline knowledge will be a useful guide for the research team.

References

Breckon J (2016) Evidence base for evidence-informed policy. Significance Mag 13:12–13

Jadad AR, Moore RA, Carroll D, Jenkinson C, Reynolds DJM, Gavaghan DJ, McQuay HJ (1996) Assessing the quality of reports of randomized clinical trials: is blinding necessary? Control Clin Trials 17(1):1–12

Khan KS, Kunz R, Kleijnen J, Antes G (2003) Five steps to conducting a systematic review. J R Soc Med 96(3):118–121

Khan S, Doi SAR, Memon MA (2016) Evidence based decision and meta-analysis with applications in cancer research studies. Appl Math Inf Sci 10(3):1–8

Langer L, Tripney J, Gough DA (2016) The science of using science: researching the use of research evidence in decision-making. UCL Institute of Education, EPPI-Centre

Melnyk BM, Fineout-Overholt E (2011) Evidence-based practice in nursing & healthcare: a guide to best practice. Lippincott Williams & Wilkins

Memon MA, Subramanya MS, Khan S, Hossain MB, Osland E, Memon B (2011) Meta-analysis of D1 versus D2 gastrectomy for gastric adenocarcinoma. Ann Surg 253(5):900–911. https://doi.org/10.1097/SLA.0b013e318212bff6

Memon MA., Khan S, Alam K, Rahman MM, Yunus RM (2020) Systematic REviews: Understanding the Best Evidences for clinical Decision-making in Health care: Pros adnd COns, Surgical Laparoscopy, Endoscopy & Percutaneous Techniques.

Moher D, Cook DJ, Eastwood S, Olkin I, Rennie D, Stroup DF (1999) Improving the quality of reports of meta-analyses of randomised controlled trials: the QUOROM statement. Quality of reporting of meta-analyses. Lancet 354(9193):1896–1900

Moher D, Cook DJ, Eastwood S, Olkin I, Rennie D, Stroup DF (2000) Improving the quality of reports of meta-analyses of randomised controlled trials: the QUOROM statement. Oncol Res Treat 23(6):597–602

Moher D, Liberati A, Tetzlaff J, Altman DG (2009) Preferred reporting items for systematic reviews and meta-analyses: the PRISMA statement. Ann Intern Med 151(4):264–269

Moher D, Hopewell S, Schulz KF, Montori V, Gøtzsche PC, Devereaux P, Altman DG (2012) CONSORT 2010 explanation and elaboration: updated guidelines for reporting parallel group randomised trials. Int J Surg 10(1):28–55

Moher D, Shamseer L, Clarke M, Ghersi D, Liberati A, Petticrew M, Stewart LA (2015) Preferred reporting items for systematic review and meta-analysis protocols (PRISMA-P) 2015 statement. Syst Rev 4:1

Sterne JA, Hernán MA, Reeves BC, Savović J, Berkman ND, Viswanathan M, Boutron I (2016) ROBINS-I: a tool for assessing risk of bias in non-randomised studies of interventions. BMJ 355:i4919

Stroup DF, Berlin JA, Morton SC, Olkin I, Williamson GD, Rennie D, Moher D, Becker BJ, Sipe TA, Thacker SB (2000) Meta-analysis of observational studies in epidemiology: a proposal for reporting. Meta-analysis of observational studies in epidemiology (MOOSE) group. JAMA 283(15):2008–2012

Yannascoli SM, Schenker ML, Carey JL, Ahn J, Baldwin KD (2013) How to write a systematic review: a step-by-step guide. Univ Pennsylvania Orthop J 23:64–69

Chapter 2
Introduction to Meta-analysis

Meta-analysis is a statistical method used to combine numerical summary results on effect size measures, extracted during the systematic review process from independent studies to synthesize a pooled result. The synthesis of a summary statistic from aggregate data in all available independent trials/studies is achieved by pooling them to find an estimate of the unknown population effect size. Meta-analysis enables us to arrive at a better estimate of the population effect size (parameter) compared to that reported in individual studies especially when results of independent studies are conflicting.

Like the systematic review, the quality of the studies is important for the robustness of results produced by meta-analyses. If the selected studies are of high quality, and the meta-analysis is appropriately conducted, then the results constitute the highest level of evidence. However, there are genuine issues related to meta-analyses that directly impact on the robustness of the final results. As a result, it is incumbent on the policy-makers, and the producers and end users of meta-analyses, to be aware of the weaknesses and strengths of the underlying processes and techniques of meta-analysis. In this chapter we introduce the fundamental concepts and different methods used in meta-analysis. We also critically examine the pros and cons of the different methods to provide insightful guidance to help professionals who are engaged in evidence-based decision-making via meta-analysis.

2.1 The Effect Size in Meta-analysis

In a systematic review we may extract numeric or quantitative data on a specific intervention from the selected independent studies. Often these are aggregate summary statistics (e.g. mean and standard deviation for continuous outcome variables and odds/risk ratios for binary/categorical outcome variables) as measures of an underlying effect size. These effect sizes are calculated based on the sample data in different primary studies as estimates of the unknown common population effect size. Unfortunately, the sample effect size differs from study to study and the study-specific

© Springer Nature Singapore Pte Ltd. 2020
S. Khan, *Meta-Analysis*, Statistics for Biology and Health,
https://doi.org/10.1007/978-981-15-5032-4_2

values of the estimated effect size are not only different but also may have opposite direction (sign), producing conflicting results and misleading evidence. In the face of inconclusive or conflicting evidence from different primary studies, the challenge is to reconcile the results to come up with a single valid estimate of the population effect size. In other words, it is about pooling the summary effects from different selected studies to estimate a common effect size. This is where the statistical meta-analytical methods are essential to combine the evidence from independent primary studies.

If the raw data (e.g. individual patient data) from all selected studies are available then one could analyse the individual-patient-data (IPD) using mega-analysis methods. Unfortunately, in reality, it is almost impossible to access the raw data from different authors, and hence almost universally evidence is computed from the summary results or statistics via aggregate meta-analysis methods.

Due to the increased use of evidence-based decision-making the application of meta-analysis has become more widespread (Khan and Doi 2015). This increased demand for meta-analysis has also attracted statisticians to come forward in addressing the statistical issues related to the current methods and come up with new methods to deal with the existing and emerging complexities to improve the quality of meta-analysis. See http://www.statsoc.org.au/general/statistical-meta-ana lysis-potential-for-new-research-opportunities/.

The forest plot

A common way to represent the results of meta-analyses is via a graph called the forest plot. This graph shows the confidence intervals on the unknown effect size based on the estimates of the individual studies and the pooled estimate on the same chart. A forest plot contains a plot of confidence intervals of the effect size against the study identifier. A typical forest plot of risk ratio (RR) is presented in Fig. 2.1.

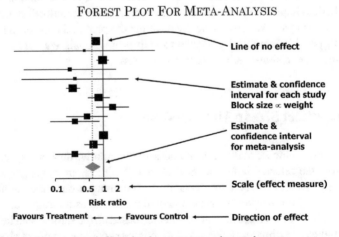

Fig. 2.1 A typical forest plot of effect size for treatment and control groups

Explanations of Forest Plot

A forest plot is a graph of 95% confidence intervals (horizontal lines bounded by the limits) of population effect size against the study identifier of each primary study separately and their synthesis (as meta-analysis) along with two vertical lines representing no-effect (black solid line at RR = 1) and point estimate of the pooled effect (dotted line through the middle of the diamond).

The point estimate of the effect size of each primary study is indicated by the middle most point of the respective black square. The size/area of the square represents the relative weight of the individual studies in the meta-analysis. The length of the horizontal lines on both sides of the black square represent the width of the 95% confidence interval.

The diamond near the bottom of the graph represents the 95% confidence interval and the point estimate for population effect size calculated by pooling results from all individual studies. The middle most point of the diamond represents the pooled point estimate of the population effect size and the two pointed horizontal ends represent the limits of the 95% confidence interval for the common effect size.

The measurement scale of the effect size is represented by the horizontal axis at the bottom of the forest plot. The values of the estimated effect size to the left side of the no-effect vertical line (at RR = 1 here) favours the treatment and the right side favours the control. If the diamond touches (or crosses) the no-effect vertical line then the treatment is not significant (at the 5% level of significance).

In a primary study each subject or patient is the study unit from which data is collected. But in meta-analysis each study/trial is the study unit, and the summary statistics come from study-level results/data.

2.2 Statistical Background for Meta-analysis

Meta-analysis is conducted based on a number of statistical methods and models. It uses summary statistics from independent studies as the data to synthesize the results from primary studies. It also contains results of statistical hypothesis test. Hence basic knowledge of statistical inference—estimation and test—are essential for the understanding and interpretation of results produced by meta-analyses.

In every meta-analyses, the interest is to estimate the common population effect size of an intervention—outcome association through the effect size (e.g. mean difference). Apart from the understanding of some elementary statistical concepts and descriptive statistics meta-analyses involve inferential statistics, estimation of parameters and test of hypotheses. The most commonly used statistical concepts, methods and techniques are covered below.

2.2.1 Basic Statistical Concepts

In statistics, the collection of all elements, items, cases or subjects on which an outcome variable is measured is called a *population*. Any numerical characteristic of a population of an outcome variable is called a *parameter*. For example, population mean (μ) and standard deviation (σ) are parameters. Often the word population refers to the distribution of a random or outcome variable, and the underlying parameters of the distribution specify the population. The parameters are often unknown and are estimated from sample data.

A *sample* is a representative part of a population that retains the characteristics of the population. This requires the samples to be randomly selected so that every elements in the population has equal chance to be included in the sample. Results from any non-random sample are usually biased and can't be extended beyond the observed data and hence it is of no use for any inferences.

Any function (e.g. sum) of a random sample from an outcome variable is called a statistic or *estimator* which is used to estimate a related unknown parameter. An estimator or a statistic (e.g. formula for sample mean) is a *rule* that is used to calculate any characteristic of the sample data.

For example, if Y (emphasis is on upper case Y) is an outcome variable with population mean μ, then based on a random sample of size n, from the population Y, the statistic $\bar{Y} = (Y_1 + Y_2 + \ldots + Y_n)/n$ (uppercase Y's) sets up the *rule* that instructs one to 'add all the sample realizations and divide the sum by the number of values'. This statistic (sample mean) is often used as an estimator of the population mean μ. Any numerical quantity calculated from an observed sample is a realized (and hence known) value of a statistic or estimator. This is called an *estimate* (a fixed quantity). For example, if (y_1, y_2, …, y_n) represents the values of n sample obsevations from the population Y then the observed value of $\bar{Y}$ becomes $\bar{y}$ $= (y_1 + y_2 + \ldots + y_n)/n$ (lowercase y's) which is an estimate of the population mean μ. Note that the uppercase letters represent random variables and its function is also a random variable (or estimator), whereas the lowercase letters represent fixed values and its function is an estimate. So, $\bar{Y}$ is a random variable (estimator) and it follows a distribution. But its observed value $\bar{y}$ is a fixed value (and is a point estimate).

Since any estimator or statistic is a random variable it has a distribution, and its distribution is called the *sampling distribution*. If an outcome variable Y follows a normal distribution with mean $\mu_Y = \mu$ and *standard deviation* $\sigma_Y = \sigma$, then for a random sample of size n, the statistic $\bar{Y}$ also follows a normal distribution with mean $\mu_{\bar{Y}} = \mu$ and *standard deviation* $\sigma_{\bar{Y}} = \sigma/\sqrt{n}$. Clearly the spread (variability) of the sampling distribution of $\bar{Y}$ becomes smaller as the sample size *n* grows larger. Note that the sample standard deviation of an estimator or statistic is called *standard error*. If the population standard deviation of the variable Y, σ is estimated by the sample standard deviation s (that is, $\hat{\sigma} = s$) based on a random sample of size n, then the estimated standard deviation, that is, *standard error* of $\bar{Y}$ is $\hat{\sigma}_{\bar{Y}} = s/\sqrt{n}$.

2.2.2   Confidence Interval (CI)

Confidence intervals are used to estimate unknown parameters (e.g. mean, μ) using the sample data. Every confidence interval has a confidence level, usually $(1 - \alpha) \times 100\%$ (and for $\alpha = 0.05$ the confidence level becomes 95%). The level of confidence impacts on the critical value of the underlying sampling distribution such as the z-score. Higher the level of confidence, larger is the critical value such as the z-score.

If the population mean μ of an outcome variable Y is estimated by the sample mean $\bar{Y}$ then the later is a point estimate of μ. As you may imagine (in repeated sampling of the same sample size from the same population) the sample mean changes from one sample to another, and it is unlikely that any of the sample means would be exactly the same as the population mean μ. But as the sample size increases the sample mean is likely to be closer to the population mean. However, any point estimate is uncertain and does not best represent the population parameter.

An interval estimate, such as confidence interval (CI), is often preferred over a point estimate as the CI provides a range of likely values of the parameter (within the lower and upper limits) with an associated confidence level (usually 95%). In most of the meta-analyses the confidence interval is about a parameter (population effect size) whose estimator follows a normal distribution. Hence the confidence intervals are based on the critical value (z-score) of the standard normal distribution.

A $(1 - \alpha) \times 100\%$ confidence interval for the population mean μ is given by

$$\bar{y} \pm z_{\frac{\alpha}{2}} \times SE(\bar{Y}) \text{ or } \bar{y} \pm z_{\frac{\alpha}{2}} \times \hat{\sigma}_{\bar{Y}} \text{ or } \bar{y} \pm z_{\frac{\alpha}{2}} \times \frac{\hat{\sigma}}{\sqrt{n}},$$

where n is the sample size
SE is the standard error
$\bar{y}$ is the sample mean
$\hat{\sigma} = s$ is the sample standard deviation
$(1 - \alpha) \times 100\%$ is the confidence level
$z_{\frac{\alpha}{2}}$ is the critical value of the standard normal distribution (z) such that $P(Z > z_{\frac{\alpha}{2}}) = \frac{\alpha}{2}$ and
'$\pm$' represents the plus and minus signs.

Note that here z-score and the standard error of $\bar{Y}$ are used in the computation of the confidence interval because the sampling distribution of $\bar{Y}$ is normal with standard error $\hat{\sigma}/\sqrt{n}$.

A confidence interval is represented by two limits (or bounds)—the lower limit (LL) and upper limit (UL):

$$LL = \bar{y} - z_{\frac{\alpha}{2}} \times \frac{\hat{\sigma}}{\sqrt{n}} \text{ and } UL = \bar{y} + z_{\frac{\alpha}{2}} \times \frac{\hat{\sigma}}{\sqrt{n}}$$

The term $z_{\frac{\alpha}{2}} \times \frac{\hat{\sigma}}{\sqrt{n}}$ is called the *margin of error* (ME). The width of any two-sided confidence interval is twice its margin of error. The larger is the margin of error, the wider is the interval. The margin of error increases as the confidence level and/or the spread/variability increases, and it decreases as the sample size increases.

In the context of meta-analysis, the value of α is set at 5%, so that the confidence level becomes $(1 - 0.05) \times 100\% = 95\%$. In that case, the critical value becomes $z_{\frac{0.05}{2}} = 1.96$ (some people use a closer round number 2.00). Then we get

$$LL = \bar{y} - 1.96 \times \frac{\hat{\sigma}}{\sqrt{n}} \text{ and } UL = \bar{y} + 1.96 \times \frac{\hat{\sigma}}{\sqrt{n}}.$$

The *width* of a (two-sided) confidence interval is twice its margin of error or difference between the upper limit and the lower limit. That is, width of a two-sided $(1 - \alpha) \times 100\%$ confidence interval is $Width = 2 \times \left[z_{\frac{\alpha}{2}} \times \frac{\hat{\sigma}}{\sqrt{n}} \right]$.

Comment: The width of the confidence interval depends on three factors

(a) Confidence level—the width of the confidence interval increases as the confidence level grow larger (e.g. from 90% with $z = 1.645$ to 95% with $z = 1.96$).
(b) Sample size—the width of the confidence interval decreases as the sample increases.
(c) Sample variance (as a consequence the standard error)—the width of the confidence interval increases as the sample variance increases.

2.2.3 Test of Hypothesis

Another commonly used statistical method in meta-analysis is the test of hypotheses, especially the significance of the effect size. If the population effect size of an outcome variable denoted by Y with unknown mean μ and standard deviation σ then the hypotheses to be tested are, the null hypothesis

$H_0 : \mu = \mu_0 = 0$ (mean effect size is zero) against the alternative hypothesis
$H_A : \mu \neq 0$ (mean effect size is NOT zero) if the test is two sided
or
$H_A : \mu > 0$ (mean effect size is greater than zero) if the test is one sided, upper tailed.

From the population of Y, select a random sample of size n, $(y_1, y_2, \ldots, y_n)$, find the sample mean $\bar{y}$ and sample standard deviation $\hat{\sigma}$. Since the sampling distribution of the estimator of μ, say $\bar{Y}$, follows a normal distribution with mean $\mu_{\bar{Y}} = \mu$ and standard error $\hat{\sigma}_{\bar{Y}} = \hat{\sigma} / \sqrt{n}$, the statistic $Z^* = \frac{\bar{Y} - \mu_0}{\sigma / \sqrt{n}}$, where μ_0 is a specific value of μ assigned by the null hypothesis (in the case of zero mean effect $\mu_0 = 0$), follows a standard normal distribution.

Since σ is unknown, it is estimated by the sample standard deviation $\hat{\sigma} = s$. Then another statistic $T = \frac{\bar{Y} - \mu_0}{\hat{\sigma} / \sqrt{n}}$ is defined using the estimate of the unknown standard deviation σ. This statistic follows a Student-t distribution with $(n - 1)$ degrees of freedom. However, if the sample size is large (that is, $n \geq 30$), the Student-t distribution will have large number of degrees of freedom, $(n - 1) \geq 29$. In that case the distribution of the T statistic can be approximated by the normal distribution (by the Central Limit Theorem). For this reason, in almost all meta-analyses, the statistic T (or Z^*) is modified to define the following statistic $Z = \frac{\bar{Y} - \mu_0}{\hat{\sigma} / \sqrt{n}}$ which follows an approximate normal distribution.

Hence to test $H_0 : \mu = \mu_0 = 0$, against a two-sided alternative, reject the null hypothesis at the α level of significance if the observed absolute value of Z (ignore the negative sign) is larger than or equal to the critical value of Z, that is, $z_{\frac{\alpha}{2}}$.

Here $z_{\frac{\alpha}{2}}$ is such that the following probability statement holds:

$P\left(|Z| \geq z_{\frac{\alpha}{2}}\right) = 1 - \alpha$ or equivalently,

$$P\left(Z \leq -z_{\frac{\alpha}{2}}\right) + P\left(Z \geq z_{\frac{\alpha}{2}}\right) = 2 \times P\left(Z \leq -z_{\frac{\alpha}{2}}\right) = 2 \times P\left(Z \geq z_{\frac{\alpha}{2}}\right) = 1 - \alpha.$$

The P-value is often used to decide whether to reject a null hypothesis or not. A P-value is the probability of observing sample data as extreme or more extreme than that produced by the observed sample, if the null hypothesis is true. In notation, for a two-sided test based on the Z statistic,

P-value $= P(|Z| > z_0 | H_0 : \mu = \mu_0)$, where z_0 is the observed value of the test statistic Z calculated from the sample data, that is, $z_0 = \frac{\bar{Y} - \mu_0}{s/\sqrt{n}}$. For any given value of the level of significance, α, the null hypothesis is rejected if the P-value of the test is less than or equal to α.

Comment: The P-value is the calculated **probability** of finding the observed, or more extreme, sample results when the null hypothesis of a study is true. Further the observed result (sample statistic) away from the value of the relevant parameter under the null hypothesis smaller is the P-value. That is, as the difference between the value of the parameter under the null hypothesis and its estimate from the sample, $(\bar{Y} - \mu_0)$ increases the value of the Z statistic increases and hence the P-value decreases (as a result the credibility of the null hypothesis decreases leading to its rejection).

For a two-sided test (when the alternative hypothesis is two-sided) the P-value is sum of the areas from both the tails of the distribution of the test statistic.

Decision Roles

Critical value approach: Reject H_0 at the α level of significance if the calculated/observed value of the Z statistic (say z_0) satisfies $|z_0| \geq z_{\alpha/2}$, where $z_{\alpha/2}$ is the $\alpha/2$ level upper cut-off point of the standard normal distribution; otherwise don't reject the null hypothesis.

P-value approach: Alternatively, reject H_0 at the α level of significance if the P-value is less than or equal to a preselected significance level, α; otherwise don't reject the null hypothesis.

Remark Another distribution used in meta-analysis is the chi-squared distribution. This is a skewed to the right distribution with degrees of freedom as the only parameter. In testing the heterogeneity of effect size among the independent studies Cochran's Q statistic is used which follows a chi-squared distribution.

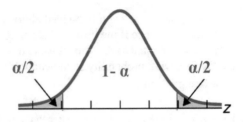

Fig. 2.2 Normal distribution curve showing $\frac{\alpha}{2}$ area at each tail and $(1 - \alpha)$ area in the middle

2.2.4 Transformation of Effect Sizes for Binary Outcomes

For the confidence interval (and test of significance) of the population effect size it is essential to know the sampling distribution of the estimator of effect size along with its standard error. For the continuous outcome variables, if the sample size is large, the distribution of the sample mean is approximately normally distributed by the well-known central limit theorem (CLT). Therefore normal distribution of the estimator of effect sizes based on sample mean (and differences of two sample means) is used for statistical inference within meta-analysis.

Unfortunately the sampling distribution of the estimator of the population effect size based on the binary or categorical outcome variables (e.g. odds ratio (OR) or risk ratio (RR)) are not readily available. However, the natural logarithm of the OR/RR (that is, lnOR or lnRR) is approximately normally distributed, and hence the distribution of lnOR (or lnRR) is used to for the statistical inference including calculating or finding the critical value (z-score) of the confidence interval (and for the testing of significance of effect size). Based on the standard normal distribution, for a 95% confidence interval the critical value is z = 1.96. By convention, this critical value is used for all confidence intervals in meta-analysis.

While testing significance of effect size (e.g. population RR or OR) the test statistic is based on the log transformation. Therefore, the test statistic is defined as the ratio of the sample ln RR/OR and the standard error of it. All calculations are based on the ln RR/OR and hence the confidence limits are found in log scale of the RR or OR. For reporting, the confidence interval, calculated from the lnOR (or lnRR), is usually transformed to the original scale using the reverse (or back) transformation, exp[lnOR] = OR.

The distribution of OR/RR and the log transformation of OR/RR are displayed in Fig. 2.3.

2.3 Effect Size Measures for Meta-analysis

The effect size is the name given to a family of indices that measure the magnitude of a treatment or intervention effect. Depending on the type of study there are various measures that can be used to determine the effect size for the intervention of interest.

LOG TRANSFORMATION OF RR AND OR

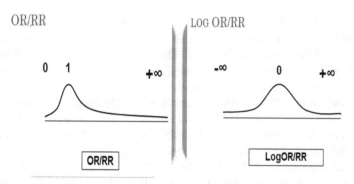

Fig. 2.3   The distribution of RR/OR and that of log transformation of RR/OR

While the effect size is independent of sample size, we can perform statistical signif-icance tests to find if any effect size is different from the null or if the difference between two or more effect sizes (e.g. across groups) is significantly different or not.

The effect size measure broadly depends on the type of outcome variables involved. There are two major categories of effect measures in meta-analysis based on the kind of outcome variable used to determine the effect size. There are those based on binary or categorical outcome variables such as the proportion, relative risks (RR) or odds ratios (OR). The other category is those effect measures for continuous outcome variables such as the standardised mean difference (SMD), weighted mean difference (WMD), and Pearson's product moment correlation coefficient.

Effect size is the foundation block for any meta-analysis. Every meta-analysis combines effect size of an intervention which is measured based on a specific under-lying outcome variable from selected independent studies to estimate the unknown common effect size for all the studies.

The popular effect size measures for meta-analyses based on continuous outcome variables include **Cohen's d** (Cohen 1969), **Hedges' g** (Hedges 1981) and **Glass' Δ** (Glass et al. 1981) statistics. Details on these are covered in Chap. 9.

2.3.1   Relationship Between Effect Size Measures

The relationship between the standardised mean difference (d), log odds ratio (ln OR), and correlation coefficient (r) allows us to convert one effect measure to another one. The following relationships are useful.

From ln OR to d: $d = \ln \text{OR} \times \frac{\sqrt{3}}{\pi}$, where $\pi = \frac{22}{7}$ is a mathematical constant.
From d to ln OR: $\ln \text{OR} = \frac{d\pi}{\sqrt{3}}$.
From r to d: $d = \frac{2r}{\sqrt{1-r^2}}$.

2.4   Inverse Variance Method and Redistribution of Weights

The main objective of any meta-analysis is to pool effect size statistics (e.g. sample mean, OR) from independent studies with a view to synthesising them to calculate an estimate of the common effect size. This is essentially a process of weighted averaging and different methodologies use different formulae to generate the weights for weighted averaging of individual studies in computing the pooled estimate. The simplest case is that of the arithmetic mean, where the weights for each study are equal to $1/k$ if there are k studies in the meta-analysis. The weight $1/k$ is termed as the natural weight and is equal for every study. This arithmetic mean estimator is unbiased, but in meta-analysis we aim to sacrifice unbiasedness for decrease in squared error in order to increase accuracy of the pooled estimator. The arithmetic mean or the estimate based on the equal weights is not optimal as it does not minimise the variance of the estimator, and hence it is not used in meta-analysis. Figure 2.2 diplays the normal distribution curve.

Conventionally, the inverse variance weights have been used in meta-analysis. This empirical weight generates the best trade-off between bias and variance. It is well known that the sample variance is inversely related to the sample/study size (n), and hence larger studies (with higher sample size) will receive higher weights under the principle of inverse variance weight than the smaller studies. But this redistribution of weights only considers random error, and systematic error is ignored and thus may lead to allocating higher than appropriate weight to the lower quality larger studies and vice versa.

There are other methods for creating empirical weights as well such as the inverse variance heterogeneity model, the random effects model and the quality effects model and these will be discussed later. It is a fact that the model that generates the weights must also have a mechanism for generating the appropriate error estimation (variance) around the point estimate that maintains nominal coverage of relevant confidence interval, and different weighting models may or may not achieve correct error estimation.

2.5   Meta-analytic Models for Non-heterogeneous Studies

Different statistical models have been used for meta-analyses under different conditions or circumstances. The main difference among the models is the way they allocate the empirical weights to the individual studies. The objective of redistribution of weights among the studies is to minimise squared error of the estimator of the pooled effect size to achieve an estimate with improved accuracy (closest to the population parameter).

Since meta-analyses are based on the summary statistics of individual studies, the between study variation must be taken into account in the analysis. So it is essential to check if heterogeneity is present in the data. This requires testing the equality of effect sizes of the studies. [If the effect sizes are not significantly different there is no heterogeneity in the data]. If the between studies variation is not significant, the meta-analysis becomes simple and straightforward. In such cases the fixed effect (FE) model is appropriate to meta-analyse the data.

The FE meta-analytic model assumes that there is a common unknown true effect size for all the studies under investigation and the study effects depart from this true effect due to random error alone. For the FE model the observed effect size for any study i is represented by $\hat{\theta}_i = \theta + \varepsilon_i$, where error term ε_i is the difference between the common true effect size, θ and the observed sample effect size for study i, $\hat{\theta}_i$. The errors are assumed to be independent and follow normal distribution with mean 0 and variance σ_i^2, that is, $\varepsilon_i \sim N(0, \sigma_i^2)$ for $i = 1,2, \ldots, k$. The fixed effect model assumes that there is only one source of variation, the within-study variation, which is the estimation error ε_i. The variance of the estimation error for the ith study, σ_i^2 is estimated by the sample variance, that is, $\hat{\sigma}_i^2 = v_i$. For very large studies the sampling errors become very small. Under the FE model, the common effect size θ is estimated by using the inverse variance weight, $\hat{\theta}_{FE} = \sum_{i=1}^{k} w_i \hat{\theta}_i \Big/ \sum_{i=1}^{k} w_i$, where $w_i = \frac{1}{v_i}$, is the weight in which v_i is the sample variance. The variance of the estimator of θ is estimated by $Var(\hat{\theta}_{FE}) = \left(\sum_{i=1}^{k} \frac{1}{v_i} \right)^{-1}$. The confidence interval and test of hypothesis for the effect size θ are based on the critical value of the standard normal distribution. However the variance expression above is known to grossly underestimate the actual variance and may lead to inflated Type 1 errors under heterogeneity. Thus when testing the significance of the meta-analytic effect there is the possibility of spurious significance if the studies are not homogeneous, and this method therefore is limited to meta-analysis of homogeneous studies (Fig. 2.4).

2.6 Meta-analytic Models for Heterogeneous Studies

Heterogeneity

In many meta-analytical studies the between studies variation is significant, that is, heterogeneity among the effect sizes of the independent studies is significant. In such cases the meta-analysis must take care of this fact in computing the pooled effect size and the confidence interval. Different approaches are available to address the issue of heterogeneity in the context of meta-analysis. Obviously, not all of them are equally effective and provide real remedy to the problem.

As in the main stream statistics literature, the heterogeneity issue has prompted many discussions in meta-analysis literature. Some of the commonly used methods to overcome the heterogeneity problem are discussed below.

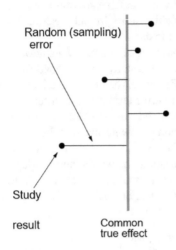

Fig. 2.4 Graphical illustration of fixed effect model

2.6.1 Assessing Heterogeneity

The assessment of the presence of heterogeneity among the study-level effect size measure is conducted by performing statistical test of hypothesis. That is, by testing $H_0 : \theta_1 = \theta_2 = \ldots = \theta_k$ against H_a : not all $\theta_i's$ are equal. The test of heterogeneity is based on the Cochrane's Q-statistic defined as

$$Q = \sum_{i=1}^{k} w_i \hat{\theta}_i^2 - \frac{\left[\sum_{i=1}^{k} w_i \hat{\theta}_i\right]^2}{\sum_{i=1}^{k} w_i}.$$

The Q-statistic follows a chi-squared distribution with $(k-1)$ degrees of freedom (df) under the null hypothesis of equality of means. The main problem with this statistic is that its value increases as the number of studies in the meta-analysis grows larger. Another statistic that quantifies heterogeneity is $I^2 = ([Q - df]/Q) \times 100\%$, and is viewed as the proportion of between studies variation and total variation (within studies plus between studies variation).

Comment: Different approaches and methods are used for meta-analysis if heterogeneity is present in the data. These include use of different statistical models, meta-regression, subgroup analysis, sensitivity analysis etc. Section 2.7 of this chapter elaborates on them.

2.6.2 Random Effects (REs) Model

The commonly used model to handle heterogeneity is the random effects (REs) model. Proposed by (DerSimonian and Laird 1986), the REs model uses weights that try to parameterize extraneous variation beyond random error alone. In so doing the model assumes that the observed treatment effect for a study is a combination of a treatment effect common to all studies (the average of true effects) and a 'random effect' specific to that study alone. The REs model re-distributes the weights to the individual studies in computing the pooled or synthesised estimate of the common effect size using two (within and between study) sources of variation.

The two sources of error/variation in the REs model are the within-study, or estimation or random error, and between-study or variation of the true effect size. Under the REs model, the observed effect size for any study i is represented by $\hat{\theta}_i = \theta + \zeta_i + \varepsilon_i$, where $\zeta_i = \theta_i - \theta$ and $\varepsilon_i = \hat{\theta}_i - \theta_i$ represent the two sources of variation with the assumption that both follow normal distribution, $\zeta_i \sim N(0, \tau^2)$ and $\varepsilon_i \sim N(0, \sigma_i^2)$ for $i = 1, 2, ..., k$. The sample estimates of τ^2 is $\hat{\tau}^2$. The combined variance of study i, that is, $\sigma_i^{2*} = \left(\sigma_i^2 + \tau^2\right)$ is estimated by $v_i^* = \left(v_i + \hat{\tau}^2\right)$, and then the weight for study i under the REs model becomes $w_i^* = \left(v_i + \hat{\tau}^2\right)^{-1}$. The pooled effect size estimator under the RE model is

$$\hat{\theta}_{RE} = \frac{\sum_{i=1}^{k} w_i^* \hat{\theta}_i}{\sum_{i=1}^{k} w_i^*}, \text{ and } Var(\hat{\theta}_{RE}) = \left(\sum_{i=1}^{k} w_i^*\right)^{-1}.$$

Under the REs model more weights are redistributed from larger to smaller studies as heterogeneity increases. Thus, the REs model method of synthesising the pooled mean effect size takes away weights from the larger studies and re-distributes them to smaller studies. With gross heterogeneity this may lead to the estimator moving towards the arithmetic mean (Fig. 2.4).

The random effects model (unjustifiably) assumes that the studies in the meta-analysis are a random sample from a population of studies. Thus the validity of the results of the REs model is dependent on meeting this assumptions of the model, which is unrealistic in practice. Unfortunately, hardly anyone ever checks the validity of the assumptions, but accepts the results for granted. The consequence is that this model though aiming to be more conservative than the FE model fails to be so and even the larger variance under the model comes with a higher squared error thus suffering from over-dispersion and faulty error estimation.

2.6.3 Inverse Variance Heterogeneity Model

Recently, (Doi et al. 2015a) introduced the inverse variance heterogeneity (IVhet) model. It emphasises that the fixed effect model based estimator variance can be

Random-effects model

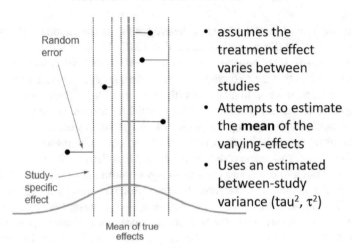

- assumes the treatment effect varies between studies
- Attempts to estimate the **mean** of the varying-effects
- Uses an estimated between-study variance (tau^2, τ^2)

Fig. 2.5 Graphical illustration of random effects model

made closer to the observed variance by modelling over-dispersion through a quasi-likelihood approach. This implies that the meta-analysis is performed under a fixed effect assumption ($\tau^2 = 0$) and the variance of the estimator is inflated to account for the heterogeneity. This has the advantage of being based purely on the variance-to-mean relationship rather than on distributional assumptions with variance appropriately inflated using a scale parameter, ψ_i. The latter can be defined by interpreting the multiplicative factor as an intra-class correlation (ICC) as described by (Kulinskaya and Olkin 2014), where the $ICC_i = \tau^2 / (\tau^2 + v_i)$ and the scale parameter is defined as $\psi_i = v_i^{-1}\sigma_i^2 = (1 - ICC_i)^{-1}$.

The expression of the variance of any weighted mean estimator $\hat{\theta}_w$ represented by $var(\hat{\theta}_w)$, for the ith study, is expressed as $w_i^2 var(\hat{\theta}_i)$ which is then inflated to $w_i^2 var(\hat{\theta}_i)\psi_i$ based on expression of ψ_i above, and this inflation of the inverse variance weights using a quasi-likelihood approach.

The IVhet estimate of the common effect size θ is given by $\hat{\theta}_{IVhet} = \sum_{i=1}^{k} w_i\hat{\theta}_i$ and

$$Var(\hat{\theta}_{IVhet}) = \sum_{i=1}^{k}\left[\left(\frac{1}{v_i} \middle/ \sum_{i=1}^{k}\frac{1}{v_i}\right)^2 (v_i + \hat{\tau}^2)\right].$$

Through extensive simulations (Doi et al. 2015c) showed that the IVhet model performs better than the REs model under varieties of conditions (Fig. 2.5).

Note that ϕ_j^2 is the additional variance contribution from internal study biases.

IVhet model

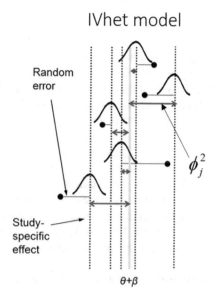

- assumes all studies are measuring the same average treatment effect (true plus beta)
- estimates that effect
- if not for random **and systematic** error, all results would have been identical – apart from a little diversity
- Beta is the super-population systematic error across studies

Fig. 2.6 Graphical illustration of inverse variance heterogeneity model

2.6.4 Advantages of IVhet Model Over REs Model

The IVhet model has clear advantages over the REs model as it resolves the two main problems of the latter model. The first advantage of the IVhet model is that the coverage (probability) of the confidence interval remains at the nominal (usually 95%) level, unlike that of the REs model for which the coverage drops significantly with increasing heterogeneity. The second advantage is that the IVhet model maintains the inverse variance weights of individual studies, unlike the REs model which allocates more weights to the small studies (and therefore less weights to larger studies) with increasing heterogeneity. The latter property of the IVhet model means that its squared error is less than the REs model estimator.

In the presence of larger heterogeneity, the individual study weights under the REs model become equal and thus the REs model estimator returns to the arithmetic mean of the individual effect sizes rather than the intended weighted average. The IVhet model does not suffer from this side-effect of the REs model. Thus it differs from the REs model estimate in two ways: (1) larger trials contribute more (weights) to the pooled estimates (as opposed to penalising larger trials in the REs model), and (2) yields confidence intervals that maintain the nominal coverage (probability) under uncertainty due to increased heterogeneity. In addition, no distributional assumptions on the estimator of the effect size is required for the IVhet model, and hence it provides a robust statistical method compared to the REs model with less squared error.

2.6.5 Quality Effects Model

Doi and Thalib (2008) introduced a quality-effects (QE) approach that combines evidence from a series of trials comparing two interventions. This approach incorporates the heterogeneity of effects in the analysis of the overall interventional efficacy. However, unlike the random-effects model based on observed between-trial heterogeneity, it suggests adjustment based on measured methodological heterogeneity between studies.

The QE model was updated by Doi et al. (2015b) to improve two specific aspects of the model. First, over-dispersion observed with the initial estimator has been corrected using an intra-class correlation based multiplicative scale parameter. Second, the quality scores are relative to the best study in the meta-analysis and thus rescaled between 0 and 1 by dividing by the maximum value of the scores within the meta-analysis before it is input into the model. This still keeps the scores in the 0–1 range but allows them to reflect the relative nature of these scores, relative to the best study in the meta-analysis.

The IVhet estimator is actually the QE estimator when quality information set to uninformative (equal). Under the QE model study quality is allowed to vary and the estimator of the pooled effect size θ is given by

$$\hat{\theta}_{QE} = \sum_{i=1}^{k} w_i' \hat{\theta}_i, \text{ where the modified weight } w_i' = \left(\frac{Q_i}{v_i} + \hat{\tau}_i\right) \bigg/ \sum_{i=1}^{k} \left(\frac{Q_i}{v_i} + \hat{\tau}_i\right).$$

For the explanation of the notations, expression of variance of the estimator and other details please refer to the Appendix A of (Doi et al. 2015b).

2.7 Dealing with Heterogeneity

In the presence of heterogeneity, different meta-analytical methods are used to assess reasons for this. Some of the most popular ones are discussed below. Details on the methods and interpretation of results will be provided in the forthcoming chapters.

2.7.1 Meta-Regression

In the presence of heterogeneity sometime meta-regression method is used if additional data on related variables are available.

Meta-regression is a moderator (or covariate) analysis method that refers to using a regression method in an attempt to find and account for systematic differences in the size of the effect of interest. The meta-regression is conducted by regressing the observed effect sizes on one or multiple study characteristics. For heterogeneous effect sizes the meta-regression may explain why heterogeneity occurred in the first place. However, in many studies there is insufficient information on any useful moderator variables as reporting them may not have been a part of the focus of individual primary studies.

In the absence of appropriate good moderator characteristics of all individual studies meta-regression would be either impossible or ineffective or misleading. Sometimes even if there are moderator variables they may not be the causes of heterogeneity and hence unhelpful to explain the diversity of variation among the studies. Any association evident from meta-regression are observational having no causal impact on the interpretation of the effect size estimate. This method is covered in Chap. 11.

2.7.2 Subgroup Analysis

Another way to explain moderator effects in meta-analytic studies is to group the studies based on the value of a moderator variable. Separate meta-analyses are conducted on each of the subgroups and this allows within subgroup results to be examined. This is exactly the same as meta-regression and is used when a single categorical moderator is of interest. This method is illustrated in Sects. 4.7, 5.7 and 9.7.

2.7.3 Sensitivity Analysis

Sensitivity analysis is useful to check the impact on the result of changing selection criteria of the studies on the pooled effect size. It provides some useful insight into the robustness of the results and how sensitive they are to inclusion/exclusion criteria. One variant is the exclusion sensitivity analysis which examines if individual studies impact on the meta-analysis result unduly.

2.8 Issues in Meta-analysis

In this section some important issues in the implementation, analysis and interpretation of results of meta-analyses are discussed.

2.8.1 Reporting Variation of Summary Statistics

The summary statistics on the outcome variables are reported in the individual studies often using different scale and/or unit of measurement. Depending on the type of the outcome variable the summary statistics could be mean and standard deviation, or correlation coefficient (for quantitative outcome variables) and odds/risk ratio/difference (for categorical outcome variables) along with the sample size. For the computation of any confidence interval for the unknown population effect size, the point estimate of the same for each of the individual studies along with their standard deviation and sample/study size are essential. Also, the distribution of the estimator of the population effect size must be identifiable in order to be able to determine the *critical value* of the underlying statistic at a predetermined confidence level.

In many cases authors of different articles selected for meta-analysis use different effect measures and units of measurement. For example, instead of reporting mean and standard deviation of the quantitative outcome variables some authors report median and inter quartile range (IQR) or median and minimum/maximum or range statistics. This kind of variation of unit of measurement makes it difficult (but not impossible) to include them in the synthesis process. Therefore, before undertaking any meta-analysis the effect size of all selected studies must be converted to one single effect measure with the same unit of measurement. See Hozo et al. (2005) for details on some useful transformation formulae on this problem.

2.8.2 Publication and Reporting Bias in Meta-Analysis

Publication bias is a serious problem in meta-analysis. It arises because of reporting bias as studies with negative or non-significant effects are not normally accepted for publication in profession journals. Also, the sponsors of research projects and the authors often prefer not to publish results of the studies that do not support their intended outcome. Either way, results from some studies are published which are identified in systematic reviews and included in the meta-analysis, but many other studies remain unreported/unpublished and hence excluded. This phenomenon impacts on the ultimate results of the meta-analysis, sometimes without realising the extent of the exclusion and their potential impact on the final results.

The language bias is also a reality. Most of the articles are published in English language journals or other publications. As a results often publications in other languages remain undetected or are overlooked.

The *funnel plot* is used to assess the publication bias in a meta-analysis. It is used primarily as a visual aid for detecting or systematic heterogeneity. A funnel plot is a scatterplot of treatment effect against a measure of study precision such as the estimated standard error or sample size of each of the studies. Asymmetry in funnel plots may be due to publication bias in meta-analysis (among other reasons including chance), but the shape of the plot in the presence of bias is sometimes difficult to ascertain. Certain P-value based tests exist to quantify asymmetry of the funnel plot but have poor power. For details on effect of selecting various study sizes see Sterne and Egger (2001).

Doi plot is another graphical method to identify the publication bias. This method also comes with the LFK index quantifying the degree of asymmetry in the plot. The Doi plot has a much less ambiguous visual appearance and the LFK index has much greater power than the corresponding tests used for the funnel plot. Illustration of both the plots is found in Sects. 4.9, 5.9 and 8.8. Details on publication bias are covered in Chap. 12.

2.8.3 Presentation and Reporting of Main Results

The usual way to present the results of meta-analyses is to show the confidence intervals of individual studies and the combined meta-analysis on the same graph in the form of a forest plot. The middle of the confidence intervals of the individual studies is marked by dark squares and the size/area of the associated squares represents the level of weight of the study. For the meta-analysis of the common effect size, the confidence interval is represented by a diamond. The horizontal edges of the diamond represent the limits of the confidence interval. The relative location of the diamond with respect to the no-effect vertical line indicates which intervention is supported by the data. If appropriate, subgroup analyses are also included in the forest plot along with the combined meta-analysis.

2.9 A Brief Appraisal of Meta-analysis

The term meta-analysis was formally coined by Glass (1976) as a statistical procedure to re-analyse the published statistical analyses from a large number of independent studies for the purpose of synthesising and integrating the findings in the context of educational research. Referring to the oversupply of information, he noted that some had termed it as a predicament "the misinformation explosion". But his view was that we face an abundance of information, and problem is to find the knowledge in the information by introducing methods for the orderly summarization of studies so that knowledge can be extracted from the myriad individual researches. His choice of the term came from the spirit of meta-mathematics, meta-psychology, meta-evaluation etc. Since then statistical meta-analysis has been extensively used in medical/health sciences, psychology, education, agriculture, and many other areas of evidence-based decision-making including government departments and businesses.

The strengths and limitations of meta-analysis are briefly noted below. For further discussion on the topic refer to Khan et al. (2019).

2.9.1   Strengths of Meta-Analysis

Meta-analysis is a scientifically valid statistical method with solid mathematical foundation. The results of meta-analyses are correct if the underlying model assumptions are met and there is no bias in the selection of studies and no error in the extraction of data.

Meta-analysis provides more statistical power due to increased sample size than that of any single study. So the results produced by meta-analyses are more precise and reliable.

Meta-analysis is a statistical method that produces objective results. The outcomes of meta-analyses are solely based on the summary data from the systematic reviews.

Meta-analysis is the only method capable of combining quantitative data of every individual studies to estimate the pooled effect size in any systematic reviews.

Because of its ability to combine data from individual studies it is able to produce the synthesised pooled estimate of the common effect size even if the results of the individual studies are inconclusive, conflicting (with opposing directions) and diversity of values.

Due to the pooling of summary statistics from many primary studies the meta-analysis improves the statistical precision of the point estimate, width of the confidence interval, and power of the test of the common mean effect size.

When needed, meta-analysis can be performed to estimate the common effect size for a subset of the selected studies sharing certain common characteristics or time period under the provision of subgroup analysis.

Meta-analyses based on well-conducted randomized controlled trials provides the highest levels of evidence by controlling extraneous variation and bias.

The selection and implementation of correct statistical model for the meta-analyses produce accurate statistics and appropriate confidence intervals leading to the high quality evidence.

Inconclusive meta-analyses may suggest the need for further independent trials or studies to help produce decisive results.

2.9.2   Limitations of Meta-Analysis

Like many other statistical methods, meta-analysis is a very powerful technique for synthesising summary statistics, even with conflicting quantitative data, from individual studies, to reach decisive conclusions. But, it is equally venerable and open for abuse by people who are not evidence-informed or ignorant or with ill-motive. Because there are many situations when this highly effective method can be abused or misused if the research team is not careful or aware of the problems that would invalidate the results of meta-analyses.

Although, meta-analysis method only depends on the input data or summary statistics of the independent studies, the quality of the results of meta-analyses are dependent on the quality of the trials/studies included in the synthesis, presence of reporting or publication bias, and presence of heterogeneity.

Meta-analysis is inappropriate if there is no common underlying effect size that each of the independent studies is attempting to estimate. If different individual studies are estimating different effects, there will be no common effect size and hence synthesis by meta-analysis *must not* be attempted.

Meta-analysis must not be used if the effect size measure of outcome variables are not the same for all studies. Mixing of different effect size measures or same measure with different scale or unit of measurement in a meta-analysis is like combining apples and oranges.

Whatever data values are feed into the meta-analysis software the computer will produce some results based on the selected procedure regardless of the quality of the data. However, the appropriateness and correctness of the results must be verified before using them for any decision-making. Inappropriate procedure and/or wrong input data will never produce any good evidence.

Meta-analysis can be inconclusive if there are conflicting evidences from different studies or trials. This may suggest no significant effect of the intervention or the need for further investigations or trials.

The presence of bias in the individual studies is a serious consideration for any inclusions in meta-analysis. Inclusion of studies with significant bias in the meta-analysis will definitely lead to the misleading results. It will not only produce incorrect results and complicate the analysis but also seriously limit any useful interpretation.

Selection of wrong model, especially to deal with the heterogeneity among the studies, means that the results of the meta-analysis is likely to be misleading.

Obviously, in the presence of significant publication bias or reporting anomalies or both the results of meta-analysis will not be accurate.

2.10   Concluding Remarks

Meta-analysis is a powerful tool to combine diverse quantitative results of independent studies and synthesise the results of individual primary studies to find the pooled estimate of population effect size. Meta-analytical methods could provide much needed high quality evidence for making appropriate decisions if the underlying processes, protocols and methods are properly and strictly observed. However, every step in a systematic review and meta-analysis must be scrutinized for potential bias, from the formulation of the research question to the interpretation and discussion of the results, to ensure the quality and applied value of the final product (Bernard 2014).

References

Bernard RM (2014) Things I have learned about meta-analysis since 1990: reducing bias in search of "The Big Picture". Can J Learn Technol 40(3):n3

Cohen J (1969) Statistical power analysis for the behavioral sciences. Academic Press, New York

DerSimonian R, Laird N (1986) Meta-analysis in clinical trials. Control Clin Trials 7(3):177–188

Doi SA, Barendregt JJ, Khan S, Thalib L, Williams GM (2015a) Advances in the meta-analysis of heterogeneous clinical trials I: the inverse variance heterogeneity model. Contemp Clin Trials 45(Pt A):130–138. https://doi.org/10.1016/j.cct.2015.05.009

Doi SA, Barendregt JJ, Khan S, Thalib L, Williams GM (2015b) Advances in the meta-analysis of heterogeneous clinical trials II: the quality effects model. Contemp Clin Trials 45(Pt A):123–129. https://doi.org/10.1016/j.cct.2015.05.010

Doi SA, Barendregt JJ, Khan S, Thalib L, Williams GM (2015c) Simulation comparison of the quality effects and random effects methods of meta-analysis. Epidemiology 26(4):e42–44

Doi SAR, Thalib L (2008) A quality-effects model for meta-analysis. Epidemiology 19(1):94–100

Glass GV (1976) Primary, secondary, and meta-analysis of research. Educ Researcher 5(10):3–8

Glass GV, Smith ML, McGaw B (1981) Meta-analysis in social research. Sage Publications, Incorporated

Hedges LV (1981) Distribution theory for Glass's estimator of effect size and related estimators. J Educ Stat 6(2):107–128

Hozo SP, Djulbegovic B, Hozo I (2005) Estimating the mean and variance from the median, range, and the size of a sample. BMC Med Res Methodol 5(1):13

Khan S, Doi SAR (2015) Statistical meta-analysis: potential for new research opportunities. From Statistical Society of Australia Inc. http://www.statsoc.org.au/general/statistical-meta-analysis-potential-for-new-research-opportunities/

Khan S, Memon B, Memon MA (2019) Meta-analysis: a critical appraisal of methodology, benefits and drawbacks. Br J Hosp Med 80(11):636–641. https://doi.org/10.12968/hmed.2019.80.11.636

Kulinskaya E, Olkin I (2014) An overdispersion model in meta-analysis. Stat Modell 14(1):49–76

Sterne JA, Egger M (2001) Funnel plots for detecting bias in meta-analysis: guidelines on choice of axis. J Clin Epidemiol 54(10):1046–1055

Part II
Meta-Analysis for Binary Outcomes

Chapter 3
Introduction to Ratio Measures

Fundamental concepts, definitions, calculating formulae and interpretations of risks and odds as well as the risk ratio and odds ratio are introduced in this chapter. The meta-analytical methods of these two very important and frequently used effect size measures, risk ratio and odds ratio, are covered in Chaps. 4 and 5.

3.1 Introduction

Most of the meta-analyses endeavor to estimate the unknown common population effect size and present the results in forest plots. In this chapter we introduce the effect size measures, namely risk ratio and odds ratio, to study the degree of association between two categorical or binary outcome variables. Here both the intervention (e.g. exposure and non-exposure) and outcome (e.g. cases or non-cases) are categorical.

Effect size
The effect size is the common name to a family of indices that measure the magnitude of a treatment or intervention effect. Depending on the type of study there are various measures that can be used to determine the effect size for the intervention of interest.

The effect size measure depends on the type of outcome variable of interest. For binary (categorical) outcome variables relative risk or risk ratio (RR) and odds ratio (OR) are used as effect size measure.

Effect measures such as a single proportion (of incidences) or difference between two proportions (also called risk difference) are also applicable to binary outcome variables. [See Chaps. 6 and 7 for details.] For continuous outcome variables the effect size is measured by standardised mean difference (SMD) or weighted mean difference (WMD), and correlation coefficient for linear relationship between two quantitative outcome variables. [These are covered in Chaps. 8–10.]

When the outcome of interest is a binary or categorical variable, ratio measures are used to investigate the association between the two variables. The most popular ratio

© Springer Nature Singapore Pte Ltd. 2020
S. Khan, *Meta-Analysis*, Statistics for Biology and Health,
https://doi.org/10.1007/978-981-15-5032-4_3

measures are the relative risk or risk ratio (RR) and odds ratio (OR). Both the RR and OR are used as effect size measures for binary outcome variables. The choice of a particular ratio measure is a decision of the researchers based on the type of study and objective of the investigation. McNutt et al. 2003 used the RR in cohort studies and clinical trials of common outcomes. Some exploration on the relationship between RR and OR are found in Shrier and Steele 2006 and a conversion formula of RR from OR is provided by Zhang and Yu 1998. Further discussions on the choice of effect measure for epidemiological data are found in Walter 2000 and Barger 2018.

In this chapter we introduce the concept, computational method and interpretation of risk ratio (RR) and odds ratio (OR) as a prelude to meta-analytical methods when they are dealt with as appropriate effect size measures in the forthcoming chapters.

3.2 Relative Risk or Risk Ratio (RR) and Odds Ratio (OR)

The risk ratio (or relative risk) and odds ratio are used to assess the association between two binary (categorical) variables, namely the explanatory variable (factor, e.g. Intervention or Treatment and Control, or Exposure and No Exposure) and outcome variable (Success and Failure, or Cases and No Cases, or Disease and No Disease, or Event and No Event). Although the purpose of the two ratios, RR and OR, is the same, they are not the same, and hence they should not be used as synonymous.

3.2.1 Root Causes for Differences in RR and OR

To appreciate the difference between the RR and OR it is important to carefully understand the difference between proportion and ratio. Although both have numerator and denominator, there are fundamental differences in the definition and interpretation of the two ratios.

Ratio: In mathematics, the ratio is described as the comparison of the size of two quantities of the same unit, which is expressed in terms of times i.e. the number of times the first value contains the second. The ratio is used to compare the quantities of two different categories like the *ratio of men to women* in a population. For example, in a study of 10 mens and 20 womens, the ratio of men to women is $10/20 = 1/2 = 0.5$.

Proportion: Proportion is a mathematical concept, which states the equality of two ratios or fractions. A proportion is the quantity of one category over the total, like the proportion of men out of total people living in a population. For example, in a study of 10 men and 20 women, the *proportion of men to women* is $10/(10 + 20) = 1/3$ or 0.3333, that is, 33.33%.

Odds: In statistics, the odds for or odds of some event reflects the likelihood that the event will take place, while odds against reflects the likelihood that it will not.

An odds is a number that is obtained by dividing one number (e.g. cases or events) by another (e.g. noncases or no events), both measuring the same outcome variable. For example, in a study of 10 men and 20 women, the *odds of men* is $10/20 = 0.5$ relative to women.

Probability: Probability is a numerical description of how likely an event is to occur. For example, in a study of 10 men and 20 women, the *probability* of randomly selecting a man is $10/30 = 0.3333$ or 33.33%. This is the same as the proportion of men in the study.

Clearly, odds is different from proportion and, or, probability. Proportion is often used a synonymous to risk and probability. Both odds and risk (probability) have the same numerator but different denominator, that is, they are on different scales.

3.2.2 Reasons for Differences Between RR and OR

Conceptually there is a fundamental difference between the risk (proportion) and odds, as the definitions are different, and hence, in general, the RR and OR are not the same. The risk of an intervention is defined as the ratio of number of cases/events relative to the total number of subjects (combining cases and non-cases) in the study, and hence it perfectly resembles probability. But the odds of an intervention is defined as the ratio of number of cases relative to the number of non-cases (excluding number of cases from total number of subjects) in the study, and hence it is different from the notion of probability. In both cases, what is common is the 'likelihood' or 'chance' (but not probability) of happening of cases/events, but relative to two different things. Often the two ratios are mixed and used synonymously by mistake because both ratios have the same numerator and represent some kind of 'likelihood' or 'change' ignoring the fact that the two ratios have totally different denominators. The RR is a ratio of two proportions (or percentages) and OR is a ratio of two odds.

To avoid confusion, make a clear note that odd reflects 'relative likelihood' or better yet 'odds', unlike risk which reflects 'probability'. The value of odds ratio is close to that of the risk ratio only if incidence (number of cases) is very small in both the exposed and the unexposed groups. If the incidence (number of cases) is high in either or both exposed and unexposed groups, then the value of RR is very different from OR.

3.2.3 Why OR is More Appropriate Than RR?

Some people do use the probability ratio, aka the relative risk (RR) to measure the effect of the intervention (X, risk factor) on the outcome (Y, disease). The disadvantage of the RR is that it is not a constant effect of X. The probability ratio changes depending on the value of X. But the OR does not change with a change in X (that is, it is constant with respect to X). The effect of X on the probability of Y has different values depending on the value of X. So if you want to know how X affects Y, odds ratio is the appropriate effect measure.

Odds is not a measure of likelihood of events out of all possible events. It's a ratio of number of events to number of non-events. You can switch back and forth between risk and odds—they will give you different information as they are on different scales. No wonder, the term 'odds' is commonplace, but not always clear, and often used inappropriately. Schmidt and Kohlmann 2008 discussed when to use the odds ratio or the relative risk in the context of epidemiological studies and emphasised that in the absence of meaningful prevalence or incidence data, the OR provides a valid effect measure.

3.2.4 Towards Defining RR and OR

The relative risk (or risk ratio) is defined based on the ratio (proportion) of two *probabilities* (or risks), and odds ratio is defined as the ratio of two *odds*. The understanding of the difference between the two different ratios depends on appreciating the basic difference in the definition of risk and odds.

Probability is the ratio of the number of times event (success) occurred compared/relative to the *total number of trials/subjects*. Probability is a number between 0 and 1. Probability $= 0.5$ implies success and failure are equally likely.

Odds is the ratio of the number of times success (*event*) occurred compared/relative to the *number of times failure occurred*. Odds is a number between 0 and ∞ (infinity). The two terms (probability and odds) are *related* but not *synonymous*, rather they are very different with the same numerator but different denominator. Equal **odds** is 1, that is, 1 success for every 1 failure.

To explain and illustrate the concepts of risk (probability) and odds, consider the following count data of binary outcomes from an hypothetical experiment on immunization for a particular disease as noted in Table 3.1.

There are two possible outcomes—disease (success/event) with count 'a' or no disease (failure/no event) with count 'b' among the participating '(a + b)' subjects. The numbers in brackets are the observed counts (number of subjects) in the call.

3.2.5 Probability

Probability of disease (success) is the *proportion* of the 'number of patients with disease' (event) relative to the '*total* number of patients (Disease plus no Disease)',

Table 3.1 Incidences of disease data

Disease	No disease	Total
a (20)	b (60)	a + b (80)

that is, $P(\text{Disease}) = a/(a+b) = 20/80 = 0.25$ and $P(\text{No Disease}) = b/(a+b) = 60/80 = 0.75$.

The occurrence of success (Disease) is complementary to the occurrence of failure (No Disease). So, $P(\text{Disease}) = 1 - P(\text{No Disease})$.

3.2.6 Risk

The risk of an event (Disease) in the Treatment group is the probability of the event. This is a proportion of 'number of events' relative to the 'total of number of events and no-events' in the Treatment group. For the data in Table 3.1, the risk of the event in the Treatment group is calculated as $R_T = a/(a+b) = 20/(20+60) = 20/80 = 1/4$ or (25%), that is $P(\text{Disease}) = 1/4$. Then $P(\text{No Disease}) = 60/80 = 3/4$. Hence $P(\text{Disease}) + P(\text{No Disease}) = 1/4 + 3/4 = 1$.

3.2.7 Odds

Odds of disease (success) is the *ratio* of the 'number of patients with *disease*' relative to the 'number of patients with *no disease*', that is, Odds (Disease) $= a/b = 20/60 = 1/3 = 0.33$. Similarly, Odds (No Disease) $= b/a = 60/20 = 3$.

Note that Odds (No Disease) $= 1/Odds(Disease)$. That is, $3 = \frac{1}{1/3}$ for the count data in the above example. Odds of Disease is reciprocal of odds of 'No Disease', and vice versa.

Remark: *Sum* of risk of Disease and risk of 'No Disease' is one. *Product* of odds of Disease and odds of 'No Disease' is one.

Odds ranges from 0 to $\propto$(infinity).

Odds (Disease) $= 1$ implies that success (Disease) and failure (No Disease) are equally likely.

Odd (Disease) > 1 implies that success (Disease) is *more* likely than failure (No Disease).

Odd (Disease) < 1 implies that success (Disease) is *less* likely than failure (No Disease).

Both relative risk or risk ratio (RR) and odds ratio (OR) assesses or measures *association* between two categorical variables, namely a binary outcome (or response) variable (Y) and a binary predictor (or explanatory) variable (X). Sometimes these two ratios are wrongly used interchangeably. They are not the same, and shouldn't be confused because they're actually defined and interpreted very differently. So it's important to keep them separate and to be precise in the language used in the interpretation of the two measures. The obvious difference is appreciated due to the fact that the odds ratio is the ratio of two *odds* whereas the risk ratio is the ratio of two *risks*.

3.2.8   Calculations of RR and OR

The concepts of RR and OR, and their differences, are explained using the following 2×2 contingency table representing an outcome variable (Y with two levels, event and non-event) and an exposure variable or intervention (X with two levels, treatment and control). The values in each of the cells in the two-way table represent the counts (frequencies) (Table 3.2).

3.3   Relative Risk (RR)

The probability (or risk) of an event (Disease) in the Treatment group is $R_T = a/(a+b)$. This is a proportion of 'number of events' relative to the 'total of number of events and non-events' in the Treatment group. It's the number of patients in the Treatment group who experienced an event (Disease) out of the total number of patients with and without event (Disease and No Disease) in the Treatment group. This is to say that if a patient was treated (vaccinated), what is the probability (or risk) of having the disease (event)?

Similarly, the probability (or risk) of an event (Disease) in the Control group is $R_C = c/(c+d)$. Again, it's just the proportion of the number of patients who had the disease (event) relative to the total number of patients with or without disease in the Control group. Although each of these probabilities (i.e., risks) is itself a

Table 3.2   Incidences of disease and vaccination data

		Y = Outcome variable		
		Event (e.g. disease)	Non event (e.g. no disease)	Row total
X = Exposure variable	Treatment (e.g. vaccinated)	a (20)	b (60)	a + b (80)
	Control (e.g. unvaccinated)	c (80)	d (20)	c + d (100)
	Column total	a + c (100)	b + d (80)	180

proportion, none of them is the risk ratio. The risk of having an event (Disease) for the subjects in the Treatment group needs be compared to that in the Control group to measure the effect of the Treatment.

The ratio of the above two probabilities (risks), RR_T and RR_C, is the relative risk or risk ratio:

$$RR = R_T / R_C = \frac{a/(a+b)}{c/(c+d)}.$$

So the RR is the ratio of the probability (risk) of the event (Disease) in the Treatment group relative to that in the Control group.

If the Treatment worked (i.e., less subjects had disease in the Treatment group), the relative risk should be smaller than one ($RR < 1$), since the risk of having disease (event) should be smaller in the Treatment group.

If the relative risk is 1, that is, $RR = 1$, the Treatment (vaccination) made no difference at all.

If it's above 1, that is, $RR > 1$ then the Treatment group actually had a higher risk (i.e., more subjects had disease in the vaccination group) than that in the Control group.

Using the count data in the above contingency table we calculate the risk of disease for the Treatment and Control groups as follows:

$$R_T = {}^a\!/(a+b) = {}^{20}\!/80 = 1/4 \text{ (or 25\%) and}$$
$$R_C = {}^c\!/(c+d) = {}^{80}\!/100 = 4/5 \text{(or 80\%).}$$

Then the relative risk (RR) of the Treatment (relative to the Control) becomes

$$RR = R_T / R_C = \frac{1/4}{4/5} = \frac{5}{16} \text{ (or 31.25\%).}$$

Since the RR is much less than 1, the Treatment reduced the risk of disease in the exposed/intervention group.

3.3.1 Interpretations of RR

Because RR is a ratio and expresses how many times more probable the outcome (Disease) is in the Treatment group, the simplest way to interpret the RR is to use the phrase "times the risk" or "times as high as" compared to those in the Control group.

If you are interpreting a risk ratio, you will always be correct by saying: "Those who received vaccine (Treatment) had RR '*times the risk*' compared to those who did not have the vaccine (Control)." Or "The risk of Disease among those who received vaccine (Treatment) was RR *'times as high as'* the risk of Disease among those who did not receive vaccine (Control)."

For the above example RR = 0.3125. Thus, the risk of disease for those who received the vaccine (Treatment) is RR = 0.3125 'times the risk' of disease for those who did not receive vaccine (Control). Since the RR is less than 1 (actually less than 1/3), there is less risk of disease in the Treatment group than that in the Control group, and hence the Treatment works. Smaller the value of RR weakest is the association between the two categorized variables.

For inference (confidence interval and hypothesis test) on RR, use the log transformation Ln(RR) with its approximate variance,

$$\text{Var}[\text{Ln}(\text{RR})] = \frac{1}{a} - \frac{1}{(a+b)} + \frac{1}{c} - \frac{1}{(c+d)}$$

and standard error

$$\text{SE}[\text{Ln}(\text{RR})] = \sqrt{\frac{1}{a} - \frac{1}{(a+b)} + \frac{1}{c} - \frac{1}{(c+d)}}.$$

For the data in the above example, the standard error becomes

$$\text{SE}[\text{Ln}(\text{RR})] = \sqrt{\frac{1}{20} - \frac{1}{(20+60)} + \frac{1}{80} - \frac{1}{(80+20)}} = \sqrt{0.04} = 0.2.$$

3.4 Odds Ratio (OR)

The odds of event (Disease) in the Treatment group is $OD_T = a/b$. This is the ratio of the number of events (Disease) relative to the number of non-events (No Disease) in the Treatment group. The numerator is the same as that of the probability, but the denominator here is different (in fact smaller). It's not a measure of events (Disease) relative to the all possible 'events and non events', rather it is relative to the non-events (No Disease) only.

Similarly, the odds of event (Disease) in the Control group is $OD_C = c/d$. This is the ratio of the number of events divided by number of non-events in the Control group.

The odds ratio (OR) of the Treatment group relative to the Control group is then defined as the ratio of the two odds, that it,

$$OR = \frac{OD_T}{OD_C} = \frac{a/b}{c/d} = \frac{a \times d}{c \times b}.$$

Now using the count data in the contingency table we calculate the odds for the Treatment and Control groups as follows:

$$OD_T = a/b = 20/60 = 1/3 \text{ and } OD_C = c/d = 80/20 = 4.00.$$

Then the odds ratio (OR) of the Treatment (against the Control) becomes

$$OR = OD_T / OD_C = \frac{1/3}{4} = \frac{1}{12}.$$

Since the OR is much less than 1, the Treatment has reduced the odds of disease in the exposed/intervention group.

3.4.1 Interpretations of OR

For the above example $OR = 1/12 = 0.0833$.

Thus, the odds ratio of event (Disease) for the vaccine (Treatment) group is 1/12 (or 0.0833). The odds of event (Disease) for those who received the vaccine (Treatment) is $OR = 0.0833$ 'times the odds' of event to those who did not receive vaccine (Control).

Since this is much less than 1, there is much less odds of event (Disease) in the Treatment group, and hence the Treatment works. This implies that the Treatment (vaccine) works to reduce the incidences of events (Disease).

For inference (confidence interval and hypothesis test) on OR, use the log transformation Ln(OR) with approximate variance,

$$\text{Var}[\text{Ln(OR)}] = \frac{1}{a} + \frac{1}{b} + \frac{1}{c} + \frac{1}{d}$$

and standard error

$$\text{SE}[\text{Ln(OR)}] = \sqrt{\frac{1}{a} + \frac{1}{b} + \frac{1}{c} + \frac{1}{d}}.$$

For the data in the above example, the standard error becomes

$$\text{SE}[\text{Ln(OR)}] = \sqrt{\frac{1}{20} + \frac{1}{60} + \frac{1}{80} + \frac{1}{20}} = \sqrt{0.129167} = 0.359398.$$

Avoid division by zero

In many cases a slightly *amended* estimator of OR is used by adding 0.5 to each cell count to avoid division by 0 as suggested by Agresti, A 1996, p. 25 and Soukri M.M 1999, p. 49. Hence, for the above example the two amended odds become

$$OD_T^* = {(a + 0.5)}/{(b + 0.5)} = {(20.5)}/{(60.5)} = 0.3388 \text{ and}$$

$$OD_C^* = {(c + 0.5)}/{(d + 0.5)} = {(80.5)}/{(20.5)} = 3.9268.$$

Then the amended odds ratio (OR*) of the Treatment (against the Control) becomes

$$OR^* = OD_T^* / OD_C^* = \frac{0.3388}{3.9268} = 0.0863.$$

Obviously, this amended $OR^* = 0.0863$ is slightly different from the original $OR = 0.0833$.

Comment: All statistical packages have this option to adjust for continuity correction. MetaXL allows a number of choices to be added to zero including 0.5.

3.4.2 Properties of OR

If $OR = 1$, the odds of event (Disease) in the Treatment group is the same as that in the Control group.

If $1 < OR < \infty$, then the odds of event (Disease) is higher in the Treatment group than in the Control group. As an example, if $OR = 4$ then the odds of evert (Disease) in the Treatment group is four 'times the odds' of event (Diseases) in the Control group. So the subjects in the Treatment group is 4 times more likely to have event (Disease) than the Control group.

If $OR = 0.25$ then the odds of event (Disease) in Treatment group is 0.25 'times the odds' of event (Disease) in the Control group.

Smaller the value of the OR weaker is the association (dependence) between the two categorical variables, exposure variable (X—Treatment or Control) and outcome variable (Y—Event and No Event).

For example, when $OR = 4$ then the association/dependence of (Exposure and Outcome variables, X and Y) is higher than when $OR = 2$ (or less). Similarly, $OR = 0.50$ indicates more dependence between (Explanatory and Outcome variables) than $OR = 0.25$ (or less).

3.5 Comparison of RR and OR

1. The RR and OR are comparable in magnitude when the event/disease studied is rare or very uncommon in both exposed and unexposed groups.
2. The OR > RR when the event/disease is more common. But OR should not be viewed as risk, it is a ratio of odds.

3. In case-control studies, risks and RR can't be calculated but OR can be calculated and use as an approximation of RR if event/disease is uncommon in the population.
4. The OR can be used to describe results of both case-control and prospective cohort studies.
5. One advantage of OR is that it is not dependent on whether we focus on the event's occurrence or its failure. That is, the OR is symmetric to which outcome level is of interest, but RR is not symmetric. That is, $Odds(Event) = \frac{1}{Odds(No-Event)}$.
6. If the OR for an event (success) deviates from 1 substantially, the OR of its non-event (failure) will also deviate from 1 substantially, although in the opposite direction.

3.5.1 When OR is Equal (or Close) to RR?

If the event (Disease) is rare, in both the exposed and unexposed groups, then the OR is closer (or equal) to the RR.

Consider the following modified count data with rare (or very small) number of events (2 for the Treatment group and 5 for the Control group) to illustrate how/when OR is closer to the RR (Table 3.3).

For the above count data, the number of events (Disease) for both the Treatment and Control groups are small, say 2 and 5 respectively, and the RR of the Treatment group is $RR_T = \frac{a/(a+b)}{c/(c+d)} = \frac{2/80}{5/100} = \frac{2 \times 100}{80 \times 5} = \frac{1}{2}$ (or 50%) and the OR of the Treatment group is $OR_T = \frac{a/b}{c/d} = \frac{2/78}{5/95} = \frac{2 \times 95}{78 \times 5} = \frac{19}{39}$ (or 0.48) which is closer to the RR of 50%.

Furthermore, if the number of events (Disease) for both the Treatment and Control groups are even smaller, say 1 for each group, that is, ($a^* = 1$, $b^* = 79$, $c^* = 1$, $d^* = 99$) then

$$RR_T = \frac{a*/(a*+b*)}{c*/(c*+d*)} = \frac{1/80}{1/100} = \frac{1 \times 100}{80 \times 1} = \frac{5}{4} \text{ (or 125.00\%) and}$$

$$OR_T = \frac{a*/b*}{c*/d*} = \frac{1/79}{1/99} = \frac{1 \times 99}{79 \times 1} = \frac{99}{79} \text{ (or 125.31) which is much closer (almost equal)}$$

to the RR of 125%.

Table 3.3 Revised incidences of disease and vaccination data

		Y = Outcome variable		
		Event (e.g. disease)	Non event (e.g. no disease)	Row total
X = Exposure variable	Treatment (e.g. vaccinated)	a (2)	b (78)	a + b (80)
	Control (e.g. unvaccinated)	c (5)	d (95)	c + d (100)
	Column total	a + c (7)	b + d (173)	180

Thus for very small number of events (Disease), in both the exposed and unexposed groups, the OR is not much different from the RR.

3.5.2 Incidence and Prevalence

Incidence and prevalence are very commonly used terms in epidemiology and public health. They may be related but very different.

Prevalence (also called prevalence rate) indicates the probability that a member of the population *has* a given condition at a point in time. So, it is the actual number of cases alive, with the disease either during a period of time (period prevalence) or at a particular date in time (point prevalence).

Incidence (also called incidence rate) is a measure of the occurrence of *new cases* of disease *during a span of time.*

The relationship between incidence and prevalence depends greatly on the natural history of the disease state being reported. In the case of a corona pandemic, the incidence may be high but not contribute to much growth of prevalence because of the high, spontaneous rate of disease resolution.

The changes in the values of RR and OR with the changes in the value of the incidence rate (I_0) at a time is presented in a graph found in Schmidt and Kohlmann 2008. In Fig. 1 of this paper the changes in the values of RR and OR with the changes in the incidence rate is displayed. Lowest (almost diagonal) line with incidence rate 0.01 represents the equality of RR and OR. The value of OR grows larger and larger as the incidence rate increases. But the value of RR becomes smaller and smaller as the incidence rate increases.

3.6 Conversion of OR to RR

There is no need to convert OR to RR if OR is properly interpreted and understood. However, some researchers try to convert OR to RR, may be to make it easily understandable to the non-specialised readers. But every researcher in the epidemiology and public health areas requires to understand odds and OR, and be prepared to interpret results based on OR.

Greenland and Holland 1991 and Zhang and Yu 1998 independently proposed a popular conversion formulas of OR to RR given by

$$RR = \frac{OR}{1 - I_C + I_C \times OR}.$$

It is interesting to note that $(1 - I_C) = 1 - \frac{c}{c+d} = \frac{d}{c+d} = I_C^0$ which is the non-incidence rate in the control group. Clearly, sum of I_C and I_C^0 is one. Similarly, for the intervention/treatment group, $(1 - I_E) = 1 - \frac{a}{a+b} = \frac{b}{a+b} = I_E^0$, and hence I_E and I_E^0 add to one.

3.7 Misuse and Misinterpretation of OR

There has been widespread unintentional misuse of odds ration (OR), especially its inappropriate interpretation as risk or probability of events. Readers may note the following examples in the epidemiological and public health literatures where *odds* is inappropriately used interchangeably with *probability* and/or risk and fails to acknowledge that odds is different from risk.

In the eight edition of the book (Merrill, 2021) notes OR as the 'relative probabilities' of disease in case-control studies without recognising that 'probabilities' are different from odds. It also recommends that odds ratios are generally interpreted as if they were risk ratios when the outcome occurs relatively infrequently (<10%). However, this 'rare disease' assumption is very infrequent.

In discussing the difference between "Probability" and "Odds" the (Boston University, 2020) notes,that the odds are defined as the *probability* that the event will occur divided by the probability that the event will not occur. Then illustrates OR with the following hypothetical pilot study on pesticide exposure and breast cancer and comes up with OR = (7/10) / (6/57) = 6.65. Interestingly, neither the numerator nor the denominator of the OR here is a probability, and that is correct because they should be odds. Yet, the definition above defines OR as ratio of probabilities.

	Diseased	Non-diseased
Pesticide Exposure	7	10
Non-exposed	6	57

Referring to (Bland & Altman, 2000), (Chen, Cohen, & Chen, 2010) report, "Odds ratio (OR) originally was proposed to determine whether the *probability* of an event (or disease) is the same or differs between the two groups, generally a high-risk group and a low-risk group."

3.8 Conclusions

The most popular ratio measures to investigate the association between two categorical variables, the RR and OR, are covered in this chapter. Meta-analyses based these effect size measures are presented in the upcoming chapters. In conducting meta-analysis for the RR or OR the log transformation of the ratio is essential. However, the final results for forest plots must be expressed in the original ratio scale by inverse/back (exponential) transformation.

Schmidt and Kohlmann 2008 note that the direct computation of RR is feasible if meaningful prevalence or incidence data is available. Cross-sectional data may serve to calculate RR from prevalence data. Cohort study designs allow for the direct calculation of RR from incidence.

The situation is more complicated for case-control studies. If meaningful prevalence or incidence data are not available, the OR provides a valid effect size measure. It describes the ratio of disease odds given exposure status. The OR for a given exposure is routinely obtained within logistic models while controlling for confounders. The availability of this approach in standard statistical software largely explains the popularity of this measure. However, it does not have as intuitive interpretation as the RR. Often people wrongly describe an OR of "2" in terms of a "double risk" of developing a disease given exposure.

Often selection of RR or OR depends on the study objective or design and choice or priority of the researcher. However, if you want to know how any exposure (e.g. smoking) affects the outcome (e.g. cancer), odds ratio is the best effect size measure.

There are some other ratio measures, such as proportion, which are covered separately in forthcoming chapters. They include single proportion and difference between two proportions (also known as risk difference).

References

Barger MK (2018) When does the odds ratio not equal the relative risk, and why should you care?(Report). J Midwifery Women's Health 63(6):648. https://doi.org/10.1111/jmwh.12919

Bland JM, Altman DG (2000) The odds ratio. Bmj, 320(7247), 1468. https://doi.org/10.1136/bmj.320.7247.1468

Boston University, So PH (2020) The Difference Between "Probability" and "Odds". Retrieved from http://sphweb.bumc.bu.edu/otlt/MPHModules/BS/BS704_Confidence_Intervals/BS704_Confidence_Intervals10.html

Chen H, Cohen P, Chen S (2010) How Big is a Big Odds Ratio? Interpreting the Magnitudes of Odds Ratios in Epidemiological Studies. Communications in Statistics–Simulation and Computation, 39(4), 860–864. https://doi.org/10.1080/03610911003650383

Greenland S, Holland P (1991) Estimating standardized risk differences from odds ratios. Biometrics 47(1):319–322. https://doi.org/10.2307/2532517

McNutt L-A, Wu C, Xue X, Hafner JP (2003) Estimating the relative risk in cohort studies and clinical trials of common outcomes.(medical research)(Author Abstract). Am J Epidemiol 157(10):940. https://doi.org/10.1093/aje/kwg074

Merrill RM (2021) Introduction to Epidemiology: Johan & Bartlett Learning.

Schmidt C, Kohlmann T (2008) When to use the odds ratio or the relative risk? Int J Public Health 53(3):165–167. https://doi.org/10.1007/s00038-008-7068-3

Shrier I, Steele R (2006) The relationship between odds ratios and relative risks: 2744. Med Sci Sports Exerc 38(Supplement):S528. https://doi.org/10.1249/00005768-200605001-03078

Walter SD (2000) Choice of effect measure for epidemiological data. J Clin Epidemiol 53(9):931–939. https://doi.org/10.1016/S0895-4356(00)00210-9

Zhang J, Yu KF (1998) What's the relative risk? A method for correcting the odds ratio in cohort studies of common outcomes.(statistical expression of risk in medical research). JAMA (Journal of the American Medical Association) 280(19):1690. https://doi.org/10.1001/jama.280.19.1690

Chapter 4
Meta-analysis of Risk Ratio

Starting from this chapter meta-analysis of each of the commonly used effect sizes is covered in seperate chapters. This chapter is devoted to exclusive meta-analysis of risk ratio (also called relative risk). It provides meta-analyses of RR under different statistical models along with subgroup analysis and detection of publication bias with illustrative examples.

4.1 Introduction

If an experiment (or a study) has two arms or interventions and the outcome of interest is a binary or categorical variable, ratio measures are used to analyse the association between the two categorical variables. The data of such experiments/studies are typically presented in a two-way contingency table of counts or frequencies. The most popular ratio measures of association are the risk ratio (RR) and odds ratio (OR). Details on the definition and interpretation of RR and OR are provided in Chap. 3. In this chapter, we cover the meta-analysis for the risk ratio (RR) as an effect size measure.

4.2 Estimation of Effect Size RR

For any experiments with binary exposure and outcome variables the association between the variables can be assessed by risk ratio (RR). In almost all cases, the population data are unavailable and hence population characteristics or parameters are unknown. In reality the unknown population parameters such as population RR is estimated from the available sample data. For any two arms experiment with binary outcome variables the sample data are presented in a contingency table of counts. The unknown population RR is then estimated from the sample data. Using the sampling

© Springer Nature Singapore Pte Ltd. 2020
S. Khan, *Meta-Analysis*, Statistics for Biology and Health,
https://doi.org/10.1007/978-981-15-5032-4_4

distribution of the estimator (statistic) of unknown parameter, RR and its standard error (SE), confidence interval is calculated for the unknown population RR.

The point estimate of the risk ratio (RR) is required to find the confidence interval (and perform hypothesis tests) for the unknown population RR (parameter). For both confidence interval and test of hypotheses, the sampling distribution of the estimator (statistic) of the parameter of interest is essential. The critical value of the statistic (e.g. z or t) in the confidence interval, and the choice of appropriate test statistic depend on the type of sampling distribution of the estimator. Refer to Chap. 2 for details.

The distribution of the estimator of population RR is not known as it does not follow any commonly known probability (statistical) distribution. However, the log transformation of RR follows an approximate standard normal distribution. Therefore, for both confidence interval and test of hypothesis the estimator (statistic) of RR is replaced by that of Ln(RR), so that the distribution of the transformed statistic can be used. Although the log transformation does not affect the outcome of the test (statistic and hence the P-value) in the hypothesis testing process, inverse (or back) transformation of the lower and upper limits are required for the limits of the confidence interval to be expressed in the original RR scale (of measurement).

For both the confidence interval and test of hypothesis, in addition to the transformed statistic Ln(RR), the standard error (SE) of the transformed statistic Ln(RR) is required (and used).

Confidence interval for RR

In meta-analysis, one of the main interest is to find the 95% confidence interval for the effect size of individual studies as well as for the common effect size by combining summary statistics from selected independent studies.

The generic form of a $(1 - \alpha) \times 100\%$ (95% if $\alpha = 0.05$ or 5%) confidence interval for the common population effect size θ is give by

$$\hat{\theta} \pm z_{\alpha/2} \times SE(\hat{\theta}),$$

where $\hat{\theta}$ is the point estimate of θ, common effect size of all studies, $z_{\alpha/2}$ is the critical value (cut-off point) of the standard normal distribution leaving $\alpha/2$ area to the upper and lower tail of the distribution, and $SE(\hat{\theta})$ is the standard error of the estimator of θ. For the ith study the confidence interval for θ_i is $\hat{\theta}_i \pm z_{\alpha/2} \times SE(\hat{\theta}_i)$ for $i = 1, 2, ..., k$.

To find the confidence interval for the unknown population parameter θ $(= RR)$ a natural log transformation, $\theta^* = \ln(\theta) = \ln(RR)$ is used. An estimator of transformed parameter θ^* is given by $\hat{\theta}^* = \ln(\hat{\theta})$ which follows an approximate normal distribution. Here $\hat{\theta}$ is the estimated RR calculated from the sample count data.

The standard error of $\hat{\theta}^* = \ln(\hat{\theta})$ is

$$SE(\hat{\theta}^*) = \sqrt{\frac{1}{a} - \frac{1}{a+b} + \frac{1}{c} - \frac{1}{c+d}}.$$

Table 4.1 Vaccination and disease data

		Y = Outcome variable		Row total
		Event (e.g. disease)	Non event (e.g. No disease)	
X = Exposure variable	Treatment (e.g. vaccinated)	a (20)	b (60)	a + b (80)
	Control (e.g. unvaccinated)	c (80)	d (20)	c + d (100)
	Column total	a + c (100)	b + d (80)	180

Then the $(1 - \alpha) \times 100\%$ confidence interval for $\theta^* = \ln(\theta)$ is represented by the lower limits: $LL^* = \hat{\theta}^* - z_{\alpha/2} \times SE(\hat{\theta}^*)$, where $z_{\alpha/2}$ is the critical value of Z for a two-sided test at the α level of significance and upper limit $UL^* = \hat{\theta}^* + z_{\alpha/2} \times SE(\hat{\theta}^*)$ in the ln RR scale, and then $LL = \exp(LL^*)$ and $UL = \exp(UL^*)$ in the original RR scale.

Example 4.1 (CI for RR) Consider the Vaccination and Disease data in Table 4.1. Find the point estimate and 95% confidence interval for the unknown population RR.

From the Vaccination and Disease data in Table 4.1 we have the point estimate of the population RR,

$$\hat{\theta} = RR = \frac{a/(a+b)}{c/(c+d)} = \frac{20/80}{80/100} = \frac{1/4}{4/5} = \frac{1 \times 5}{4 \times 4} = 5/16 = 0.3125.$$

To find the confidence interval for the population RR we need to find the log of the point estimate (lnRR) and standard error of the estimator of lnRR.

Here, the sample lnRR becomes

$$\hat{\theta}^* = \ln(\hat{\theta}) = \ln(0.3125) = -1.16315081 \text{ and}$$

$$SE(\hat{\theta}^*) = SE[\ln(RR)] = \sqrt{\frac{1}{a} - \frac{1}{a+b} + \frac{1}{c} - \frac{1}{c+d}} = \sqrt{\frac{1}{20} - \frac{1}{80} + \frac{1}{80} - \frac{1}{100}}.$$
$$= \sqrt{0.04} = 0.2.$$

Then the 95% confidence interval for the population RR, θ is given by the lower and upper limits:

$$LL^* = \hat{\theta}^* - z_{\alpha/2} \times SE(\hat{\theta}^*) = -1.16315081 - 1.96 \times 0.2 = -1.55515081 \text{ and}$$

$$UL^* = \hat{\theta}^* + z_{\alpha/2} \times SE(\hat{\theta}^*) = -1.16315081 + 1.96 \times 0.2 = -0.77115081$$

in the ln RR scale, and using the back transformation we get

$LL = \exp(LL^*) = \exp(-1.55515081) = 0.211157536$ and
$UL = \exp(UL^*) = \exp(-0.77115081) = 0.462480535$ in the original RR scale.

Thus the 95% confidence interval for θ (population RR) becomes (0.2111, 0.4625).

4.3   Significance Test on Effect Size RR

To test the significance of the population RR, θ the null hypothesis is $H_0 : \theta = 1$ (the risk is the same for the treatment and control groups) we actually need to test the null hypothesis $H_0 : \theta^* = \ln(\theta) = \ln(1) = 0$ (that is, there is no significant difference of risk for the two groups) since the sampling distribution of estimator of θ is unknown but that of θ^* is approximately normal.

The appropriate test statistic to test $H_0 : \theta^* = 0$ against $H_A : \theta^* \neq 0$ is $Z = \frac{\hat{\theta}^*}{SE(\hat{\theta}^*)}$ which follows a standard normal distribution.

Example 4.2 (Test for RR) Consider the count data in Table 4.1. Perform a test of significance on the population RR.

For the Vaccination and Disease data in Table 4.1 we have from Example 4.1.
$\hat{\theta} = RR = 5/16 = 0.3125, \hat{\theta}^* = \ln(\hat{\theta}) = \ln(0.3125) = -1.16315081$ and $SE(\hat{\theta}^*) = SE[\ln(RR)] = 0.2$.
Hence the observed value of the Z statistic becomes

$$z_0 = \frac{\hat{\theta}^*}{SE(\hat{\theta}^*)} = \frac{-1.16315081}{0.2} = -5.8157 \approx -5.82.$$

The two-sided P-value $= P(|Z| > 5.82) = P(Z < -5.82) + P(Z > 5.82) = 2 \times P(Z > 5.82) = 0$ (from the Normal Table).

Since the P-value is 0, the test is highly significant. That is, there is a very strong sample evidence against the null hypothesis of $\ln(RR) = 0$, (that is, RR = 1). Hence we reject the null hypothesis in favour of the alternative hypothesis (and conclude that there is strong association/dependency between the outcome and intervention). In other words, the incidence of disease is dependent on the intervention—treatment (vaccination) or control (no vaccination). So there is an association between the exposure variable (treatment/vaccinated or control/unvaccinated) and the outcome variable (event/disease or non-event/no-disease).

More details on the tests of hypotheses for meta-analysis and their powers are found in Hedges and Pigott (2001).

The meta-analysis method for the RR is provided in the forthcoming sections under different statistical models.

4.4 Fixed Effect (FE) Model

The fixed effect (FE) and other statistical models are applicable for meta-analysis of effect size measure of studies involving both binary and continuous outcome variables. The FE model is used if there is no significant heterogeneity of effect size among the independent studies. In this section, the FE model is presented in a general framework for the meta-analysis of RR with example. An introduction to the FE model is found in Borenstein et al. (2010) and in Chapter 11 of Borenstein et al. (2009).

Let us consider k independent studies selected for a meta-analysis after systematic review of all studies on a particular topic of interest. Let the outcome variable of interest be binary. The underlying assumption is that there is an unknown common effect size (RR), θ based on the binary outcome variable for all the independent primary studies. Meta-analysis enables us to pool results from all independent studies to estimate the common population effect size θ.

Let θ_i be the unknown true (population) study specific effect size of interest which includes systematic bias specific to the study (if no systematic bias then $\theta_i = \theta$) and σ_i^2 be the unknown population variance of the ith study for $i = 1, 2, ..., k$. The sample estimate of the population effect size for the ith primary study based on a random sample of size n_i is denoted by $\hat{\theta}_i$ and the sample variance by v_i. The unknown inverse variance population weight $\omega_i = \frac{1}{\sigma_i^2}$ of the ith study is estimated by $w_i = \frac{1}{v_i}$.

Normally, individual primary study reports the sample estimate of the effect size $\left(\hat{\theta}_i\right)$ and the sample variance (v_i) of the estimator of the population effect size along with the sample size n_i. Based on these information, a 95% confidence interval for θ_i is constructed for each of the studies if the sampling distribution of $\hat{\theta}_i$ is known. Obviously, the confidence intervals vary from one study to another, and some of the studies may even provide conflicting results (with even opposing signs). Therefore, it is important to combine the results from all the k studies by pooling the summary statistics into a single point estimate and find a confidence interval for the common effect size θ.

The fixed effect (FE) model assumes that all studies share a common effect size and attempt is made to estimate the unknown population common effect size from the sample data.

Under the FE model, the estimator of the transformed common effect size $\theta_{FE}^* = Ln(\theta_{FE})$ is given by

$$\hat{\theta}_{FE}^* = \frac{\sum_{i=1}^{k} w_i \hat{\theta}_i^*}{\sum_{i=1}^{k} w_i}, \tag{4.1}$$

where $w_i = \frac{1}{v_i}$ is the weight of the ith study. The pooled estimate under the FE model is the weighted mean of the estimated effect sizes of all the independent studies. The denominator is to ensure that the sum of the weights is 1. The sample variance of the estimator of the common effect size $\hat{\theta}_{FE}^*$ is $Var(\hat{\theta}_{FE}^*) = 1 \Big/ \sum_{i=1}^{k} w_i$. Therefore, the standard error of the estimator of the common effect size under the FE model is

$$SE(\hat{\theta}_{FE}^*) = \sqrt{\frac{1}{\sum_{i=1}^{k} w_i}}. \tag{4.2}$$

The estimator in Eq. (4.1) and standard error in Eq. (4.2) are used in the formulation of the confidence interval and test statistic.

The confidence interval
Although the distribution of $\hat{\theta}_{FE}$ is unknown, we could use its log transformation as the distribution of log of $\hat{\theta}_{FE}$ is approximately normal. Thus, first we find the confidence interval in LnRR scale (from log $\hat{\theta}_{FE}$) and then apply the back/reverse transformation to find the confidence interval in the original RR scale.

Define $\hat{\theta}_{FE}^* = \ln(\hat{\theta}_{FE})$ and standard error of LnRR $SE(\hat{\theta}_{FE}^*) = \sqrt{Var(\hat{\theta}_{FE}^*)}$. Then the $(1 - \alpha) \times 100\%$ confidence interval for LnRR is given by the limits $LL^* = \hat{\theta}_{FE}^* - z_{\alpha/2} \times SE(\hat{\theta}_{FE}^*)$ and $UL^* = \hat{\theta}_{FE}^* + z_{\alpha/2} \times SE(\hat{\theta}_{FE}^*)$.

Here $z_{\alpha/2}$ is the $\frac{\alpha}{2}$th cut-off point of standard normal distribution. For a 95% confidence interval $z_{\alpha/2} = z_{0.05/2} = 1.96$.

Now using the back/reverse transformation of LnRR on the above limits we get the confidence interval in RR scale as

$$LL = \exp(LL^*)$$
$$UL = \exp(UL^*).$$

Test of hypothesis
To test the significance of the common effect size (RR) under the FE model, test the null hypothesis, $H_0 : \theta = 0$ (null) against $H_a : \theta \neq 0$ using the test statistic

$$Z = \frac{\hat{\theta}_{FE}^* - 0}{SE(\hat{\theta}_{FE}^*)},$$

where the statistic Z follows the standard normal distribution.

Decision Rules
Critical value approach: For a two-tailed test, reject H_0 at the α level of significance if the calculated/observed value of the Z statistic (say z_0) satisfies $|z_0| \geq z_{\alpha/2}$, where $z_{\alpha/2}$ is the $\alpha/2$ level upper cut-off point of the standard normal distribution; otherwise don't reject the null hypothesis.

Table 4.2 Count data on the number of patients with **ablation** in the low-dose and high-dose groups

Study name	Treatment (high dose)			Control (low dose)		
	N1	Cases	Non-cases	N2	Cases	Non-cases
Doi (2000)	49	23	26	39	25	14
Ramacciotti (1982)	9	3	6	20	12	8
Angelini (1997)	426	226	200	180	101	79
Liu (1987)	40	14	26	20	11	9
Lin (1998)	21	6	15	25	11	14
McCowen (1976)	28	10	18	36	15	21
Maxon (1992)	37	6	31	26	6	20

P-value approach: Alternatively, for a two-tailed test, reject H_0 at the α level of significance if the P-value is less than or equal to a preselected significance level, α; otherwise don't reject the null hypothesis in Table 4.2.

Example 4.3 Consider the data in Table 4.2 on the number of patients with high dose radio-active iodine versus low dose after thyroidectomy in patients with differentiated thyroid cancer. The study looked at the risk of **ablation** (surgical removal of tissue) as the outcome variable. For illustration we consider seven independent studies as in the Table 4.2.

For the above ablation data, find the sample RR, the ln RR (LnRR), the variance of ln RR [Var(LnRR)] and the 95% confidence interval for the population RR.

Solutions
The relative risk (RR) of the Treatment (High dose) group, log of RR (LnRR), variance of LnRR, weight (W), limits of 95% confidence interval and other calculations for individual studies are shown in the following table (Table 4.3).

Example 4.4 Consider the ablation data in Example 4.3.

Under the fixed effect model, find

(i) The point estimate of the population RR
(ii) Standard error of the estimator of the population LnRR
(iii) The 95% confidence interval for the population RR and
(iv) Test the significance of the population RR.

Solution:

(i) Under the FE model the point estimate of the common effect size (RR) is

$$\hat{\theta}_{FE}^* = \frac{\sum\limits_{i=1}^{k} w_i \hat{\theta}_i^*}{\sum\limits_{i=1}^{k} w_i} = \frac{\sum\limits_{i=1}^{7} W LnRR}{\sum\limits_{i=1}^{7} W} = \frac{-29.883}{217.085} = -0.1377 \text{ in the ln RR scale,}$$

Table 4.3 Calculations for LnRR, Var(LnRR), W(LnRR), W × LnRR, 95% confidence intervals, and sum of W(LnRR) and sum of W × LNRR

Study name	RR	LnRR	Var(LnRR)	W(LnRR)	W × LnRR	95% CI LL	UL
Doi (2000)	0.7322	−0.3116	0.037429	26.7172	−8.3262	0.5012	1.0699
Ramacciotti (1982)	0.5556	−0.5878	0.255556	3.91304	−2.3	0.2063	1.4964
Angelini (1997)	0.9455	−0.0561	0.006423	155.695	−8.7295	0.808	1.1063
Liu (1987)	0.6364	−0.452	0.087338	11.4498	−5.1751	0.3566	1.1357
Lin (1998)	0.6494	−0.4318	0.169957	5.88385	−2.5405	0.2894	1.4568
McCowen (1976)	0.8571	−0.1542	0.103175	9.69231	−1.4941	0.4567	1.6087
Maxon (1992)	0.7027	−0.3528	0.267845	3.73351	−1.3173	0.2548	1.9378
				217.085	**−29.883**		

and hence the estimated effect size in the RR scale, under the FE model, becomes

$$\hat{\theta}_{FE} = \exp(\hat{\theta}^*_{FE}) = \exp(-0.1377) = 0.8714.$$

(ii) The standard error of the estimator of Ln RR is

$$SE(\hat{\theta}^*_{FE}) = \sqrt{\frac{1}{\sum_{i=1}^{k} w_i}} = \sqrt{\frac{1}{\sum_{i=1}^{7} W}} = \sqrt{0.004606} = 0.06787.$$

(iii) The 95% confidence interval for the (transformed) common effect size (θ^*) in Ln RR scale is

$$LL^* = \hat{\theta}^*_{FE} - 1.96 \times SE(\hat{\theta}^*_{FE}) = -0.1377 - 1.96 \times 0.06787 = -0.27068$$
$$UL^* = \hat{\theta}^*_{FE} + 1.96 \times SE(\hat{\theta}^*_{FE}) = -0.1377 + 1.96 \times 0.06787 = -0.00463.$$

Then the 95% confidence interval for the common effect size (θ) in the original RR scale is

$$LL = \exp(LL^*) = \exp(-0.27068) = 0.7628 \approx 0.76$$
$$UL = \exp(UL^*) = \exp(-0.00463) = 0.9954 \approx 1.00.$$

Remark: The *above* point estimate (0.87) and the 95% confidence interval (0.76, 1.00) are reported at the bottom row of the forest plot in Fig. 4.1.

(iv) To test $H_0 : \theta = 0$ (that is, LnRR = 0) against $H_a : \theta \neq 0$ the observed value of the test statistic $Z = \frac{\hat{\theta}^*}{SE(\hat{\theta}^*)}$ is $z_0 = \frac{-0.1377}{0.06787} = -2.0289 \approx -2.03$.

The two-sided P-value is $P(|Z| > 2.03) = P(Z < -2.03) + P(Z > 2.03) = 2 \times 0.0212 = 0.0424$ (<0.05). So, at the 5% significance level the RR is significant.

The effect size (RR) of ablation after thyroidectomy in patients is significantly different for the low dose and high dose patients at the 5% level of significant.

Forest plot for RR under FE model using MetaXL
The forest plot under the FE model (indicated by "IV" in the MetaXL code) is produced by using MetaXL code

=MAInputTable("Thyroid RR FE","NumRR","IV",B17:H23).

Remark: Explanations of MetaXL Code
For this type of meta-analyses in MetaXL the 'opening' code starts with MA Input Table '= MAInputTable'. This is followed by an open parenthesis inside which the first quote contains the text that appears as the 'title of the output of the forest plot' e.g. "Thyroid RR FE" in the above code (user may choose any appropriate title here, but RR is chosen to indicate the relevant effect size measure here and FE is chosen to indicate fixed effect model). Then in the second quote enter the type of effect measure, e.g. "NumRR" in the above code tells that the *outcome variable is numerical and the effect size measure is risk ratio*. Within the third quote enter the statistical model, e.g. "IV" in the above code stands for the *fixed effect* (abbreviated by FE) model. Each quotation is followed by a comma, and after the last comma enter the data area in Excel Worksheet, e.g. B17:H23 in the above code tells that the data on the independent studies are taken from the specified cells. The code ends with a closing parenthesis.

The forest plot of the meta-analysis of RR using the above MetaXL code is found to be in Fig. 4.1.

Explanations of Forest plot
The point estimate of the effect size of any individual study is represented by the middle most point of the relevant blue square, the size/area of the square indicates the redistributed study weight allocated by the model, and horizontal lines on both sides of the square represent the limits of the 95% confidence interval for the unknown effect size of the study.

The vertical solid line is the line of no effect (i.e. RR = 1, the position at which there is no clear difference between the intervention group and the control group).

If the outcome of interest is adverse (e.g. mortality), the results to the left of the vertical line favour the intervention over the control. That is, if result estimates are located to the left, it means that the outcome of interest (e.g. mortality) occurred less frequently in the intervention group than in the control group (RR < 1).

If the outcome of interest is desirable (e.g. remission), the results to the right of the vertical line favour the treatment over the control. That is, if result estimates are located to the right, it means that the outcome of interest (e.g. remission) occurred more frequently in the intervention group than in the control group (RR > 1).

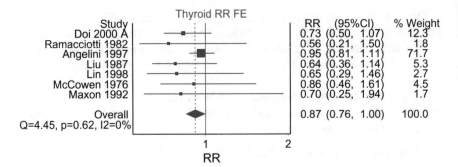

Fig. 4.1 Forest plot of RR for the ablation of low-dose and high-dose patients using fixed effect model

The diamond at the bottom represents the 95% confidence interval for the pooled common effect size. The vertical line through the middle of the diamond represents the common effect size estimate, and the two horizontal ends of the diamond represent the lower and upper limit of the 95% confidence interval.

If the diamond touches the vertical line (at RR = 1), the overall (combined) result is not statistically significant. It means that the overall outcome rate in the intervention group is much the same as in the control group (except for random variation).

Interpretation of forest plot in Fig. 4.1

From the above meta-analysis presented in the forest plot, the estimated common RR is 0.87 and the 95% confidence interval is (0.76, 1.00). The RR is not statistically significant (as RR = 1 is included in the confidence interval).

The high dose patients have lower risk of ablation compared to the patients with low dose after thyroidectomy differentiated thyroid cancer. The patients with high dose have 13% (1–0.87) less risk of ablation than those with low dose. But the result is not statistically significant.

4.4.1   Measuring Heterogeneity Between the Study Effects

Heterogeneity occurs when the values of the effect size measures across the independent studies are significantly different. It is a real concern in meta-analysis as it is common in many meta-analyses and makes the analyses much more difficult. Ignoring heterogeneity would lead to inappropriate and misleading results. It is essential for every meta-analysis to investigate the presence of heterogeneity among the individual studies so that an appropriate statistical model/method could be used to analyse the data properly. For this reason every forest plot contains results on the measure of heterogeneity such as the Cochran's Q statistic Cochran (1973) and I^2 index. For further insight into the heterogeneity measures in meta-analysis refer to Higgins et al. (2003).

Here we cover the Cochran's Q statistic and I^2 index to measure heterogeneity among the studies as most of the popular statistical packages on meta-analysis including MataXL, routinely use these measures.

To test the heterogeneity between study effect sizes, we test the null hypothesis, $H_0 : \theta_1 = \theta_2 = \ldots = \theta_k$ against the alternative hypothesis, H_a: not all θ_i's are equal for $i = 1, 2, .., k$ using the following Q statistic

$$Q = \sum_{i=1}^{k} w_i \hat{\theta}_i^2 - \frac{\left(\sum_{i=1}^{k} w_i \hat{\theta}_i \right)^2}{\sum_{i=1}^{k} w_i},$$

where Q follows a chi-squared distribution with $(k - 1)$ degrees of freedom. The value of Q statistic increases as the number of independent studies included in the meta-analysis increases. This problem is addressed by Higgin's I^2 index defined as

$$I^2 = \left(\frac{Q - df}{Q} \right) \times 100\%.$$

Example 4.5 For the ablation data in Example 4.3, find the value of the Q and I^2 statistics.

To answer this question, first the summary statistics are calculated as in Table 4.4.

For the above data, using the sums (in bold fonts) from the last row of Table 4.4 the value of the Q statistic is found as

$$Q = \sum_{i=1}^{k} w_i \hat{\theta}_i^2 - \frac{\left(\sum_{i=1}^{k} w_i \hat{\theta}_i \right)^2}{\sum_{i=1}^{k} w_i} = \sum_{1}^{7} W \times Ln\,RR^2 - \frac{\left[\sum_{1}^{7} W \times Ln\,RR \right]^2}{\sum_{1}^{7} W}$$

Table 4.4 Calculations of LnRR, Var(LnRR), W(LnRR), W × LnRR, W × LnRR², and sum of W(LnRR), sum of W × LNRR and sum of W × LNRR²

Study name	RR	LnRR	Var(LnRR)	W(LnRR)	W × LnRR	W × LnRR²
Doi (2000)	0.7322	−0.3116	0.0374	26.7172	−8.3262	2.594765
Ramacciotti (1982)	0.5556	−0.5878	0.2556	3.913043	−2.3	1.35193
Angelini (1997)	0.9455	−0.0561	0.0064	155.6954	−8.7295	0.489448
Liu (1987)	0.6364	−0.452	0.0873	11.44981	−5.1751	2.339089
Lin (1998)	0.6494	−0.4318	0.17	5.883851	−2.5405	1.096962
McCowen (1976)	0.8571	−0.1542	0.1032	9.692308	−1.4941	0.230313
Maxon (1992)	0.7027	−0.3528	0.2678	3.733506	−1.3173	0.464758
				217.0852	**−29.883**	**8.567264**

$$= 8.567264 - \frac{(-29.8827)^2}{217.0852} = 4.4538 \approx 4.45.$$

The Q statistic follows a chi-squared distribution with $(k - 1) = 7 - 1 = 6$ degrees of freedom. Then the P-value of testing equality of population effect sizes becomes $p = P(\chi_6^2 > 4.45) = 0.62$. Using chi-squired distribution table, it is found that the P-value is between 0.50 and 0.75 (which includes 0.62). Since the P-value is very large (much larger than 5%), there is insignificant heterogeneity between the study means, and we don't reject the null hypothesis.

Then, the value of the I^2 statistic becomes

$$I^2 = \left(\frac{Q - df}{Q} \right) \times 100\% = \left(\frac{4.45 - 6}{4.45} \right) \times 100\% = -0.35\% \to 0$$

(negative values of I^2 is truncated to 0). Since the value of I^2 is 0, there is no significant heterogeneity between the study effects.

Remarks: Note that I^2 is the percentage of variation across studies that is due to heterogeneity rather than chance. Higgins et al. (2003) suggest that the I^2 values of 25%, 50% and 75% indicate low, moderate and high heterogeneity respectively among the population effect sizes.

If $I^2 \leq 25\%$ studies are considered to be homogeneous, and a fixed effect model of meta-analysis can be used.

Comment: The values of Q and I^2 statistics are calculated from the sample summary data and they are not dependent on any statistical models.

4.5   Random Effects (REs) Model

Under the random effects (REs) model there is no common effect size for the k independent studies. In stead, it is assumed that every primary study has a different population effect size which is a random variable. As such, there is variation between the effect sizes of the individual studies. So, the variance of effect size under the REs model is the sum of within study and between studies variances. As suggested by DerSimonian and Laird (1986) the between studies variance is estimated by method of moments. In recent years many researchers have criticized the REs model pointing out its shortcomings including simulation comparison as in Doi et al. (2015b).

Since, under the REs model, there are two sources of variance, so the overall study error variance has two components. First, the within-study error variance, v_i and second, the between-study variance. The population between-studies variance is the variance of θ_i about θ and is denoted by τ^2 which is estimated by the variance of $\hat{\theta}_i$ about θ and is denoted by $\hat{\tau}^2$. Thus, under the REs model the estimated variance of any observed effect size $\hat{\theta}_i$ about θ is the sum of the within-study and between-study variances, that is, $v_i^* = v_i + \hat{\tau}^2$. Therefore, the weight assigned to each study is different from that in the fixed effect model, and is given by

$$w_i^* = \frac{1}{v_i + \hat{\tau}^2}$$

which is an estimate of the unknown population weight $\omega_i^* = \frac{1}{\sigma_{i*}^2}$ with $\sigma_{i*}^2 = \sigma_i^2 + \tau^2$.

The common effect size estimator under the random effects (REs) model is

$$\hat{\theta}_{RE}^* = \frac{\sum\limits_{i=1}^{k} w_i^* \hat{\theta}_i}{\sum\limits_{i=1}^{k} w_i^*} \quad \text{in the LnRR scale}$$

with the standard error of the estimator of LnRR

$$SE(\hat{\theta}_{RE}^*) = \sqrt{\frac{1}{\sum\limits_{i=1}^{k} w_i^*}}.$$

Estimation of τ^2: The between studies variance τ^2 is estimated as a scaled excess variation as follows

$$\hat{\tau}^2 = \frac{Q - df}{C},$$

where

$$Q = \sum_{i=1}^{k} w_i \hat{\theta}_i^{*2} - \frac{\left(\sum\limits_{i=1}^{k} w_i \hat{\theta}_i^*\right)^2}{\sum\limits_{i=1}^{k} w_i}, \quad C = \sum_{i=1}^{k} w_i - \frac{\sum\limits_{i=1}^{k} w_i^2}{\sum\limits_{i=1}^{k} w_i}$$

and $df = (k - 1)$ in which k is the number of studies.

Illustration of RR under REs Model

Example 4.4 Table 4.5 provides summary data on the number of patients with **heartburn** after surgery for Gastro-Esophageal Reflux Disease using Laparoscopic Anterior (LAF) versus Posterior Fundoplication (LPF). Details are found in Memon et al. (2015).

Table 4.5 Count data on number of heartburn patients after LAF and LPF surgery

Study name	N1	Cases	Non-cases	N2	Cases	Non-cases
		LAF			LPF	
Watson et al. (1999)	54	5	49	53	5	48
Hagedorn et al. (2003)	47	25	22	48	10	38
Watson et al. (2004)	60	11	49	52	2	50
Spence et al. (2006)	40	6	34	39	5	34
Khan et al. (2010)	31	7	24	29	3	26
Raue et al. (2011)	30	1	29	27	1	26
Cao et al. (2012)	49	8	41	47	8	39

Find the value of the

(i)   Q and C statistics for the heartburn data
(ii) Estimate of τ^2
(iii) Modified weight for the first study (Watson et al. 1999) under the REs model.

To answer the above questions, first calculate sample values of RR, LnRR and Var(LnRR) W × LnRR, W × LnRR^2 and W^2 as found in Table 4.6.

Illustration of calculations in the above table

For example, for the first study (Watson et al. 1999):

The risk of LAF is Risk(LAF) = 5/54 = 0.0926 and the risk of LPF is Risk(LPF) = 5/53 = 0.0943, and hence the risk ratio (of LAF relative to LPF) is RR = 0.0926/0.0943 = 0.9815. Then log of RR become LnRR = ln(0.9815) = −0.0187 (this is rounded to −0.02 in the above table).

The variance of the estimator of LnRR is

Table 4.6 Calculation of LnRR and Var(LnRR), W(LnRR), W × LnRR, W × LnRR^2 and W^2 along with the sums of W(LnRR), W × LnRR, W × LnRR^2 and W^2 for the heartburn data

Study name	RR	LnRR	Var(LnRR)	W(LnRR)	W × LnRR	W × LnRR^2	W^2
Watson et al. (1999)	0.98	−0.02	0.36261	2.75776	−0.0515	0.000964	7.60522
Hagedorn et al. (2003)	2.55	0.94	0.09789	10.2155	9.5755	8.975517	104.357
Watson et al. (2004)	4.77	1.56	0.55501	1.80176	2.8137	4.394038	3.24635
Spence et al. (2006)	1.17	0.16	0.31603	3.1643	0.4968	0.078001	10.0128
Khan et al. (2010)	2.18	0.78	0.40945	2.4423	1.9065	1.488209	5.96484
Raue et al. (2011)	0.9	−0.11	1.92963	0.51823	−0.0546	0.005753	0.26857
Cao et al. (2012)	0.96	−0.04	0.20832	4.80042	−0.2	0.008336	23.044
				25.7003	**14.486**	**14.95082**	**154.499**

$$V(LnRR) = \frac{1}{a} - \frac{1}{a+b} + \frac{1}{c} - \frac{1}{c+d} = \frac{1}{5} - \frac{1}{54} + \frac{1}{5} - \frac{1}{53} = 0.3626.$$

Now we could answer the questions as follows:

(i)   The value of the Q statistic is found to be

$$Q = \sum_{i=1}^{k} w_i \hat{\theta}_i^{*2} - \frac{\left(\sum_{i=1}^{k} w_i \hat{\theta}_i^{*}\right)^2}{\sum_{i=1}^{k} w_i} = \sum_{i=1}^{7} W \times LnRR^2 - \frac{\left(\sum_{i=1}^{7} W \times LnRR\right)^2}{\sum_{i=1}^{7} W}$$

$$= 14.9508 - \frac{(14.4863)^2}{25.7003} = 6.7854, \text{ and}$$

$$C = \sum_{i=1}^{k} w_i - \frac{\sum_{i=1}^{k} w_i^2}{\sum_{i=1}^{k} w_i} = \sum_{i=1}^{7} W - \frac{\sum_{i=1}^{7} W^2}{\sum_{i=1}^{7} W} = 25.7003 - \frac{154.4990}{25.7003} = 19.6887,$$

and $df = k - 1 = 7 - 1 = 6$.

(ii)   Then, the estimated value of τ^2 becomes

$$\hat{\tau}^2 = \frac{Q - df}{C} = \frac{6.7854 - 6}{19.6887} = 0.0399.$$

(iii)   The *modified weight* under the REs model for the first study (Watson et al. 1999).
Becomes $w_1^* = \frac{1}{v_1 + \hat{\tau}^2} = \frac{1}{0.3626 + 0.0399} = 2.4844$ (as shown in Table 4.7).

Table 4.7 Calculation of LnRR, Var(LnRR), τ^2, W*(LnRR), and W* $\times$ LnRR^2 along with the sums of W*(LnRR) and W* $\times$ LnRR^2 for the heartburn data

Study name	RR	LnRR	Var(LnRR)	τ^2	W*(LnRR)	W* $\times$ LnRR
Watson et al. (1999)	0.98	−0.02	0.3626	0.0399	2.484432	−0.0464
Hagedorn et al. (2003)	2.55	0.94	0.0979	0.0399	7.257786	6.80304
Watson et al. (2004)	4.77	1.56	0.555	0.0399	1.680942	2.62504
Spence et al. (2006)	1.17	0.16	0.316	0.0399	2.809631	0.44112
Khan et al. (2010)	2.18	0.78	0.4094	0.0399	2.225473	1.73722
Raue et al. (2011)	0.9	−0.11	1.9296	0.0399	0.507737	−0.0535
Cao et al. (2012)	0.96	−0.04	0.2083	0.0399	4.028875	−0.1679
				Sum	**20.99488**	**11.3386**

Example 4.7 Consider the heartburn data in Example 4.6.

Under the REs model, find the

(i)   estimated value of the unknown combined population LnRR
(ii)   standard error of the estimator of population LnRR
(iii) 95% confidence interval for unknown combined population LnRR
(iv)   Test the significance of unknown combined population LnRR.

To answer the above questions, we need the computations of the summary statistics as in Table 4.7. The second last column of the table gives the modified weights, W* of the LnRR which is used to calculate the pooled estimate of the common population LnRR under the REs model.

(i)   The effect size estimator of LnRR under the random effects (REs) model becomes

$$\hat{\theta}^*_{RE} = \frac{\sum_{i=1}^{k} w_i^* \hat{\theta}_i}{\sum_{i=1}^{k} w_i^*} = \frac{\sum_{i=1}^{7} W^* Ln\,RR}{\sum_{i=1}^{7} W^*} = \frac{11.3386}{20.9949} = 0.54 \text{ in LnRR scale.}$$

(ii)   The standard error is

$$SE(\hat{\theta}^*_{RE}) = \sqrt{\frac{1}{\sum_{i=1}^{k} w_i^*}} = \sqrt{\frac{1}{\sum_{i=1}^{7} W^*}} = \sqrt{\frac{1}{20.9949}} = 0.2182.$$

(iii) The 95% confidence interval for the unknown common population parameter LnRR is given by

$$LL^* = \hat{\theta}^*_{RE} - 1.96 \times SE(\hat{\theta}^*_{RE}) = 0.54 - 1.96 \times 0.2182 = 0.1123 \text{ and}$$
$$UL^* = \hat{\theta}^*_{RE} + 1.96 \times SE(\hat{\theta}^*_{RE}) = 0.54 + 1.96 \times 0.2182 = 0.9678 \text{ in LnRR scale.}$$

Then the 95% confidence interval of the pooled population RR in the original RR scale becomes

$$LL = \exp(LL^*) = \exp(0.1123) = 1.1189 \approx 1.12 \text{ and}$$
$$UL = \exp(UL^*) = \exp(0.0.9678) = 2.6322 \approx 2.63.$$

Note that the point estimate of the combined population parameter RR is

$$\hat{\theta}_{RE} = \exp(\hat{\theta}^*_{RE}) = \exp(0.54) = 1.7162 \approx 1.72.$$

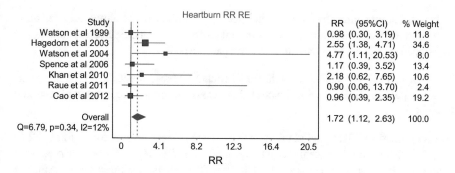

Fig. 4.2 Forest plot of RR for the ablation of heartburn for the LAF and LPF patients under the random effects model

Remark : The forest plot in Fig. 4.2 reports the above point estimate (1.72) and confidence interval (1.12, 2.63) of RR in the last row and represented by the diamond.

(iv) To test the significance of common population LnRR the null hypothesis is $H_0 : Ln\,RR = 0$ (same risk for both groups) against $H_a : Ln\,RR \neq 0$. Based on the sample data the observed value of the test statistic Z is

$$z_0 = \frac{0.54}{0.2181} = 2.4759 \approx 2.48.$$

The two-sided P-value is $P(|Z| > 2.48) = 2 \times P(Z > 2.48) = 2 \times 0.0066 = 0.0132$. Therefore the test is significant at the 5% level of significance, that is, the RR is significantly different from 1. So the chance of heartburn of patients in the LPF group is much (1.72 times) higher than that in the LAF group.

REs Meta-analysis of RR with MetaXL
In MetaXL, use the following code to produce the forest plot under the REs model:

```
=MAInputTable("Heartburn RR RE","NumRR","RE",N5:T11),
```

where "N5:T11" indicates the data area in Excel sheet, and "RE" represents REs model.

Remark: Explanations of MetaXL Code For this type of meta-analyses in MetaXL the 'opening' code starts with MA Input Table ' = MAInputTable'. This is followed by an open parenthesis inside which the first quote contains the text that appears as the 'title of the output of the forest plot' e.g. "Heartburn RR RE" in the above code (user may choose any appropriate title here). Then in the second quote enter the type of effect measure, e.g. "NumRR" in the above code tells that the *outcome variable is binary and the effect size measure is relative risk or risk ratio*. Within the third quote enter the statistical model, e.g. "RE" in the above code stands for the *random effects* (abbreviated by RE) model. Each quotation is followed by a comma, and after

the last comma enter the data area in Excel, e.g. N5:T11 in the above code tells that
the data on the independent studies are taken from the specified cells in the Excel
Worksheet. The code ends with a closing parenthesis.

The following forest plot produced by MetaXL shows the 95% confidence intervals of individual studies and the pooled effect size along with redistributed modified
weights.

Interpretation: The pooled effect size estimate of heartburn is found to be RR =
1.72 with 95% confidence interval (1.12, 2.63). The RR of heartburn for the patients
after surgery for Gastro-Esophageal Reflux Disease using Laparoscopic Anterior
(LAF) and Posterior Fundoplication (LPF) is significant (because 1 is not included
in the confidence interval). There is higher risk (1.72 times higher) of heartburn for
the patients with LPF compared to those with LAF. The risk of heartburn in the LPF
group is 72% (or 1.72 times) higher than those in the LAF group.

Aside: If fixed effect model is used for the same data the following forest
plot is produced by MetaXL with code: = MAInputTable("Heartburn RR
FE","NumRR","IV",N5:T11) (Fig. 4.3).

Remarks: Note that the value of the pooled estimate of RR under REs model is
1.72 and that under FE is 1.76. The difference in the two estimates of the RR is due
to the use of different (redistributed) weights under the two models. The width of
the confidence interval under the REs model is much higher (1.51) compared to that
of the FE model (1.40). This is due to higher variance of the REs model (0.2181)
compared to 0.06787 for the FE model. The redistribution of weights under the REs
and FE models are significantly different. The REs model allocates more weights for
smaller studies than the FE model.

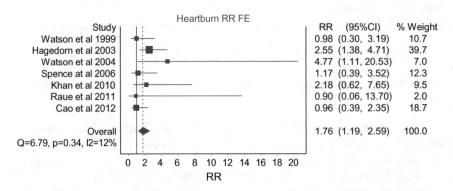

Fig. 4.3 Forest plot of RR for the ablation of heartburn for the LAF and LPF patients under the
fixed effect model

4.6 Inverse Variance Heterogeneity (IVhet) Model

The inverse variance heterogeneity (IVhet) model was proposed by Doi et al. (2015a) as a better alternative to the random effects (REs) model to deal with heterogeneous meta-analyses. The weights under the IVhet model would be identical to that of the FE model weights, and thus the form of the weighted FE estimator and weighted IVhet estimator is identical but the IVhet model derives the variance differently. Thus the IVhet model estimate of the transformed common effect size RR, LnRR ($= \theta^*$) is given by

$$\hat{\theta}^*_{IVhet} = \frac{\sum\limits_{i=1}^{k} w_i \hat{\theta}^*_i}{\sum\limits_{i=1}^{k} w_i}.$$

But the variance of the estimator of LnRR ($= \theta^*$) under the IVhet model is given by

$$Var(\hat{\theta}^*_{IVhet}) = \sum_{i=1}^{k} \left[\left(\frac{1}{v_i} \Big/ \sum_{i=1}^{k} \frac{1}{v_i} \right)^2 (v_i + \hat{\tau}^2) \right] = \sum_{i=1}^{k} \left[\left(w_i \Big/ \sum_{i=1}^{k} w_i \right)^2 (v_i + \hat{\tau}^2) \right].$$

For the computation of the confidence interval of the common effect size based on the IVhet model use the following standard error

$$SE(\hat{\theta}^*_{IVhet}) = \sqrt{Var(\hat{\theta}^*_{IVhet})}.$$

Then, the $(1 - \alpha) \times 100\%$ confidence interval for the common effect size θ under the IVhet model is given by the lower limit (LL) and upper limit (UL) in the LnRR scale as follows:

$$LL = \hat{\theta}^*_{IVhet} - z_{\alpha/2} \times SE(\hat{\theta}^*_{IVhet}) \text{ and}$$
$$UL = \hat{\theta}^*_{IVhet} + z_{\alpha/2} \times SE(\hat{\theta}^*_{IVhet}),$$

where $z_{\alpha/2}$ is the $\frac{\alpha}{2}$ th cut-off point of standard normal distribution.

Illustration of IVhet Model for Risk Ratio

Example 4.8 Table 4.8 provides summary data on the number of patients with heartburn after surgery for Gastro-Esophageal Reflux Disease using Laparoscopic Anterior (LAF) versus Posterior Fundoplication (LPF). The full data set is found in Memon et al. (2015).

Table 4.8 Count data of incidences of heartburn for the LAF and LPF surgeries of patients

Study name	LAF			LPF		
	N1	Cases	Non-cases	N2	Cases	Non-cases
Watson et al. (1999)	54	5	49	53	5	48
Hagedorn et al. (2003)	47	25	22	48	10	38
Watson et al. (2004)	60	11	49	52	2	50
Spence et al. (2006)	40	6	34	39	5	34
Khan et al. (2010)	31	7	24	29	3	26
Raue et al. (2011)	30	1	29	27	1	26
Cao et al. (2012)	49	8	41	47	8	39

Calculate the modified variances and weights for all the studies under the IVhet model.

For the above data, the effect size measure RR and its log transformation (LnRR), variance (Var), estimated value of between studies variance (τ^2), modified variance (V*) and modified weight (W*) are provided in Table 4.9.

Illustration of calculations: For the first study (Watson et al. 1999),
W(LnRR) = 1/Var(LnRR) = 1/0.362614 = 2.75776, the weight of LnRR

The modified variance, V*((LnRR) = Var(LnRR) + τ^2 = 0.362614 + 0.0399 = 0.40251, and modified weight for the IVhet model

$$ W*(\text{IVhet}) = \left[\frac{W(LnRR)}{\sum W(LnRR)} \right]^2 \times V^*(LnRR) = \left[\frac{2.75776}{25.7003} \right]^2 \times 0.40251 = 0.004635. $$

Example 4.9 Consider the heartburn data in Example 4.6.

Under the IVhet model, find the

Table 4.9 Calculations of LnRR, Var(LnRR), τ^2, V*(LnRR), W*(LnRR), and sums of W(LnRR), V*(LnRR) and W*(LnRR) of heartburn data

Study name	RR	LnRR	Var(LnRR)	τ^2	W(LnRR)	V*(LnRR)	W*(IVhet)
Watson et al. (1999)	0.98	−0.019	0.362614	0.0399	2.75776	0.40251	0.004635
Hagedorn et al. (2003)	2.55	0.9373	0.09789	0.0399	10.2155	0.13778	0.021769
Watson et al. (2004)	4.77	1.5616	0.555012	0.0399	1.80176	0.5949	0.002924
Spence et al. (2006)	1.17	0.157	0.316026	0.0399	3.1643	0.35592	0.005395
Khan et al. (2010)	2.18	0.7806	0.40945	0.0399	2.4423	0.44934	0.004058
Raue et al. (2011)	0.9	−0.105	1.92963	0.0399	0.51823	1.96952	0.000801
Cao et al. (2012)	0.96	−0.042	0.208315	0.0399	4.80042	0.24821	0.00866
					25.7003	**4.15819**	**0.048241**

Note V*(LnRR) is the sum of the within and between studies variances of LnRR

(i)   Estimate of the unknown common population LnRR (θ^*)
(ii) Standard error of the estimator of LnRR
(iii) 95% confidence interval for unknown common population LnRR (θ^*)
(iv) Test the significance of the unknown common population LnRR (θ^*)

To answer the above questions, first we need to find the statistics in Table 4.10.

(i)   The IVhet model estimate of the transformed common effect size LnRR is given by

$$\hat{\theta}^*_{IVhet} = \frac{\sum\limits_{i=1}^{k} w_i \hat{\theta}^*_i}{\sum\limits_{i=1}^{k} w_i} = \frac{14.48629}{25.7003} = 0.56366 \approx 0.56 \text{ in the LnRR scale.}$$

(ii) The variance of the estimator of LnRR under the IVhet model is given by

$$Var(\hat{\theta}^*_{IVhet}) = \sum_{i=1}^{k} \left[\left(\frac{1}{v_i} \bigg/ \sum_{i=1}^{k} \frac{1}{v_i} \right)^2 (v_i + \hat{\tau}^2) \right]$$

$$= \sum_{i=1}^{7} \left[\left(W \bigg/ \sum_{i=1}^{7} W \right)^2 (v_i + \hat{\tau}^2) \right] = 0.048241.$$

Hence the standard error becomes

$$SE(\hat{\theta}^*_{IVhet}) = \sqrt{Var(\hat{\theta}^*_{IVhet})} = \sqrt{0.048241} = 0.219638.$$

(iii) The 95% confidence interval for the common effect size LnRR under the IVhet model is given by

$$LL^* = \hat{\theta}^*_{IVhet} - 1.96 \times SE(\hat{\theta}^*_{IVhet}) = 0.5637 - 1.96 \times 0.219638 = 0.133209 \text{ and}$$
$$UL^* = \hat{\theta}^*_{IVhet} + 1.96 \times SE(\hat{\theta}^*_{IVhet}) = 0.5637 + 1.96 \times 0.219638 = 0.994199 \text{ in LnRR scale.}$$

Then the 95% confidence interval in the original RR scale becomes

$$LL = \exp(LL*) = \exp(0.133209) = 1.142487 \approx 1.14 \text{ and}$$
$$UL = \exp(UL*) = \exp(0.994199) = 2.702537 \approx 2.70.$$

The IVhet point estimate of the common effect size RR is $RR = \exp(\hat{\theta}^*_{IVhet}) = \exp(0.5637) = 1.757162 \approx 1.76$ in original RR scale.

Remark: The above point estimate (1.76) and confidence interval (1.14, 2.70) are reported at the bottom row of the forest plot in Fig. 4.4 and is represented by the diamond.

Table 4.10 Calculations of LnRR, Var(LnRR), W(LnRR), W*(LnRR), V*(LnRR), W*(IVhet) and sums of W(LnRR), W × LnRR, V*(LnRR) and W*(IVhet) of heartburn data

Study name	RR	LnRR	Var(LnRR)	W(LnRR)	W × LnRR	V*(LnRR)	W*(IVhet)
Watson et al. (1999)	0.98	−0.019	0.362614	2.75776	−0.05155	0.402507	0.004635
Hagedorn et al. (2003)	2.55	0.9373	0.09789	10.2155	9.575477	0.137783	0.021769
Watson et al. (2004)	4.77	1.5616	0.555012	1.80176	2.81372	0.594905	0.002924
Spence et al. (2006)	1.17	0.157	0.316026	3.1643	0.496807	0.355919	0.005395
Khan et al. (2010)	2.18	0.7806	0.40945	2.4423	1.906477	0.449343	0.004058
Raue et al. (2011)	0.9	−0.105	1.92963	0.51823	−0.0546	1.969523	0.000801
Cao et al. (2012)	0.96	−0.042	0.208315	4.80042	−0.20005	0.248208	0.00866
				25.7003	**14.48629**	**4.158186**	**0.048241**

(iv)   To test the significance of population LnRR, test the null hypothesis H_0 : $LnRR = 0$ (same risk for both groups) against $H_a : LnRR \neq 0$. Based on the sample data the observed value of the test statistic Z is

$$z_0 = \frac{0.56366}{0.219638} = 2.5663 \approx 2.57.$$

The two-sided P-value is $P(|Z| > 2.57) = 2xP(Z > 2.57) = 2 \times 0.00508 = 0.01016$. Therefore the test is significant at the 5% level, that is, the RR is significantly different from 1.

IVhet Meta-analysis of RR with MetaXL
In MetaXL use following code:

```
=MAInputTable("Heartburn RR IVhet","NumRR","IVhet",N5:T11),
```

where "N5:T11" indicates the data area in Excel Worksheet, and "IVhet" represents IVhet model.

Remark: Explanations of MetaXL Code
For this type of meta-analyses in MetaXL the 'opening' code starts with MA Input Table ' = MAInputTable'. This is followed by an open parenthesis inside which the first quote contains the text that appears as the 'title of the output of the forest plot' e.g. "Heartburn RR IVhet" in the above code (user may choose any appropriate title here). Then in the second quote enter the type of effect measure, e.g. "NumRR" in the above code tells that the *outcome variable is numerical and the effect size measure is risk ratio*. Within the third quote enter the statistical model, e.g. "IVhet" in the above code stands for the *inverse variance heterogeneity* (abbreviated by IVhet) model. Each quotation is followed by a comma, and after the last comma enter the data area

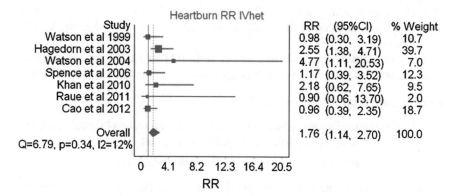

Fig. 4.4 Forest plot of RR for the ablation of heartburn for the LAF and LPF patients under the IVhet model

in Excel, e.g. N5:T11 in the above code tells that the data on the independent studies are taken from the specified cells. The code ends with a closing parenthesis.

The following forest plot, under the IVhet model, produced by MetaXL shows the 95% confidence intervals of individual studies and the pooled effect size along with redistributed weights.

Interpretation:
The estimated value of the common effect size RR under the IVhet model is 1.76 with 95% confidence interval (1.14, 2.70). The RR of heartburn is significantly different (since 1 is not included in the confidence interval) for the patients treated with LAF and LPF surgeries. The patients with LPF surgery have higher risk of heartburn compared to those with LAF surgery. There is 76% (or 1.76 times) higher risk of heartburn for the patients receiving LPF surgery than those received LAF surgery.

4.7   Subgroup Analysis

In the presence of heterogeneity often researchers look for ways to deal with the problem by dividing the studies into homogeneous subgroups. It is also used when there is an interest to compare the effect size for different regions or period/size of the studies. Subgroup analysis is a special case of meta-regression when the only explanatory (moderator) variable is categorical.

Subgroup analysis is appropriate when the studies could be divided into different groups based on some distinguishing characteristics of the studies. This is done if there is a reason to suspect real differences in the effect size estimate among the groups of studies. The procedure is explained below for the heartburn data meta-analysis.

The seven studies in the heartburn data in Example 4.4 are divided into two groups by their study period (Old studies 1999-2006, and Recent studies 2010–2012) for subgroup analyses. The aim here is to perform separate meta-analysis for each of the two subgroups and present the results of the meta-analysis of all the studies on the same forest plot to compare the effect size estimate between the subgroups and the overall studies.

Interested readers may refer to Paget et al. (2011) for an example of subgroup analysis. Some useful advices on subgroup analysis are found in Yusuf et al. (1991).

Steps in Subgroup analysis using MetaXL

Step 1: First run the following MetaXL code to create a forest plot (in cell C16, say) so that "Heartburn Subgroup RR RE" is shown on this cell.

```
=MAInputTable("Heartburn Subgroup RR RE","NumRR","re",B5:H11)
```

Step 2: Then create a table of groups (as shown below) of studies by any distinguishing characteristic, e.g. studies published before 2010 (Old studies), and those published in 2010 or later (Recent studies) in separate columns. For the current example, to illustrate the subgroup analysis in Fig. 4.5, the 'Old studies' group consists of four studies and 'Recent studies' group consists of three studies as follows:

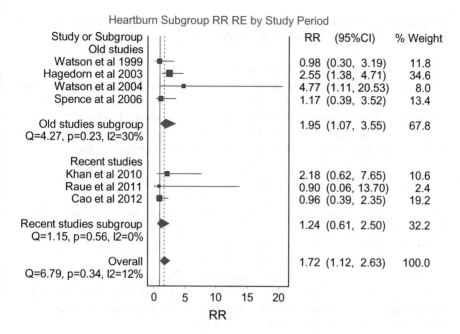

Fig. 4.5 Forest plot of subgroup analysis of old and recent studies of RR of heartburn for the LAF and LPF patients under the *random effects* model in RR scale

Old studies	Recent studies
Watson et al. (1999)	Khan et al. (2010)
Hagedorn et al. (2003)	Raue et al. (2011)
Watson et al. (2004)	Cao et al. (2012)
Spence et al. (2006)	

Step 3: Finally, run the following MetaXL code to produce the forest plot of subgroup analysis as in Fig. 4.5:

=MASubGroups("Study Period",C16, I4:J8)

Note the cell "C16" refers to the Excel Worksheet where meta-analysis of all the studies is restored, and the range of cells "I4:J8" indicates the area in the Excel Worksheet where table of subgroups is located.

The above code creates a forest plot of subgroup analysis with three subplots - one for each of the two separate study periods and another one combining all studies across the two groups.

Without conducting subgroup analysis, across all the studies, the LPF group has higher RR than the LAF group. But the subgroup analysis reveals that the 'old studies' subgroup favours the LAF as the RR for the APF patients (RR = 1.95) is much high compared to that of the 'recent studies' subgroup (pooled RR = 1.24).

Interpretation of subgroup analysis:
For the Old studies subgroup the risk of heartburn in the LPF group is 1.95 times higher than that in the LAF group. The confidence interval does not cross the vertical line at RR = 1, and hence the effect size is significant at the 5% level of significance.

But for the Recent studies subgroup, the risk of heartburn in the LPF group is 1.24 times higher than that in the LAF group. The effect size in this subgroup of Old studies is not significant as the confidence interval includes RR = 1.

The pooled results (combining all Old and Recent studies) show that the risk of heartburn is 1.72 times higher in the LAF group compared to the LPF group. The confidence interval for the pooled effect size does not cross the vertical line at RR = 1, and hence the pooled effect size is significant at the 5% level of significance.

So, the incidence of heartburn is much higher in the LPF group than the LAP group across all the time and over all the studies.

The forest plot in Fig. 4.5 is reproduced in log RR scale for better visibility as in Fig. 4.6. The confidence intervals in this forest plot are more clear than that of the RR scale, but the final results are the same. Make XL provide the flexibility to present the forest plot either in RR or log RR scale.

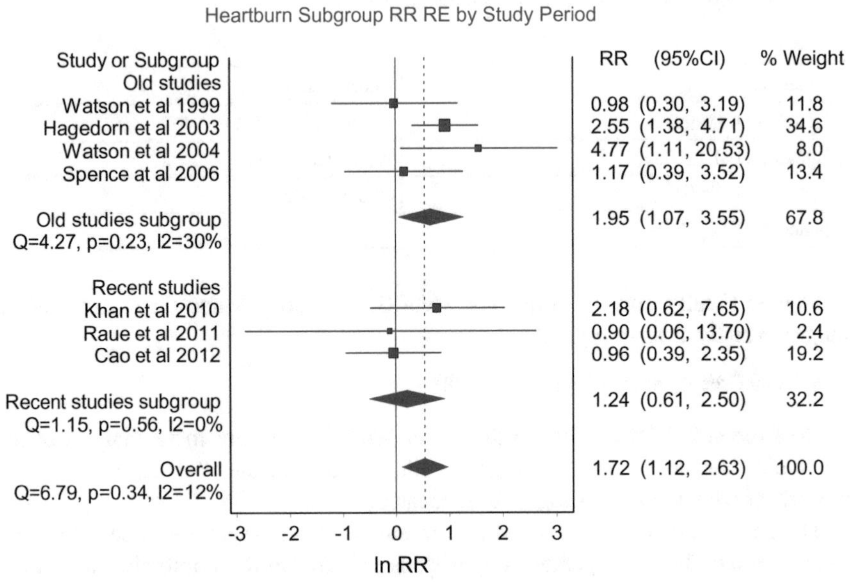

Heartburn Subgroup RR RE by Study Period

Study or Subgroup	RR	(95%CI)	% Weight
Old studies			
Watson et al 1999	0.98	(0.30, 3.19)	11.8
Hagedorn et al 2003	2.55	(1.38, 4.71)	34.6
Watson et al 2004	4.77	(1.11, 20.53)	8.0
Spence at al 2006	1.17	(0.39, 3.52)	13.4
Old studies subgroup	1.95	(1.07, 3.55)	67.8
Q=4.27, p=0.23, I2=30%			
Recent studies			
Khan et al 2010	2.18	(0.62, 7.65)	10.6
Raue et al 2011	0.90	(0.06, 13.70)	2.4
Cao et al 2012	0.96	(0.39, 2.35)	19.2
Recent studies subgroup	1.24	(0.61, 2.50)	32.2
Q=1.15, p=0.56, I2=0%			
Overall	1.72	(1.12, 2.63)	100.0
Q=6.79, p=0.34, I2=12%			

ln RR

Fig. 4.6 Forest plot of subgroup analysis of old and recent studies of RR of heartburn for the LAF and LPF patients under the *random effects* model in ln RR scale

4.8 Discussions and Comparison of Results

The forest plots can be displayed in the Ln RR scale for better exposure of the confidence intervals as in Figs. 4.7, 4.8, and 4.9. These plots only change the second column (panel containing scatterplot of confidence intervals) of the forest plot keeping the study names in the first column, point estimates and confidence intervals in the third and fourth columns and weights in the fifth column the same (as it is in the forest plot of original RR scale).

As always, the point estimate of the common effect size RR is the same (1.76) for the FE and IVhet models. But the confidence interval for the FE is (1.19, 2.59) and that for the IVhet is (1.14, 2.70) with the same redistribution of weights among the studies. Thus the IVhet model meta-analysis enables higher width (2.70 – 1.44 = 1.66) of the confidence interval than the FE model (width, 2.59 – 1.19 = 1.40) by allowing for higher variance in the way of inclusion of between studies variation.

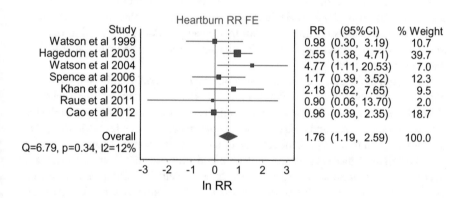

Fig. 4.7 Forest plot of RR of heartburn data for FE model in LnRR scale

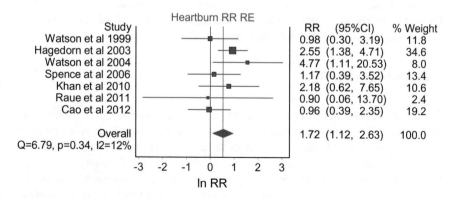

Fig. 4.8 Forest plot of RR of heartburn data for REs model in LnRR scale

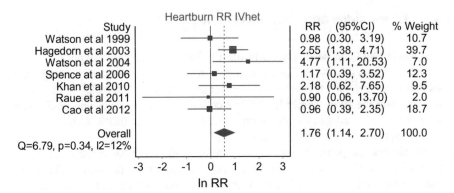

Fig. 4.9 Forest plot of RR of heartburn data for IVhet model in LnRR scale

For the REs model, the point estimate of the combined effect size RR is 1.72 with confidence interval (1.12, 2.63). The redistribution of weights among the studies under this model is very different from that under the IVhet model. Contradictory to common logic, under the REs model, the smaller studies receive higher weights than the larger studies.

The width of the confidence interval under the REs model (2.63 − 1.12 = 1.51) is wider than that under the FE model (1.40) but shorter than that under the IVhet model (1.66). Note that because of the shorter width, the coverage probability under the REs model is compromised and falls short of the nominal confidence level (of 95%). This does not happen to the IVhet model which maintains the nominal confidence level.

Under all three models the common/combined effect size RR is significant (higher RR of heartburn for higher LPF group). The heterogeneity is insignificant as the value of $I^2 = 12\%$ and the P-value of the Q statistic is 0.34. Note that the Q statistic and the I^2 index are note, dependent on any statistical model.

Obviously, the point estimates and confidence intervals of all individual studies remain the same in the forest plot regardless of the statistical model of analysis. Only changes are in the pooled estimate and confidence interval due to the different redistributed study weights under different models.

4.9 Publication Bias

For various reasons not all research studies, including randomised control trials, are published and hence results or summary statistics on the research question of interest are not always publicly accessible for meta-analysis. Absence or unavailability of some studies that from meta-analysis causes publication bias. One major reason for publication bias is the results of intervention that are not significant are not usually published due to the choice of the journal editor or as a result of the instructions of funding agency to avoid publishing negative or unfavourable results. Sometimes studies published in non-English literatures are not included in meta-analysis causing publication bias. There are methods to identify or assess and deal with publication bias. This topic is covered in details in Chap. 12.

The publication bias is a real and serious problem, and hence received considerable attention among the researchers including Sterne et al. (2000); Elvik (2011, 2013); Mathew and Charney (2009); and Uesawa et al. (2010).

4.9.1 The Funnel Plot

Publication bias is usually detected by using funnel plot. A funnel plot is a scatter plot of standard error of the studies against effect size (or transformed effect size). If a funnel plot is symmetrical about the vertical line in the middle, then there is no publication bias. However, if the funnel plot is asymmetrical there is publication bias in the study. There are some methods in the literature to deal with the impact of publication bias. The two graphical methods to identify and assess publication bias are described in this section.

The funnel plot is not dependent on any of the statistical models. But is it produced as part of fixed effect model meta-analysis procedure by MetaXL.

Interpretation:
From the funnel plot in Fig. 4.10 it is evident that there is publication bias in the study as the plot is asymmetrical. There are more (four) studies/points on the left side of the "no effect" vertical line than on the right. Also there is one study with very small value of standard error on the left side of the vertical line.

4.9.2 The Doi Plot

Another graphical method to study publication bias is the Doi plot. It is a scatter plot of absolute z-score of the value of effect size versus the effect size (or transformed

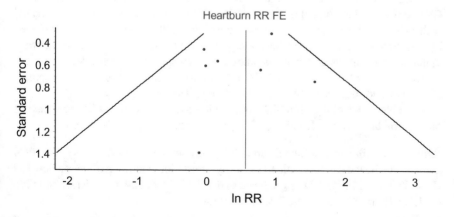

Fig. 4.10 Funnel plot of Ln RR of heartburn data

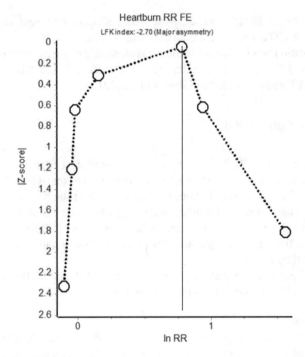

Fig. 4.11 Doi plot of RR of heartburn

effect size). The individual dots on the graph are then connected with a continuous curve. Details are found in Doi (2018), and Furuya-Kanamori et al. (2018).

Like the funnel plot, the Doi plot is used to alert researchers to possible publication bias, but the Doi plot is more sensitive than the funnel plot. The interpretation, however, is much like that of the funnel plot: a symmetrical plot gives no reason to suspect publication bias, an asymmetrical one does.

Smaller less precise trials will produce an effect size (ES) that scatters increasingly widely, and the absolute Z-score will gradually increase for both smaller and larger ES's on either side of that of the precise trials. Thus, a symmetrical triangle is created with a Z-score close to zero at its peak. If the trials are homogeneous and not affected by selection or other forms of bias, the plot will therefore resemble a symmetrical mountain with similar number of studies and equal spread on each side.

The Doi plot also displays the LFK index of asymmetry, including an assessment of severity and suggesting 'No' or 'Minor' or 'Major' asymmetry.

The above Doi plot in Fig. 4.11 is showing asymmetry indicating presence of publication bias. The LFK index (−2.70) also suggests major asymmetry.

Remark: Similar to the funnel plot, Doi plot does not depend on any statistical models, and hence can be obtained from any forest plot regardless of the model. The above Doi plot in Fig. 4.11 is produced under the FE model, but the REs and IVhet models will produce the same Doi plot and funnel plot.

Appendix 4—Stata Codes for Risk Ratio (RR) Meta-analysis

A4.1 Thyroid ablation data

Study_name	TrN1	TrCases	TrNon-cases	ConN2	ConCases	ConNon-cases
Doi (2000)	49	23	26	39	25	14
Ramacciotti (1982)	9	3	6	20	12	8
Angelini (1997)	426	226	200	180	101	79
Liu (1987)	40	14	26	20	11	9
Lin (1998)	21	6	15	25	11	14
McCowen (1976)	28	10	18	36	15	21
Maxon (1992)	37	6	31	26	6	20

A4.2 Stata code for meta-analysis of ablation data

ssc install admetan

FE model meta-analysis

admetan TrCases TrNoncases ConCases ConNoncases, **rr** model(**fixed**) study(study_name) effect(Relative Risk)

REs model meta-analysis

admetan TrCases TrNoncases ConCases ConNoncases, rr model(random) study(study_name) effect(Relative Risk)

IVhet model meta-analysis

admetan TrCases TrNoncases ConCases ConNoncases, rr model(ivhet) study(study_name) effect(Relative Risk)

A4.3 Heartburn data

Study_name	TrN1	TrCases	TrNon-cases	ConN2	ConCases	ConNon-cases
Watson et al. (1999)	54	5	49	53	5	48
Hagedorn et al. (2003)	47	25	22	48	10	38
Watson et al. (2004)	60	11	49	52	2	50
Spence et al. (2006)	40	6	34	39	5	34
Khan et al. (2010)	31	7	24	29	3	26
Raue et al. (2011)	30	1	29	27	1	26
Cao et al. (2012)	49	8	41	47	8	39

A4.4 Stata code for heartburn data

FE model meta-analysis

admetan TrCases TrNoncases ConCases ConNoncases, **rr** model(fixed) study(study_name) effect(Relative Risk)

REs model meta-analysis

admetan TrCases TrNoncases ConCases ConNoncases, rr model(random)
study(study_name) effect(Relative Risk)

IVhet model meta-analysis

admetan TrCases TrNoncases ConCases ConNoncases, rr model(ivhet)
study(study_name) effect(Relative Risk)

References

Borenstein M, Hedges LV, Higgins JP, Rothstein HR (2010) A basic introduction to fixed-effect
  and random-effects models for meta-analysis. Res Synth Methods 1(2):97–111
Borenstein M, Larry H, Higgins J, Rothstein H (2009) Introduction to meta-analysis. Wiley-
  Blackwell, Oxford
Cochran WG (1973) Experiments for nonlinear functions (R.A. Fisher Memorial Lecture). J Am
  Stat Assoc 68(344):771–781. https://doi.org/10.1080/01621459.1973.10481423
DerSimonian R, Laird N (1986) Meta-analysis in clinical trials. Control Clin Trials 7(3):177–188
Doi AS (2018) Rendering the plot properly in meta-analysis. Int J Evid-Based Healthc 16(4):242–
  243. https://doi.org/10.1097/XEB.0000000000000158
Doi SA, Barendregt JJ, Khan S, Thalib L, Williams GM (2015a) Advances in the meta-analysis
  of heterogeneous clinical trials I: the inverse variance heterogeneity model. Contemp Clin Trials
  45(Pt A):130–138. https://doi.org/10.1016/j.cct.2015.05.009
Doi SA, Barendregt JJ, Khan S, Thalib L, Williams GM (2015b) Simulation comparison of the
  quality effects and random effects methods of meta-analysis. Epidemiology 26(4):e42–44
Elvik R (2011) Publication bias and time-trend bias in meta-analysis of bicycle helmet efficacy: a
  re-analysis of Attewell, Glase and McFadden, 2001. Accid Anal Prev 43(3):1245–1251
Elvik R (2013) Corrigendum to: "Publication bias and time-trend bias in meta-analysis of bicycle
  helmet efficacy: a re-analysis of Attewell, Glase and McFadden, 2001". Accid Anal Prev 60:245–
  253
Furuya-Kanamori JL, Barendregt ARJ, Doi ARS (2018) A new improved graphical and quantitative
  method for detecting bias in meta-analysis. Int J Evid-Based Healthc 16(4):195–203. https://doi.
  org/10.1097/XEB.0000000000000141
Hedges LV, Pigott TD (2001) The power of statistical tests in meta-analysis. Psychol Methods
  6(3):203–217
Higgins JP, Thompson SG, Deeks JJ, Altman DG (2003) Measuring inconsistency in meta-analyses.
  BMJ 327(7414):557–560
Mathew SJ, Charney DS (2009) Publication bias and the efficacy of antidepressants. Am J Psychiatry
  166(2):140–145
Memon MA, Subramanya MS, Hossain MB, Yunus RM, Khan S, Memon B (2015) Laparoscopic
  anterior versus posterior fundoplication for gastro-esophageal reflux disease: a meta-analysis and
  systematic review. World J Surg 39(4):981–996. https://doi.org/10.1007/s00268-014-2889-0
Paget MA, Chuang-Stein C, Fletcher C, Reid C (2011) Subgroup analyses of clinical effectiveness
  to support health technology assessments. Pharm Stat 10(6):532–538
Sterne JA, Gavaghan D, Egger M (2000) Publication and related bias in meta-analysis: power of
  statistical tests and prevalence in the literature. J Clin Epidemiol 53(11):1119–1129
Uesawa Y, Takeuchi T, Mohri K (2010) Publication bias on clinical studies of pharmacokinetic
  interactions between felodipine and grapefruit juice. Pharmazie 65(5):375–378
Yusuf S, Garg R, Zucker D (1991) Analyses by the intention-to-treat principle in randomized trials
  and databases. Pacing Clin Electrophysiol 14(12):2078–2082

Chapter 5
Meta-analysis of Odds Ratio

Odds ratio is an appropriate measure of association between two categorical variables (intervention and outcome). The meta-analysis of odds ratio is covered in this chapter. Meta-analysis under different statistical models along with subgroup analysis and detection of publication bias are also covered.

5.1 Odds Ratio (OR)

For two arms experiments or studies, if the outcome variable of interest is binary or categorical, ratio measures are used to analyse the association between the two variables. The most popular ratio measures are the odds ratio (OR) and risk ratio (RR). The choice between the OR and RR depends on the objective of the study and to be decided by the researchers. Formal definition, example, computation and interpretation of OR are covered in Chap. 3. This chapter provides detailed on the meta-analysis methods of independent studies when odds ratio (OR) is the appropriate effect size measure.

5.2 Estimation of Effect Size OR

The point estimate of OR (from the sample data) is required to find confidence interval (and perform hypothesis tests) for the unknown population OR (parameter). For both confidence intervals and test of hypotheses, the sampling distribution and standard error of the estimator of the population OR are essential. The critical value of appropriate statistic (e.g. z) is required for the confidence interval and the choice of appropriate test statistic depends on the sampling distribution of the estimator of OR.

© Springer Nature Singapore Pte Ltd. 2020
S. Khan, *Meta-Analysis*, Statistics for Biology and Health,
https://doi.org/10.1007/978-981-15-5032-4_5

The distribution of the estimator of population OR is not known as it does not follow any commonly known probability (statistical) distribution. However, the natural log transformation of the estimator of OR follows an approximate normal distribution (see Chap. 2 for details). Therefore, for both confidence interval and test of hypothesis the point estimate of OR is replaced by Ln(OR), and the distribution of the transformed statistic is used. Although the log transformation does not effect the value of the test statistic (and hence the P-value) in the hypothesis testing process, inverse (or back) transformation of the lower and upper limits of the confidence interval is required to express the limits in the original scale (of OR).

For both the confidence interval and test of hypothesis, in addition to the transformed statistic Ln(OR), the standard error of the transformed statistic is also required. This is true for all statistical models of meta-analysis.

Let the population effect size measured by OR be denoted by θ. Then its log transformation is defined as $\theta^* = \ln(\theta)$. For the inference on the population OR this transformed parameter θ^* is used as the distribution of the estimator of the transformed parameter, say $\hat{\theta}^*$, is known to follow an approximate normal distribution.

Confidence interval for population OR

To find the 95% confidence interval for $\theta = $ OR, the log transformation, $\theta^* = \ln(\theta) = \ln(OR)$ is used.

An estimator of the population $\theta = $ OR is defined as (the sample OR)

$$\hat{\theta} = OR = \frac{a/b}{c/d} = \frac{a \times c}{b \times d},$$

where a, b, c and d are the cell counts in the contingency table (see Table 5.1 below).

Hence an estimator of the transformed population OR (θ^*) becomes

$$\hat{\theta}^* = \ln(\hat{\theta}).$$

The standard error of $\hat{\theta}^*$ is given by

$$SE(\hat{\theta}^*) = \sqrt{\tfrac{1}{a} + \tfrac{1}{b} + \tfrac{1}{c} + \tfrac{1}{d}}.$$

Then the $(1-\alpha) \times 100\%$ confidence interval for $\theta^* = \ln(\theta) = \ln(OR)$ is represented by the lower and upper limits as follows:

$LB^* = \hat{\theta}^* - z_{\alpha/2} \times SE(\hat{\theta}^*)$ and

$UB^* = \hat{\theta}^* + z_{\alpha/2} \times SE(\hat{\theta}^*)$

in the LnOR scale, and then using the back transformation

$LL = \exp(LL^*)$ and

$UL = \exp(UL^*)$

in the original OR scale.

Table 5.1 Vaccination and disease data

		Y = Outcome variable		
		Event (e.g. Disease)	Non event (e.g. No disease)	Row total
X = Exposure or Explanatory variable	Treatment (e.g. Vaccinated)	a (20)	b (60)	a + b (80)
	Control (e.g. Unvaccinated)	c (80)	d (20)	c + d (100)
	Column total	a + c (100)	b + d (80)	180

Example 5.1 (CI for OR) Consider the count data on Vaccination and Disease from Table 5.1.

Find the (i) point estimate of θ and θ^* (ii) standard error of estimator of θ^* and (iii) 95% confidence intervals for θ^* and θ.

Solution:

(i) For the above Vaccination and Disease data in Table 5.1 we have the point estimate of the population OR of Disease in the Treatment/Vaccination group,

$$\hat{\theta} = OR = \frac{a/b}{c/d} = \frac{20/60}{80/20} = \frac{1/3}{4/1} = 1/12 = 0.083333.$$

So, $\hat{\theta}^* = \ln(\hat{\theta}) = \ln(0.083333) = -2.48490665$.

(ii) The standard error of $\hat{\theta}^*$ is $SE(\hat{\theta}^*) = \sqrt{\frac{1}{20} + \frac{1}{60} + \frac{1}{80} + \frac{1}{20}} = 0.359397644$.

(ii) The 95% confidence interval for the population $\theta^* = \ln(\theta)$ is given by

$$LL^* = \hat{\theta}^* - z_{\alpha/2} \times SE(\hat{\theta}^*) = -2.48490665 - 1.96 \times 0.359397644 = -3.18932603 \text{ and}$$
$$UL^* = \hat{\theta}^* + z_{\alpha/2} \times SE(\hat{\theta}^*) = -2.48490665 + 1.96 \times 0.359397644 = -1.78048727$$

in the ln OR scale, and that of θ, obtained by back transformation, as

$LL = \exp(LL^*) = \exp(-3.18932603) = 0.041199629$ and
$UL = \exp(UL^*) = \exp(-1.78048727) = 0.168555995$ in the original OR scale.
Thus the 95% confidence interval for $\theta = OR$ becomes $(0.0412, 0.1686)$.

5.3 Significance Tests on OR

To test the significance of the population OR, θ the null hypothesis is $H_0 : \theta = 1$(the odds is the same for the treatment and control groups) we actually need to test the null hypothesis $H_0 : \theta^* = \ln(\theta) = \ln(1) = 0$ since the sampling distribution of estimator of θ is unknown but that of θ^* is approximately normal. Note that testing $\theta = 1$ is the same as testing $\theta^* = \ln(1) = 0$.

The appropriate test statistic to test $H_0 : \theta^* = 0$ against $H_A : \theta^* \neq 0$ is $Z = \frac{\hat{\theta}^*}{SE(\hat{\theta}^*)}$ which follows a standard normal distribution.

Example 5.2 (Test for OR) Consider the count data on the Vaccination and Disease in Table 5.1.

Test the significance of $\theta^* = \ln(\theta)$.

Solution:

From the above count data we have

$\hat{\theta} = OR = 1/12 = 0.083333$, $\hat{\theta}^* = \ln(\hat{\theta}) = \ln(0.083333) = -2.48490665$ and $SE(\hat{\theta}^*) = 0.359397644$.

Hence the observed value of the test statistic Z is

$$z_0 = \frac{\hat{\theta}^*}{SE(\hat{\theta}^*)} = \frac{-2.48490665}{0.359397644} = -6.914.$$

The P-value $= P(|Z| > 6.914) = P(Z < -6.914) + P(Z > 6.914) = 0$.

So, the test is highly significant. That is, there is very strong sample evidence against the null hypothesis of $\ln(OR) = 0$, that is, $OR = 1$. Hence we reject the null hypothesis in favour of the alternative hypothesis (and conclude that there is strong association/dependency between the outcome and exposure/intervention).

Comment There is a strong association between the two categorical variables (intervention or exposure) and outcome (disease or non disease). The same conclusion is arrived by either testing the RR or OR. However, the test for OR yields a larger absolute (ignoring sign) value of Z statistic (-6.914) than the test on RR (with z $= -5.82$ in Chap. 4), and hence the test on OR is more significant than that on RR.

5.4 Fixed Effects (FEs) Model

The fixed effect (FE) and other statistical models are applicable for meta-analysis of studies involving both binary and continuous outcome variables. In this section, the FE model is presented in the context of meta-analysis for odds ratio (OR). But the FE model can also be used for the meta-analyses of all kind of effect sizes regardless of types of outcome variables. The FE model is used for meta-analysis if the between studies variation is insignificant.

A basic introduction to the FE model meta-analysis is found in Borenstein et al. 2010 and in Chap. 11 of Borenstein et al. (2009).

Let us consider k independent primary studies selected for a meta-analysis after systematic review of all studies on a particular topic of interest. The underlying assumption is that there is an unknown common effect size (OR), θ for all the independent studies included in the investigation. Meta-analysis enables us to pool results from all independent studies to estimate the common effect size. Meta-analysis provides a method to combine the effect size measure of all the studies to get a more accurate estimate of the common effect size.

The ith individual study measures the common effect size θ by the individual effect size θ_i. Then the unknown population parameter θ_i is estimated by the sample effect size, $\hat{\theta}_i$ which includes errors (combination of sampling error and errors due to individual study bias), $\theta_i = \theta + \varepsilon_i$. Let σ_i^2 be the unknown (within) population variance of the ith study for $i = 1, 2, \ldots, k$. The sample estimate of the population effect size for the ith primary study based on a random sample of size n_i is denoted by $\hat{\theta}_i$ and the sample variance by v_i. Then the unknown inverse variance population weight $\omega_i = \frac{1}{\sigma_i^2}$ of the ith study is estimated by the sample weight $w_i = \frac{1}{v_i}$.

Normally, the ith individual study reports the sample estimate of the effect size, ($\hat{\theta}_i$) the sample variance (v_i) of the estimator of effect size and the sample size n_i. Based on these information, a 95% confidence interval for θ_i is constructed for each of the studies if the sampling distribution of $\hat{\theta}_i$ is known. Obviously, the confidence intervals vary from one study to another, and some of them may even provide conflicting results. Therefore, it is important to combine the results from all the k studies by pooling the summary statistics data into a single point estimate and find a confidence interval for the common effect size θ.

The fixed effect (FE) model assumes that the errors follow a normal distribution with mean 0 and variance σ_i^2. Hence θ_i is also distributed normally with mean θ and variance σ_i^2. So, under the FE model all studies share a common effect size and attempt is made to estimate the unknown population common effect size from the sample data. Under the FE model, the common effect size estimator for the log OR, $\theta^* = Ln\,OR$ is given by

$$\hat{\theta}_{FE}^* = \frac{\sum\limits_{i=1}^{k} w_i \hat{\theta}_i^*}{\sum\limits_{i=1}^{k} w_i} \tag{5.1}$$

which is the weighted mean of the estimated effect sizes of all the independent studies. The denominator in Eq. (5.1) ensures that the sum of the weights is 1. The variance of the estimator of the common effect size θ^* is

$Var(\hat{\theta}_{FE}^*) = \dfrac{1}{\sum\limits_{i=1}^{k} w_i}$. Therefore, the standard error of the estimator of the common

effect size under the FE model is $SE(\hat{\theta}_{FE}^*) = \sqrt{\dfrac{1}{\sum\limits_{i=1}^{k} w_i}}$.

The confidence interval under FE model

The $(1 - \alpha) \times 100\%$ confidence interval for the transformed effect size θ^* under the FE model is given by the lower limit (LL) and upper limit (UL) as follows:

$LL^* = \hat{\theta}_{FE}^* - z_{\alpha/2} \times SE(\hat{\theta}_{FE}^*)$ and

$UL^* = \hat{\theta}_{FE}^* + z_{\alpha/2} \times SE(\hat{\theta}_{FE}^*)$ in ln OR scale, and then

$LL = \exp(LL^*)$ and

$LU = \exp(LU^*)$ in the original OR scale.

Here $z_{\alpha/2}$ is the $\frac{\alpha}{2}$ th cut-off point of standard normal distribution. For a 95% confidence interval $z_{\alpha/2} = z_{0.05/2} = 1.96$.

Test of hypothesis

To test the significance of the common effect size, θ^* under the FE model, of all studies, test the null hypothesis

$H_0 : \theta^* = 0$ (that is, LnOR = 0) against $H_a : \theta^* \neq 0$ using the test statistic

$$Z = \frac{\hat{\theta}^*}{SE(\hat{\theta}^*)},$$

where the test statistic Z follows the standard normal distribution.

Decision Rules:

Critical value approach: For a two-tailed test, reject H_0 at the α level of significance if the calculated/observed value of the Z statistic (say z_0) satisfies $|z_0| \geq z_{\alpha/2}$, where $z_{\alpha/2}$ is the $\frac{\alpha}{2}$ level upper cut-off point of the standard normal distribution; otherwise don't reject the null hypothesis.

P-value approach: For a two-tailed test, reject H_0 at the α level of significance if the P-value is less than or equal to α; otherwise don't reject the null hypothesis.

Illustration of FE model for OR

Example 5.3 Consider the data on the number of patients with high dose radioactive iodine versus low dose after thyroidectomy in patients with differentiated thyroid cancer. The study looked at the risk of ablation (surgical removal of tissue) as the outcome variable. For illustration we consider seven independent studies as in Table 5.2 below.

Find the (i) point estimate and (ii) standard error of the estimator, (iii) 95% confidence interval, and (iv) test the significance of the population OR under the FE model.

Table 5.2 Count data on the number of thyroid cancer patients with ablation in the low-dose and high-dose groups

Study name	Treatment (High dose)			Control (Low dose)		
	N1	Cases	Non-cases	N2	Cases	Non-cases
Doi (2000)	49	23	26	39	25	14
Ramacciotti (1982)	9	3	6	20	12	8
Angelini (1997)	426	226	200	180	101	79
Liu (1987)	40	14	26	20	11	9
Lin (1998)	21	6	15	25	11	14
McCowen (1976)	28	10	18	36	15	21
Maxon (1992)	37	6	31	26	6	20

Solution:

The odds ratio (OR) of the Treatment (high dose) group, log of OR (LnOR), variance of log OR, weight (W), 95% confidence levels and other calculations for individual studies are shown in Table 5.3 below.

Using the summary statistics in Table 5.3 we answer the above questions as follows:

(i) The point estimate of the common pooled effect (OR) under the FE model is found as

$$\hat{\theta}^*_{FE} = \frac{\sum_{i=1}^{7} w_i \hat{\theta}^*_i}{\sum_{i=1}^{7} w_i} = \frac{-15.364}{49.694} = -0.3092 \text{ in the LnOR scale, and hence the estimated}$$

effect size in the OR scale under the FE model becomes

$$\hat{\theta}_{FE} = \exp(\hat{\theta}^*_{FE}) = \exp(-0.3092) = 0.73406.$$

Table 5.3 Calculations and summary statistics for the thyroid cancer with ablation data for the FE model

Study name	OR	LnOR	Var(LnOR)	W(OR)	WxLnOR	95% CI LL	UL
Doi (2000)	0.4954	−0.7024	0.1934	5.1715	−3.6326	0.2092	1.1729
Ramacciotti (1982)	0.3333	−1.0986	0.7083	1.4118	−1.551	0.064	1.7349
Angelini (1997)	0.8839	−0.1235	0.032	31.266	−3.8599	0.6225	1.2549
Liu (1987)	0.4406	−0.8197	0.3119	3.206	−2.628	0.1474	1.3164
Lin (1998)	0.5091	−0.6751	0.3957	2.5274	−1.7063	0.1484	1.7468
McCowen (1976)	0.7778	−0.2513	0.2698	3.7059	−0.9313	0.281	2.1529
Maxon (1992)	0.6452	−0.4383	0.4156	2.4062	−1.0545	0.1824	2.2825
				49.694	**−15.364**		

(ii)   The standard error of the estimator of population lnOR under the FE model is

$$SE(\hat{\theta}_{FE}^*) = \sqrt{\frac{1}{\sum\limits_{i=1}^{7} w_i}} = \sqrt{\frac{1}{49.694}} = 0.141856.$$

(iii)   The 95% confidence interval for the common effect size in ln OR scale is

$$LL^* = \hat{\theta}_{FE}^* - 1.96 \times SE(\hat{\theta}_{FE}^*) = -0.3092 - 1.96 \times 0.141856 = -0.5872 \text{ and}$$
$$UL^* = \hat{\theta}_{FE}^* + 1.96 \times SE(\hat{\theta}_{FE}^*) == -0.3092 + 1.96 \times 0.141856 = -0.03113$$

Then the 95% confidence interval in the OR scale is

$$LL = \exp(LL^*) = \exp(-0.5872) = 0.5559 \text{ and}$$
$$UL = \exp(UL^*) = \exp(-0.03113) = 0.9693.$$

Hence the 95% confidence interval for the population OR of ablation is (0.56, 0.97).

Comment The above point estimate 0.73 (rounded) and confidence limits 0.56 and 0.97 are reported in the last row of the forest plot in Fig. 5.1.

(iv)   To test $H_0 : \theta = 0$ (that is, LnOR $= 0$) against $H_a : \theta \neq 0$ the observed value of the test statistic

$$Z = \frac{\hat{\theta}^*}{SE(\hat{\theta}^*)} \text{ is}$$

$$z_0 = \frac{-0.3092}{0.148156} = -2.1794 \approx -2.18.$$

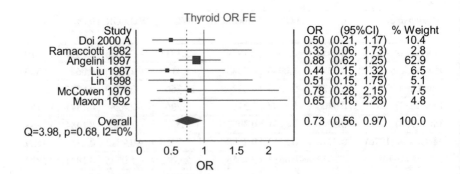

Fig. 5.1 Forest plot of OR for Thyroid data under the FE model using MetaXL

The two-sided P-value is $P(|Z| > -2.18) = 2 \times P(Z < -2.18) = 2 \times 0.0146 = 0.0292 \ (< 0.05)$. So, at the 5% significance level the OR is significant.

The effect size (OR) of ablation after thyroidectomy is significantly different for the low dose and high dose patients.

Measuring Heterogeneity of between study ORs

In many statistical analyses heterogeneity is a major problem. This is more so for meta-analysis. In the presence of heterogeneity in the data special methods are required for the analysis. So, it is essential for every meta-analysis to investigate the heterogeneity before selecting any specific statistical model.

In meta-analysis, the heterogeneity among the studies are measured by Cochran's Q statistic Cochran 1973 and Higgin's I^2 index. Higgins et al. (2003) provides further insight into the heterogeneity measures in meta-analysis.

To test the heterogeneity among population effect size (θ_i), test the null hypothesis, $H_0 : \theta_1 = \theta_2 = \ldots = \theta_k$ against the alternative hypothesis H_a : not all θ_i's are equal for $i = 1, 2, \ldots, k$ using the test statistic defined as

$$Q = \sum_{i-1}^{k} w_i \hat{\theta}_i^{*2} - \frac{\left(\sum_{i=1}^{k} w_i \hat{\theta}_i^* \right)^2}{\sum_{i=1}^{k} w_i} \quad \text{using the ln OR as the effect measure.}$$

Example 5.4 Consider the ablation data in Exercise 5.3.

Calculate the value of the Q and I^2 statistics for the effect size OR.

Solution:

For the above data set in Example 5.3, using the summary statistics from the Table 5.4, we get

Table 5.4 Calculations and summary statistics for the thyroid cancer with ablation data for Q and I^2 statistics

Study name	OR	LnOR	Var(LnOR)	W(LnOR)	WxLnOR	WxLnOR^2
Doi (2000)	0.4954	−0.70242	0.193368	5.17148	−3.6326	2.551581
Ramacciotti (1982)	0.3333	−1.09861	0.708333	1.41176	−1.551	1.703928
Angelini (1997)	0.8839	−0.12346	0.031984	31.2656	−3.8599	0.476524
Liu (1987)	0.4406	−0.81971	0.31191	3.20605	−2.628	2.154223
Lin (1998)	0.5091	−0.67513	0.395671	2.52735	−1.7063	1.151964
McCowen (1976)	0.7778	−0.25131	0.269841	3.70588	−0.9313	0.23406
Maxon (1992)	0.6452	−0.43825	0.415591	2.40621	−1.0545	0.462154
				49.6944	**−15.364**	**8.734434**

$$Q = \sum_{i=1}^{7} w_i \hat{\theta}_i^{*2} - \frac{\left(\sum_{i=1}^{7} w_i \hat{\theta}_i^*\right)^2}{\sum_{i=1}^{7} w_i} = \sum_{i=1}^{7} WLnOR^2 - \frac{\left(\sum_{i=1}^{7} WLnOR\right)^2}{\sum_{i=1}^{7} W}$$

$$= 8.734434 - \frac{(-15.3636)^2}{49.69437} = 3.984578 \approx 3.98.$$

The above Q statistic follows a chi-squared distribution with $(k-1) = 7-1 = 6$ degrees of freedom. Then the P-value of testing equality of population effect sizes (OR) becomes

$$p = P\left(\chi_6^2 > 3.98\right) = 0.68.$$

Using chi-squired distribution table, it is found that the P-value of the test is between 0.50 and 0.75 (which includes 0.68). The exact critical value of the chi-squared statistic is rarely found from the chi-squared Table but can easily be obtained by using any statistical package.

Since the P-value is very large, there is insignificant heterogeneity between the study effect sizes.

The value of the I^2 statistic is found to be

$$I^2 = \left(\frac{Q - df}{Q}\right) \times 100\% = \left(\frac{3.98 - 6}{3.98}\right) \times 100\% = -0.51\% \rightarrow 0\%$$

(negative values of I^2 statistic is truncated to 0%). Hence there is no significant heterogeneity between the study effects.

Comment The I^2 statistic above represents the percentage of variation across studies that is due to systematic heterogeneity rather than chance.

Forest plot for OR using MetaXL:
The forest plot under the FE model (indicated by "IV" in the code) is produced by using MetaXL code
    =MAInputTable("Thyroid OR FE","NumOR","IV",B17:H23),
    where "B17:H23" refers to the data area in Excel sheet.

Remark: Explanations of MetaXL Code
For this type of meta-analyses in MetaXL the 'opening' code starts with MA Input Table " = MAInputTable". This is followed by an open parenthesis inside which the first quote contains the text that appears as the 'title of the output of the forest plot' e.g. "Thyroid OR FE" in the above code (user may choose any appropriate title here). Then in the second quote enter the type of effect measure, e.g. "NumOR" in the above code tells that the *outcome variable is numerical and the effect size*

measure is odds ratio. Within the third quote enter the statistical model, e.g. "IV" in the above code stands for the *fixed effect* (inverse variance is abbreviated by IV) model. Each quotation is followed by a comma, and after the last comma enter the data area in Excel Worksheet, e.g. B17:H23 in the above code tells that the data on the independent studies are taken from the specified cells in the Excel Worksheet. The code ends with a closing parenthesis.

The forest plot of the meta-analysis of OR using the above MetaXL code is given in Fig. 5.1.

Comment For the explanations and components on the forest plot please see the FE model forest plot of RR in Chap. 4.

Interpretation:
From the forest plot of meta-analysis in Fig 5.1, the odds of ablation of thyroid patients with low dose of after thyroidectomy differentiated thyroid cancer is 0.73 relative to the high dose patients. The patients with high dose have 0.27 times less odds of ablation than those with low dose.

Aside: The use of the term 'probability' for the word 'odds' is inappropriate since by definition the two terms are very different. Hence the two terms are not interchangeable.

The 95% confidence interval (0.56, 0.97) does not include OR = 1 (odds are no different) indicating the effect size is significant at the 5% level of significance. This is also evidenced by the fact that the diamond does not cross the vertical line at OR = 1.

The value of the Q statistic is 3.98 with P-value = 0.68 indicating absence of heterogeneity among the population effect sizes. The 0% value of the I^2 statistic also leads to the same conclusion of no heterogeneity in the data.

5.5 Random Effects (REs) Model

General discussions on the random effects (REs) model are found in Chap. 2. Under the REs model, the assumption is that there is no common effect size for the k independent studies. In stead, it is assumed that every primary study has a different population effect size which is a random variable, and follows normal distribution. As such, there is variation between the effect sizes of the individual studies. So, the variance of effect size under the REs model is the sum of within study and between studies variances. As suggested by DerSimonian and Laird (1986), the between studies variance is estimated by method of moments. Some serious flaws of the REs model have been discussed by many authors and the shortcomings of REs model has been explained by simulation comparison as in Doi et al. (2015b).

The REs model assumes, $\hat{\theta}_i = \theta + \varsigma_i + \varepsilon_i$ in which $\varsigma_i = \theta_i - \theta$ is distributed normally with mean 0 and variance τ^2 and $\varepsilon_i = \hat{\theta}_i - \theta_i$ follows a normal distribution with mean 0 and variance σ_i^2.

Since, under the REs model, there are two sources of variation, the overall study error variance has two components. First, the within-study error variance, and second, the between-study variance. The population between-studies variance is the variance of θ_i about θ and is denoted by τ^2 which is estimated by the sample variance of $\hat{\theta}_i$ about θ and is denoted by $\hat{\tau}^2$. Thus, under the REs model the estimated variance of any observed effect size $\hat{\theta}_i$ about θ is the sum of the within-study and between-study variances, that is, $v_i^* = v_i + \hat{\tau}^2$. Therefore, the weight assigned to the ith study under the REs model is given by

$$w_i^* = \frac{1}{v_i + \hat{\tau}^2}$$

which is an estimate of the unknown population weight $\omega_i^* = \frac{1}{\sigma_{i*}^2}$ with $\sigma_{i*}^2 = \sigma_i^2 + \tau^2$.

The combind effect size (LnOR $= \theta^*$) estimator under the random effects (REs) model is

$$\hat{\theta}_{RE}^* = \frac{\sum\limits_{i=1}^{k} w_i^* \hat{\theta}_i^*}{\sum\limits_{i=1}^{k} w_i^*} \tag{5.2}$$

with standard error

$$SE(\hat{\theta}_{RE}^*) = \sqrt{\frac{1}{\sum\limits_{i=1}^{k} w_i^*}}.$$

Estimation of τ^2

The between-studies variance is estimated as a scaled excess variation as follows

$$\hat{\tau}^2 = \frac{Q - df}{C},$$

where

$$Q = \sum_{i=1}^{k} w_i \hat{\theta}_i^2 - \frac{\left(\sum\limits_{i=1}^{k} w_i \hat{\theta}_i\right)^2}{\sum\limits_{i=1}^{k} w_i}, \ldots C = \sum_{i=1}^{k} w_i - \frac{\sum\limits_{i=1}^{k} w_i^2}{\sum\limits_{i=1}^{k} w_i}$$

and $df = (k - 1)$ in which k is the number of studies.

Table 5.5 The count data for the heartburn of patients

Study name	LAF			LPF		
	N1	Cases	Non-cases	N2	Cases	Non-cases
Watson et al. (1999)	54	5	49	53	5	48
Hagedorn et al. (2003)	47	25	22	48	10	38
Watson et al. (2004)	60	11	49	52	2	50
Spence et al. (2006)	40	6	34	39	5	34
Khan et al. (2010)	31	7	24	29	3	26
Raue et al. (2011)	30	1	29	27	1	26
Cao et al. (2012)	49	8	41	47	8	39

Illustration of Random Effects Model for OR

Example 5.5 The Table 5.5 provides summary data on the number of patients with heartburn after surgery for Gastro-Esophageal Reflux Disease using Laparoscopic Anterior (LAF) versus Posterior Fundoplication (LPF). Reference Memon et al. (2015).

Find the estimated value of the between studies variance τ^2 for the heartburn data.

Solution:

From the data, the calculated sample values of OR, LnOR, Var(LnOR) and other statistics are found in Table 5.6.

Illustration of calculations:
For example, for the first study (Watson et al. 1999):

The odds of LAF is OD(LAF) = 5/49 = 0.10204 and the odds of LPF is OD(LPF) = 5/48 = 0.10417, and hence the odds ratio (odds of LAF relative to LPF) is OR = 0.10204/0.10417 = 0.9796 or 0.98 (rounded). Then log of OR become LnOR = ln(0.9796) = −0.0206 or −0.021 (rounded).

The variance of the estimator of LnOR is
$V(LnOR) = \frac{1}{a} + \frac{1}{b} + \frac{1}{c} + \frac{1}{d} = \frac{1}{5} + \frac{1}{49} + \frac{1}{5} + \frac{1}{48} = 0.4412.$

To estimate the value of between studies variance, τ^2 we need to find the values of following statistics (note that the sample value of LnOR for the ith study is $\hat{\theta}_i$ in the formulae) below:

$$Q = \sum_{i=1}^{7} w_i \hat{\theta}_i^2 - \frac{\left(\sum\limits_{i=1}^{7} w_i \hat{\theta}_i\right)^2}{\sum\limits_{i=1}^{7} w_i} = \sum W \times LnOR^2 - \frac{\sum (W \times LnOR)^2}{\sum W(LnOR)} \text{(from notations in}$$

Table 5.6).

That is, $Q = 16.4568 - \frac{(11.46928)^2}{16.53557} = 8.50158 \approx 8.502$ and

Table 5.6 Calculations for the heartburn data to find $\hat{\tau}^2$ for REs model

Study name	OR	LnOR	Var(LnOR)	W(LnOR)	WxLnOR	WxLnOR^2	W^2
Watson et al. (1999)	0.98	−0.021	0.44124	2.26633	−0.0467	0.000964	5.13626
Hagedorn et al. (2003)	4.32	1.463	0.21177	4.7221	6.9076	10.10474	22.2982
Watson et al. (2004)	5.61	1.725	0.63132	1.58399	2.7323	4.71309	2.50902
Spence et al. (2006)	1.2	0.182	0.42549	2.35023	0.4285	0.078124	5.52358
Khan et al. (2010)	2.53	0.927	0.55632	1.79753	1.6669	1.545806	3.23112
Raue et al. (2011)	0.9	−0.109	2.07294	0.48241	−0.0527	0.005752	0.23272
Cao et al. (2012)	0.95	−0.05	0.30003	3.33299	−0.1667	0.008336	11.1088
				16.5356	**11.469**	**16.45681**	**50.0397**

$$C = \sum_{i=1}^{k} w_i - \frac{\sum_{i=1}^{k} w_i^2}{\sum_{i=1}^{k} w_i} = \sum W(LnOR) - \frac{\sum [W(LnOR)]^2}{\sum W(LnOR)}$$

$$= 16.53557 - \frac{50.03969}{16.53557} = 13.50939 \approx 13.51.$$

Then, the estimated value of τ^2 becomes

$$\hat{\tau}^2 = \frac{Q - df}{C} = \frac{8.502 - 6}{13.51} = 0.1852,$$

where df $= k - 1 = 7 - 1 = 6$.

Example 5.6 Consider the heartburn data in Example 5.5

Under the REs model, find the (i) point estimate and (ii) standard error of the estimator, (iii) 95% confidence interval and (iv) test the significance of the population effect size OR for the heartburn data.

To answer the above questions, we need to use the calculations of summary statistics in Table 5.7.

In Table 5.7, Tau^2 represents estimated value of τ^2, Var* represents the combined variance as the sum of Var and Tau^2, and W* is the modified weight calculated as the inverse of Var*.

For the illustration of computations, note that the modified variance for the ith study under the REs model becomes.

$w_i^* = \frac{1}{v_i + \hat{\tau}^2}$ which is $W_i^* = \frac{1}{Var_i^* + Tau^2}$ in the table notation.

For example, for the first study (Watson et al. 1999) the modified weight, under REs model, based on modified variance becomes

$$w_1^* = \frac{1}{v_1 + \hat{\tau}^2} = \frac{1}{Var_1 + Tau^2} = \frac{1}{0.4412 + 0.1852} = 1.5963.$$

Table 5.7 Calculations for REs model meta-analysis of OR for the heartburn data

Study name	OR	LnOR	Var(LnOR)	Tau^2	Var*	W*	W*xLnOR
Watson et al. (1999)	0.98	−0.021	0.44124	0.1852	0.6264	1.596318	−0.03291
Hagedorn et al. (2003)	4.32	1.463	0.21177	0.1852	0.397	2.51908	3.684997
Watson et al. (2004)	5.61	1.725	0.63132	0.1852	0.8165	1.224714	2.112571
Spence et al. (2006)	1.2	0.182	0.42549	0.1852	0.6107	1.637491	0.29855
Khan et al. (2010)	2.53	0.927	0.55632	0.1852	0.7415	1.348584	1.250596
Raue et al. (2011)	0.9	−0.109	2.07294	0.1852	2.2581	0.442841	−0.04836
Cao et al. (2012)	0.95	−0.05	0.30003	0.1852	0.4852	2.060873	−0.10307
						10.8299	**7.162376**

Using the summary statistics in Table 5.7 the answers to the questions Example 5.6 are provided as follows:

(i) The point estimate of the common effect size estimate of LnOR under the random effects (REs) model is

$$\hat{\theta}^*_{RE} = \frac{\sum_{i=1}^{k} w_i^* \hat{\theta}_i}{\sum_{i=1}^{k} w_i^*} = \frac{\sum W^* \times LnOR}{\sum W^*} = \frac{7.162376}{10.8299} = 0.6614, \text{ in ln OR scale.}$$

Then, the point estimate of population OR becomes $\hat{\theta}_{RE} = OR = \exp\left(\hat{\theta}^*_{RE}\right) = \exp(0.6614) = 1.937503 \approx 1.94$ in original OR scale.

(ii) The standard error is found as

$$SE(\hat{\theta}^*_{RE}) = \sqrt{\frac{1}{\sum_{i=1}^{k} w_i^*}} = \sqrt{\frac{1}{\sum W^*}} = \sqrt{\frac{1}{10.8299}} = 0.30387.$$

(iii) The 95% confidence interval for the unknown population parameter LnOR is given by

$LL^* = \hat{\theta}^*_{RE} - 1.96 \times SE(\hat{\theta}^*_{RE}) = 0.66 - 1.96 \times 0.30387 = 0.064415$ and
$UL^* = \hat{\theta}^*_{RE} + 1.96 \times SE(\hat{\theta}^*_{RE}) = 0.54 + 1.96 \times 0.30387 = 1.255585$ in ln OR scale.
Then the 95% confidence interval in the original RR scale becomes

$$LL = \exp(LL^*) = \exp(0.064415) = 1.067 \approx 1.07 \text{ and}$$
$$UL = \exp(UL^*) = \exp(1.255585) = 3.50989 \approx 3.51.$$

Remark The above value of the point estimate (1.94) and the confidence interval (1.07, 3.51) of the population OR are reported in the bottom row of the forest plot and represented by the diamond as in Fig. 5.2.

(iv) To test the significance of population OR the null hypothesis is $H_0 : OR = 1$ (same odds for both groups) against $H_a : OR \neq 1$. That is, test $H_0 : \ln OR = 0$ versus $H_1 : \ln OR \neq 0$. Based on the heartburn data the observed value of the test statistic, Z is

$$z_0 = \frac{\hat{\theta}^*_{RE}}{SE\left(\hat{\theta}^*_{RE}\right)} = \frac{0.6616}{0.30387} = 2.17659 \approx 2.18.$$

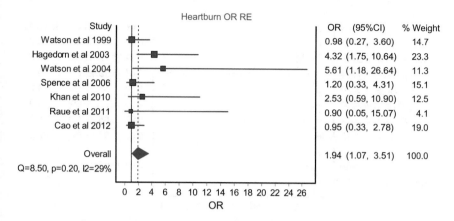

Fig. 5.2 Forest plot of OR for heartburn data under REs model using MetaXL

The two-sided P-value is $P(|Z| > 2.18) = 2 \times P(Z > 2.18) = 2 \times 0.0146 = 0.0292$. Therefore the test is significant at the 5% level, that is, the RR is significantly different from 1.

REs Model Working with MetaXL for OR
In MetaXL use following code:
=MAInputTable("Heartburn OR RE","NumOR","RE",N5:T11),
where "N5:T11" indicates the data area in Excel sheet, and "RE" represents REs model.

Remark: Explanations of MetaXL Code
For this type of meta-analyses in MetaXL the 'opening' of the code starts with '= MAInputTable'. This is followed by an open parenthesis inside which the first quote contains the text that appears as the 'title of the output of the forest plot' e.g. "Heartburn OR RE" in the above code (user may choose any appropriate title here). Then in the second quote enter the type of effect measure, e.g. "NumOR" in the above code tells that the *outcome variable is numerical and the effect size measure is odds ratio*. Within the third quote enter the statistical model, e.g. "RE" in the above code stands for the *random effects* (abbreviated by RE) model. Each quotation is followed by a comma, and after the last comma enter the data area in Excel, e.g. N5:T11 in the above code tells that the data on the independent studies are taken from the specified cells. The code ends with a closing parenthesis.

Interpretation
The estimated value of the combined effect size OR under the REs model is 1.94. The odds of heartburn in the LAF group is 1.94 times the odds of LPF group. So the LPF group has much (1.94 times) higher odds than the LAF group.

The 95% confidence interval is (1.07, 3.51) which does not contain 1 (equal odds of heartburn for LAP and LPF group patients). Since the 95% confidence interval does not include OR = 1, the effect size is significant at the 5% level of significance.

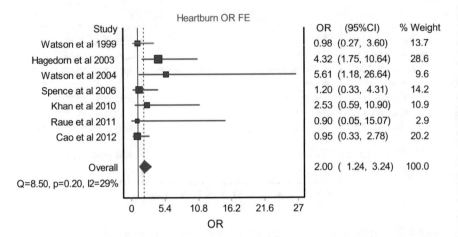

Fig. 5.3 Forest plot of OR for the heartburn data under FE model using MetaXL

The Q statistic is not significant as the P-value is (0.20) large. Similarly, the value of $I^2 = 29\%$ is low, indicating no significant heterogeneity among the studies.

Aside: Compare FE model results
If fixed effect (FE) model is used for the same heartburn data the in Fig. 5.3 forest plot is produced by MetaXL with code:

=MAInputTable("Heartburn OR FE","NumOR","IV",N5:T11)

Comparative Interpretations
From Fig. 5.3, the estimated value of the combined effect size OR under the FE model is 2.00 with the 95% confidence interval (1.24, 3.24).

From Fig. 5.2, the estimated value of the combined effect size OR under the REs model is 1.94 with 95% confidence interval is (1.07, 3.51).

Although, under both FE and REs models the effect size is significant, the value of the point estimate is higher (2.00) for the FE model than that under the REs model (1.94), the 95% confidence interval is much wider under the REs model than the FE model.

As always, the values of Q and I^2 statistics are unchanged under the two models. In fact, the two statistics are not dependent on any statistical models.

5.6 Inverse Variance Heterogeneity (IVhet) Model

The inverse variance heterogeneity (IVhet) model is a better alternative to the random effects (REs) model to deal with heterogeneous meta-analyses. As explained in Doi et al. (2015a, 2015b) the IVhet model has much better statistical properties than the REs model.

Here we adopt the model to analyse the odds ratio (OR) as an effect size measure. The IVhet estimate of the transformed common effect size LnOR $(= \theta^*)$ is given by

$$\hat{\theta}^*_{IVhet} = \frac{\sum\limits_{i=1}^{k} w_i \hat{\theta}^*_i}{\sum\limits_{i=1}^{k} w_i}.$$

Then the variance of the transformed estimator under the IVhet model is given by

$$Var(\hat{\theta}^*_{IVhet}) = \sum_{i=1}^{k} \left[\left(\frac{1}{v_i} \middle/ \sum_{i=1}^{k} \frac{1}{v_i} \right)^2 (v_i + \hat{\tau}^2) \right] = \sum_{i=1}^{k} \left[\left(w_i \middle/ \sum_{i=1}^{k} w_i \right)^2 (v_i + \hat{\tau}^2) \right].$$

For the computation of the confidence interval of the common effect size, θ^*, based on the IVhet model use the following standard error

$$SE(\hat{\theta}^*_{IVhet}) = \sqrt{Var(\hat{\theta}^*_{IVhet})}.$$

Then, the $(1 - \alpha) \times 100\%$ confidence interval for the transformed common effect size $\theta^* = \ln OR$ under the IVhet model is given by the lower limit (LL*) and upper limit (UL*) as follows:

$LL^* = \hat{\theta}^*_{IVhet} - z_{\alpha/2} \times SE(\hat{\theta}^*_{IVhet})$ and

$UL^* = \hat{\theta}^*_{IVhet} + z_{\alpha/2} \times SE(\hat{\theta}^*_{IVhet})$ in lnOR scale,

where $z_{\alpha/2}$ is the $\frac{\alpha}{2}$ th cut-off point of standard normal distribution.

So, the $(1 - \alpha) \times 100\%$ confidence interval for the common effect size $\theta = OR$ under the IVhet model is given by the lower limit (LL) and upper limit (UL) as follows:

$LL = \exp(LL^*)$ and

$UL = \exp(UL^*)$, in original OR scale.

Test of significance

To test the significance of population OR the null hypothesis is $H_0 : OR = 1$ (same odds for both groups) against $H_a : OR \neq 1$. Under the IVhet model, the test statistic is

$Z = \dfrac{\hat{\theta}^*_{IVhet}}{SE(\hat{\theta}^*_{IVhet})}$ which follows the standard normal distribution under the null hypothesis.

Illustration of IVhet Model for OR

Example 5.7 Consider the heartburn data in Example 5.5.

Under the IVhet model, find the (i) point estimate and (ii) standard error of the estimator, (iii) 95% confidence interval and (iv) test the significance of the population effect size OR for the heartburn data.

Solution:

To answer the above questions, we need to use the calculations of the summary statistics in Table 5.8 below.

For the first study (Watson et al. 1999), weight of LnOR is

$W(LnOR) = 1/Var(LnOR) = 1/0.441241 = 2.26633$, the modified variance of LnOR is $V^*((LnOR) = Var(LnOR) + Tau^2 = 0.441241497 + 0.185173 = 0.626414497$, and the modified weight under the IVhet model is

$$W^*(IVhet) = \left[\frac{W(LnOR)}{\sum W(LnOR)}\right]^2 \times V^*(LnOR) = \left[\frac{2.26633}{16.5356}\right]^2 \times 0.62641 = 0.011767.$$

To find the estimated value of the population LnOR under the IVhet model the sums of columns of $W(LnOR)$ and $W \times LnOR$, that is, $\sum W(LnOR) = 16.5356$ and $\sum W \times LnOR = 11.46928$, from Table 5.8 are required.

Now, using the summary statistics in Table 5.8 we answer the questions in the above example.

(i)   The point estimate of the transformed common effect size LnOR under the IVhet model is given by

$$\hat{\theta}^*_{IVhet} = \frac{\sum_{i=1}^{7} w_i \hat{\theta}^*_i}{\sum_{i=1}^{7} w_i} = \frac{\sum W \times LnOR}{\sum W(LnOR)} = \frac{11.46928}{16.5356} = 0.693611 \approx 0.69 \text{ in the LnOR scale.}$$

So, the point estimate of OR in the original OR scale is given by $\hat{\theta}_{IVhet} = OR_{IVhet} = \exp\left(\hat{\theta}^*_{IVhet}\right) = \exp(0.693611) = 2.000928 \approx 2.00$.

(ii)   The variance of the estimator of LnOR $= \theta^*$ under the IVhet model is given by the sum of the last column of the above table, that is,

$$Var(\hat{\theta}^*_{IVhet}) = \sum_{i=1}^{7} \left[\left(\frac{1}{v_i} \middle/ \sum_{i=1}^{7} \frac{1}{v_i}\right)^2 (v_i + \hat{\tau}^2)\right] = \sum_{i=1}^{7} \left[\frac{W_i}{\sum W_i}\right] \times V_i^* = 0.094364.$$

Hence the standard error becomes

$$SE(\hat{\theta}^*_{IVhet}) = \sqrt{Var(\hat{\theta}^*_{IVhet})} = \sqrt{0.094364} = 0.307187.$$

(iii)   Then, the 95% confidence interval for the transformed common effect size LnOR under the IVhet model is given by

Table 5.8 Calculations for IVhet model meta-analysis of OR for the heartburn data

Study name	OR	LnOR	Var(LnOR)	W(LnOR)	Wx(LnOR)	V*(LnOR)	W*(IVhet)
Watson et al. (1999)	0.98	−0.02.6	0.441241	2.26633	−0.04673	0.62641	0.011767
Hagedorn et al. (2003)	4.32	1.46283	0.21177	4.7221	6.907646	0.39694	0.032371
Watson et al. (2004)	5.61	1.72495	0.631317	1.58399	2.732304	0.81649	0.007492
Spence et al. (2006)	1.2	0.18232	0.42549	2.35023	0.428498	0.61066	0.012336
Khan et al. (2010)	2.53	0.92734	0.556319	1.79753	1.666923	0.74149	0.008762
Raue et al. (2011)	0.9	−0.1092	2.072944	0.48241	−0.05268	2.25812	0.001922
Cae et al. (2012)	0.95	−0.05	0.300031	3.33299	−0.16668	0.4852	0.019713
				16.5356	**11.46928**	**5.93532**	**0.094364**

Note that the modified variance, V*(LnOR) is the sum of the within and between studies variances of LnOR for the individual studies

$LL^* = \hat{\theta}^*_{IVhet} - 1.96 \times SE(\hat{\theta}^*_{IVhet}) = 0.6931 - 1.96 \times 0.307187 = 0.09101$ and
$UL^* = \hat{\theta}^*_{IVhet} + 1.96 \times SE(\hat{\theta}^*_{IVhet}) = 0.6931 + 1.96 \times 0.307187 = 1.29519$
in ln OR scale.

Then the 95% confidence interval in the original OR scale becomes
$LL = \exp(LL*) = \exp(0.09101) = 1.09528 \approx 1.10$ and
$UL = \exp(UL*) = \exp(1.29519) = 3.65168 \approx 3.65.$

Remark The above point estimate (2.00) of the pooled OR and confidence interval
(1.10, 3.65) are reported in the forest plot in the last row in Fig. 5.4 with the diamond
representing the values.

IVhet Meta-analysis of OR with MetaXL
In MetaXL use following code:

```
=MAInputTable("Heartburn OR IVhet","NumOR","IVhet",N5:T11),
```

where "N5:T11" indicates the data area in Excel sheet, and "IVhet" represents IVhet
model.

Remark: Explanations of MetaXL Code
For this type of meta-analyses in MetaXL the 'opening' code starts with MA Input
Table ' = MAInputTable'. This is followed by an open parenthesis inside which the
first quote contains the text that appears as the 'title of the output of the forest plot'
e.g. "Heartburn OR IVhet" in the above code (user may choose any appropriate title
here). Then in the second quote enter the type of effect measure, e.g. "NumOR" in the
above code tells that the *outcome variable is numerical and the effect size measure
is odds ratio*. Within the third quote enter the statistical model, e.g. "IVhet" in the
above code stands for the *inverse variance heterogeneity* (abbreviated by IVhet)
model. Each quotation is followed by a comma, and after the last comma enter the

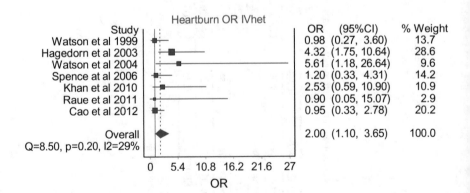

Fig. 5.4 Forest plot of OR of heartburn under inverse variance heterogeneity model using MetaXL

data area in Excel, e.g. N5:T11 in the above code tells that the data on the independent studies are taken from the specified cells. The code ends with a closing parenthesis.

The following forest plot produced by MetaXL shows the 95% confidence intervals of individual studies and the pooled effect size along with redistributed weights.

Interpretation
Under the IVhet model, the point estimator of OR is (2.00) and the 95% confidence interval is (1.10, 3.65). Since the 95% confidence interval of the OR of heartburn is significantly different for the patients treated with LAF and LPF surgeries. The patients with LPF surgery have higher odds of heartburn compared to those with LAF surgery. There is 2 'times higher odds' of heartburn for the patients receiving LPF surgery than those received LAF surgery.

The P-value of the Q statistic is not small (0.20) and hence the heterogeneity among the studies is not significant. This is also supported by the $I^2 = 29\%$.

5.7 Subgroup Analysis

Subgroup analysis is appropriate when the studies could be divided into different groups based on some distinguishing characteristics of the studies. This is done if there is a reason to suspect real differences in the effect size estimate among the groups of studies. Subgroup analysis is also conducted if there are significant heterogeneity among the studies. It provides an opportunity to compare the results among different subgroups and also with the pooled results of all studies. Subgroup analysis is a special case of meta-regression when the only explanatory (moderator) variable is categorical.

Interested readers may refer to Paget et al. (2011) for an example of subgroup analysis. Moreover, some useful advices on subgroup analysis are found in Yusuf et al. (1991).

The subgroup analysis method and procedure are illustrated and explained below for the heartburn data meta-analysis using MetaXL.

Steps in Subgroup analysis using MetaXL
Step 1: First run the following MetaXL code to create a forest plot (in cell C16, say) so that "Heartburn Subgroup OR RE" is shown on this cell.
    =MAInputTable("Heartburn Subgroup OR RE","NumOR","RE",B5:H11)
Step 2: Then create a table of subgroups of studies (as below) by study period e.g. studies published before 2010 (Old studies), and those published in 2010 or later (Recent studies) in separate columns. For the current example, to illustration the subgroup analysis in Fig. 5.5, the 'Old studies' group consists of four studies and 'Recent studies' group consists of three studies as shown in Table 5.9 below.
Step 3: Finally, run the following MetaXL codes to produce the forest plot of subgroup analysis as in Fig. 5.5:

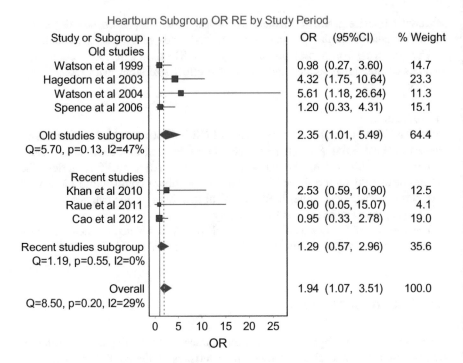

Fig. 5.5 Forest plot of OR for subgroup analysis heartburn data under REs model using MetaXL

Table 5.9 Distribution of studies in two subgroups

Old studies	Recent studies
Watson et al. (1999)	Khan et al. (2010)
Hagedorn et al. (2003)	Raue et al. (2011)
Watson et al. (2004)	Cao et al. (2012)
Spence et al. (2006)	

=MASubGroups("Study Period",C16, I4:J8)

The seven studies in the heartburn data example are grouped by study period (4 Old studies 1999–2006 and 3 Recent studies 2010–2012) for subgroup analyses.

Without conducting subgroup analysis, across all the studies the LPF has 1.94 times higher odds than the LAF. But, as in Fig. 5.5, the subgroup analysis reveals that the 'Old studies' subgroup favours the LAF as the OR for the APF patients (pooled OR = 2.35) is much high compared to that of the 'Recent studies' subgroup (pooled OR = 1.29).

Interpretation of subgroup analysis:

For the Old studies subgroup the odds of heartburn in the LPF group is 2.35 times higher than that in the LAF group. The confidence interval (1.01, 5.49) does not cross

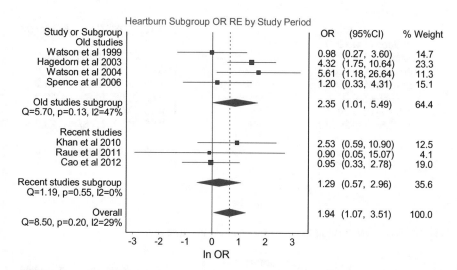

Fig. 5.6 Forest plot of OR of heartburn data with graphical display of confidence intervals in ln OR for subgroup analysis under REs model using MetaXL

the vertical line at OR = 1, and hence the effect size is significant at the 5% level of significance.

But for the Recent studies subgroup, the odds of heartburn in the LPF group is 1.29 times higher than that in the LAF group. The effect size of this group is not significant as the confidence interval (0.57, 2.96) includes OR = 1.

The pooled results (combining all Old and Recent studies) show that the odds of heartburn is 1.94 times higher in the LAF group compared to the LPF group. The confidence interval (1.07, 3.51) for the pooled effect size does not cross the vertical line at OR = 1, and hence the effect size is significant at the 5% level of significance.

So, the incidence of heartburn is much higher in the LPF group than the LAP group across all the time periods and over all the studies.

Forest plot in ln OR scale
The forest plot in Fig. 5.5 used the horizontal axis in OR scale, but in Fig. 5.6 it is in the ln OR scale. The graphical display of confidence intervals represented in ln OR (scale) as in the forest plot in Fig. 5.6 is much clearer than that in original OR (scale) in Fig. 5.5.

5.8 Discussions and Comparison of Results

The forest plots with graphical display of confidence intervals in ln OR scale better display the graph of the confidence intervals as in Figs. 5.7, 5.8, 5.9. These plots, in ln OR scale, only changes the second column (panel containing scatterplot of

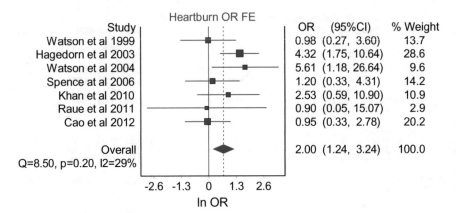

Fig. 5.7 Forest plot of OR of heartburn for FE model in LnOR scale

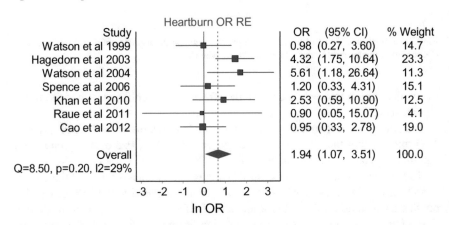

Fig. 5.8 Forest plot of OR of heartburn for REs model in LnOR scale

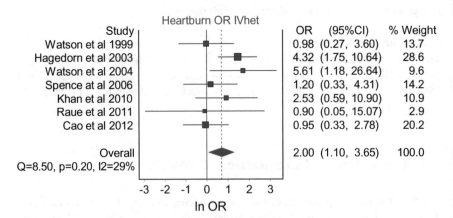

Fig. 5.9 Forest plot of OR of heartburn for IVhet model in LnOR scale

confidence intervals) of the forest plot keeping the study names in the first column, point estimates and confidence intervals in the third and fourth columns and weights in the fifth column the same (as it is in the forest plot of original OR scale).

From the definition, the point estimate of the common effect size OR is the same (2.00) for the FE and IVhet models. But the confidence interval for the FE is (1.24, 3.24) shorter than that for the IVhet is (1.10, 3.65), but with the same redistribution of weights among the studies. Thus the IVhet model meta-analysis enables higher width of the confidence interval than the FE model by allowing for higher variance in the way of inclusion of between studies variation.

For the REs model, the point estimate of the common effect size OR is 1.94 with confidence interval (1.07, 3.51). The redistribution of weights among the individual studies under this model is very different from those under the IVhet model. Contradictory to common logic, under the RE model, the smaller studies receive higher redistributed weights than the larger studies.

Under all three models the common effect size OR is significant (higher OR of heartburn for higher dose group). The heterogeneity under all the models is small/insignificant as the P-value of he Q statistic is 0.20 and the value of $I^2 = 29\%$.

The point estimate of the population OR (2.00) is the same under the FE and IVhet model regardless of the level of heterogeneity. The redistributed weights in both FE and IVhet models are about the same. However, the 95% confidence interval under FE model (1.24, 3.24) is shorter than that under the IVhet model (1.10, 3.65).

The redistributed weights are very different for the REs model than the FE or IVhet model. As a result the point estimate (1.94) under the REs model is different from the FE and IVhet models. The 95% confidence interval under the REs model (1.07, 3.51) with width 2.44 is wider than that of the FE model (1.24, 3.24) with width 2.00, but shorter than that of the IVhet model (1.10, 3.65) with width 2.55.

Obviously, the point estimates and confidence intervals of all individual studies remain the same in the forest plot regardless of the statistical model of analysis. Only changes are in the pooled estimate and confidence interval due to the different redistributed study weights under different statistical models.

5.9 Publication Bias

Publication bias is detected by using funnel plot and Doi plot. A funnel plot is a scatter plot of standard error of the studies against respective effect size. If a funnel plot is symmetrical about the vertical line, then there is no publication bias. However, if the funnel plot is asymmetric there is publication bias in the study.

The publication bias is a real and serious problem, as it has the potential to produce misleading results and hence received considerable attention among the researchers including Sterne et al. (2000), Elvik (2011) and Elvik (2013), Mathew and Charney (2009) and Uesawa et al. (2010).

Chapter 13 covers the publication bias issue in details with illustrative examples.

5.9.1   The Funnel Plot

From the funnel plot below it is evident that there is publication bias in the meta-analysis as the plot is asymmetric. One particular study (at the bottom) with very large standard error stands out from rest of the studies (Figs. 5.10 and 5.11).

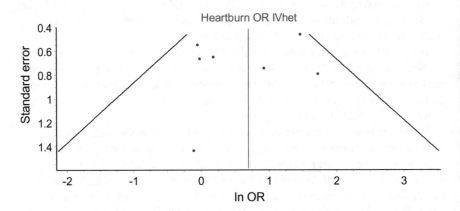

Fig. 5.10   Funnel plot of OR (in LnOR scale) showing slight asymmetry in the heartburn data study

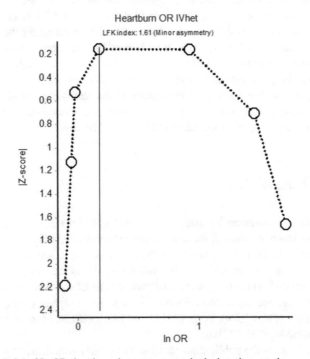

Fig. 5.11   Doi plot of LnOR showing minor asymmetry in the heartburn study

5.9.2   The Doi Plot

Another graphical method to study publication bias is the Doi plot. It is a scatter plot of absolute z-score of the value of effect size versus the effect size (or transformed effect size). The individual dots on the graph are then connected with a continuous curve. Details on Doi plot are found in Doi (2018) and Furuya-Kanamori et al. (2018).

The Doi plot below shows presence of publication bias. The LFK index (1.61) indicates minor asymmetry in the study.

Appendix 5—Stata Codes for Odds Ratio Meta-analysis

A5.1 Thyroid ablation data

Study_name	TrN1	TrCases	TrNon-cases	ConN2	ConCases	ConNon-cases
Doi (2000)	49	23	26	39	25	14
Ramacciotti (1982)	9	3	6	20	12	8
Angelini (1997)	426	226	200	180	101	79
Liu (1987)	40	14	26	20	11	9
Lin (1998)	21	6	15	25	11	14
McCowen (1976)	28	10	18	36	15	21
Maxon (1992)	37	6	31	26	6	20

A5.2 Stata code for meta-analysis of ablation data

ssc install admetan

FE model meta-analysis
   admetan TrCases TrNoncases ConCases ConNoncases, or model(**fixed**) study(study_name) effect(Relative Risk)

REs model meta-analysis
   admetan TrCases TrNoncases ConCases ConNoncases, or model(random) study(study_name) effect(Relative Risk)

IVhet model meta-analysis
   admetan TrCases TrNoncases ConCases ConNoncases, or model(ivhet) study(study_name) effect(Relative Risk)

A5.3 Heartburn data

Study_name	TrN1	TrCases	TrNon-cases	ConN2	ConCases	ConNon-cases
Watson et al. (1999)	54	5	49	53	5	48
Hagedorn et al. (2003)	47	25	22	48	10	38
Watson et al. (2004)	60	11	49	52	2	50
Spence et al. (2006)	40	6	34	39	5	34
Khan et al. (2010)	31	7	24	29	3	26
Raue et al. (2011)	30	1	29	27	1	26
Cao et al. (2012)	49	8	41	47	8	39

A5.4 Stata code for heartburn data

FE model meta-analysis

    admetan TrCases TrNoncases ConCases ConNoncases, or model(fixed) study(study_name) effect(Relative Risk)

REs model meta-analysis

    admetan TrCases TrNoncases ConCases ConNoncases, or model(random) study(study_name) effect(Relative Risk)

IVhet model meta-analysis

    admetan TrCases TrNoncases ConCases ConNoncases, or model(ivhet) study(study_name) effect(Relative Risk)

A5.5 Subgroup analysis

A5.5.1 Heartburn data for subgroup analysis

Study_name	Study_period	LafCases	LafNon-cases	LpfCases	LpfNon-cases	OR	LnOR	SELnOR
Watson et al. (1999)	Old studies	5	49	5	48	0.98	−0.021	0.6643
Hagedorn et al. (2003)	Old studies	25	22	10	38	4.318	1.4628	0.4602
Watson et al. (2004)	Old studies	11	49	2	50	5.612	1.725	0.7946
Spence et al. (2006)	Old studies	6	34	5	34	1.2	0.1823	0.6523
Khan et al. (2010)	New studies	7	24	3	26	2.528	0.9273	0.7459
Raue et al. (2011)	New studies	1	29	1	26	0.897	−0.109	1.4398
Cao et al. (2012)	New studies	8	41	8	39	0.951	−0.05	0.5478

A5.6 Stata code for subgroup analysis of heartburn data

admetan   LnOR   SELnOR,   eform   model(random)   by(study_period) study(study_name) effect(Odds Ratio)

References

Borenstein M, Hedges LV, Higgins JP, Rothstein HR (2010) A basic introduction to fixed-effect and random-effects models for meta-analysis. Res Synth Methods 1(2):97–111

Borenstein MH, Larry H, Julian H, Hannah R (2009) Introduction to meta-analysis. Wiley-Blackwell, Oxford

Cochran WG (1973) Experiments for nonlinear functions (R.A. Fisher Memorial Lecture). J Am Stat Assoc 68(344):771–781. https://doi.org/10.1080/01621459.1973.10481423

DerSimonian R, Laird N (1986) Meta-analysis in clinical trials. Control Clin Trials 7(3):177–188

Doi AS (2018) Rendering the Doi plot properly in meta-analysis. Int J Evidence-Based Healthcare 16(4):242–243. https://doi.org/10.1097/XEB.0000000000000158

Doi SA, Barendregt JJ, Khan S, Thalib L, Williams GM (2015a) Advances in the meta-analysis of heterogeneous clinical trials I: the inverse variance heterogeneity model. Contemp Clin Trials 45(Pt A):130–138. https://doi.org/10.1016/j.cct.2015.05.009

Doi SA, Barendregt JJ, Khan S, Thalib L, Williams GM (2015b) Advances in the meta-analysis of heterogeneous clinical trials II: the quality effects model. Contemp Clin Trials 45(Pt A):123–129. https://doi.org/10.1016/j.cct.2015.05.010

Elvik R (2011) Publication bias and time-trend bias in meta-analysis of bicycle helmet efficacy: a re-analysis of Attewell, Glase and McFadden, 2001. Accid Anal Prev 43(3):1245–1251

Elvik R (2013) Corrigendum to: "Publication bias and time-trend bias in meta-analysis of bicycle helmet efficacy: a re-analysis of Attewell, Glase and McFadden, 2001". Accid Anal Prev 60:245–253

Furuya-Kanamori JL, Barendregt ARJ, Doi ARS (2018) A new improved graphical and quantitative method for detecting bias in meta-analysis. Int J Evidence-Based Healthcare 16(4):195–203. https://doi.org/10.1097/XEB.0000000000000141

Higgins JP, Thompson SG, Deeks JJ, Altman DG (2003) Measuring inconsistency in meta-analyses. BMJ 327(7414):557–560

Mathew SJ, Charney DS (2009) Publication bias and the efficacy of antidepressants. Am J Psychiatry 166(2):140–145

Paget MA, Chuang-Stein C, Fletcher C, Reid C (2011) Subgroup analyses of clinical effectiveness to support health technology assessments. Pharm Stat 10(6):532–538

Sterne JA, Gavaghan D, Egger M (2000) Publication and related bias in meta-analysis: power of statistical tests and prevalence in the literature. J Clin Epidemiol 53(11):1119–1129

Uesawa Y, Takeuchi T, Mohri K (2010) Publication bias on clinical studies of pharmacokinetic interactions between felodipine and grapefruit juice. Pharmazie 65(5):375–378

Yusuf S, Garg R, Zucker D (1991) Analyses by the intention-to-treat principle in randomized trials and databases. Pacing Clin Electrophysiol 14(12):2078–2082

Chapter 6
Meta-analysis on One Proportion

Proportion is an appropriate effect size measure when we are interested in the incidence or prevalence of certain disease in a population. Meta-analysis under different statistical models along with subgroup analysis is covered here with illustrative examples.

6.1 Introduction to Proportion

The majority of meta-analyses are devoted to establishing the effects of exposures or interventions, and therefore the aim is to get a pooled estimate of effect size based on the difference between two groups. However, meta-analytical methods can be useful to get a more precise estimate of disease frequency, such as disease incidence and prevalence proportions. Unlike the ratio measures, proportion as such is not a realistic measure of effect size to measure association between two categorical variables representing exposure and control groups. But proportion is an appropriate effect size measure when we are interested in the prevalence of a disease in a specific population. In this chapter, meta-analysis of single proportion is considered.

6.2 Estimation of Effect Size

Let the population proportion of prevalence (of any disease) in a single intervention group be π. This population proportion is a parameter and usually unknown. Based on a random sample of size n, π can be estimated by the sample proportion p. Here p is a point estimate of the unknown population proportion π, that is, $\hat{\pi} = p$. If x is the number of people with the prevalence in the sample, then the sample proportion of prevalence is $p = \frac{x}{n}$, where n is the total number of people in the sample. Here

© Springer Nature Singapore Pte Ltd. 2020
S. Khan, *Meta-Analysis*, Statistics for Biology and Health,
https://doi.org/10.1007/978-981-15-5032-4_6

p is the sample effect size (prevalence proportion) which estimates the unknown population effect size π.

The variance of the estimator of π is given by Var $(p) = \frac{p(1-p)}{n}$.

For the ith study, the estimate of the effect size (π_i) is denoted by p_i and the variance of the estimator of π_i is given by Var $(p_i) = \frac{p_i(1-p_i)}{n_i}$ for i $= 1, 2, ..., k$. For the inverse variance weighting method, the weight for the ith study becomes $w_i = \frac{1}{Var(p_i)}$.

Then the pooled sample prevalence (proportion) of all studies is obtained as

$$p = \frac{\sum\limits_{i=1}^{k} w_i p_i}{\sum\limits_{i=1}^{k} w_i} \text{ with standard error of the estimator,}$$

$$SE(p) = \sqrt{\frac{1}{\sum\limits_{i=1}^{k} w_i}}.$$

Remark: The sampling distribution of the estimator of population proportion π, the sample proportion, p follows an approximate normal distribution with mean $\mu(p) = \pi$ and variance $Var(p) = \frac{\pi(1-\pi)}{n}$ if the sample size, n is large (usually 30 or more). Since the distribution of the estimator of population effect size, p is known (normal), there is no need to transform the effect size to make inferences about π.

Example 6.1 For a single experiment involving one group of human subjects the sample size for the group is $n = 80$. The observed number of prevalence in the sample is 48. [Adapted from Hartung et al. (2008), p. 18].

Find the (i) point estimate of the effect size (population proportion) and (ii) standard error of its estimator.

Solution:

(i) The point estimate of the effect size $\theta (= \pi)$ is $\hat{\theta} = p = \frac{48}{80} = 0.60$.

(ii) The variance of the estimator of π is $Var(p) = \frac{p(1-p)}{n} = \frac{0.60 \times 0.40}{80} = 0.003$ and hence the standard error becomes $SE(p) = \sqrt{Var(p)} = \sqrt{0.003} = 0.054772$.

The confidence interval

The confidence interval for the unknown population effect size (π) based on the sample prevalence proportion (p) is given by the lower limit (LL) and upper limit (UL) as follows:

$$LL = p - z_{\alpha/2} \times SE(p) \text{ and}$$
$$UL = p + z_{\alpha/2} \times SE(p).$$

Here $z_{\alpha/2}$ is the $\frac{\alpha}{2}$th cut-off point of the standard normal distribution and $SE(p) = \sqrt{Var(p)}$.

Example 6.2 Consider the prevalence data in Example 6.1

Find the 95% confidence interval for the unknown effect size (population proportion), π.

Solution:

From Example 6.1, we have p = 0.6 and SE(p) = 0.0548. So, the 95% confidence interval for the effect size π is found by calculating the lower limit (LL) and upper limit (UL) as follows:

$$LL = p - z_{\alpha/2} \times SE(p) = 0.6 - 1.96 \times 0.0548 = 0.49 \text{ and}$$
$$UL = p + z_{\alpha/2} \times SE(p) = 0.6 + 1.96 \times 0.0548 = 0.71.$$

So the 95% confidence interval for π is (0.49, 0.71). Note the 95% confidence interval does not include 0 (null effect size), and hence the effect size π is statistically significant.

6.3 Tests on Effect Size

To test the null hypothesis that the population proportion, π (effect size) is zero, that is,

$H_0 : \pi = 0$ against the alternative hypothesis, $H_a : \pi \neq 0$ use the test statistic $Z = \frac{p-0}{SE(p)}$ which follows standard normal distribution under the null hypothesis.

Example 6.3 Consider the prevalence data in Example 6.1

Test the significance of the unknown effect size (population proportion), π at the 5% level of significance.

Solution:

Here to test,

$H_0 : \theta = \pi = 0$ against $H_a : \pi \neq 0$ calculate the value of the test statistic Z,

$$z_0 = \frac{p-0}{SE(p)} = \frac{0.6-0}{0.0548} = 10.949.$$

Then the P-value is $p = P(|Z| > 10.949) = 2 \times P(Z > 10.949) = 0$, so we reject the null hypothesis at the 5% significance level. Since the P-value is too small, there is very strong sample evidence to reject the null hypothesis (that the population proportion $\pi = 0$).

6.4   Fixed Effect (FE) Model

The fixed effect (FE) model assumes that all studies share a common effect size and attempt is made to estimate the unknown population effect size from the sample data. Refer to Borenstein et al. (2010), Chapter 11 of Borenstein et al. (2009), Doi et al. (2015a, b, c) for fixed effect and other statistical meta-analytic models.

For the common effect size of population proportion, let the parameter is $\theta = \pi$, be estimated by the sample proportion, $\hat{\theta} = p$.

Under the fixed effect (FE) model the estimate of the common effect size, base on k independent studies, is given by the pooled estimate

$$\hat{\theta}_{FE} = \frac{\sum\limits_{i=1}^{k} w_i \hat{\theta}_i}{\sum\limits_{i=1}^{k} w_i} = \frac{\sum\limits_{i=1}^{k} w_i p_i}{\sum\limits_{i=1}^{k} w_i} = p_{FE} \qquad (6.1)$$

which is the weighted mean of the estimated effect size of all the independent studies. The denominator $\left(\sum w_i\right)$ in Eq. (6.1) is to ensure that the sum of the weights is 1. The variance of the estimator of the common effect size is $Var(\hat{\theta}_{FE}) = \frac{1}{\sum\limits_{i=1}^{k} w_i} = Var(p_{FE})$.

Therefore, the standard error of the estimator of the common effect size is $SE(\hat{\theta}_{FE}) = \sqrt{\frac{1}{\sum\limits_{i=1}^{k} w_i}} = SE(p_{FE})$.

The confidence interval
The $(1 - \alpha) \times 100\%$ confidence interval for the common effect size $\theta(=\pi)$, under the FE model, based on the sample estimates from independent studies is given by the lower limit (LL) and upper limit (UL) as follows:

$$LL = \hat{\theta}_{FE} - z_{\alpha/2} \times SE(\hat{\theta}_{FE}) = p_{FE} - z_{\alpha/2} \times SE(p_{FE}) \text{ and}$$
$$UL = \hat{\theta}_{FE} + z_{\alpha/2} \times SE(\hat{\theta}_{FE}) = p_{FE} + z_{\alpha/2} \times SE(p_{FE}).$$

Here $z_{\alpha/2}$ is the $\frac{\alpha}{2}$th cut-off point of standard normal distribution. For a 95% confidence interval $z_{\alpha/2} = z_{0.05/2} = 1.96$.

Test of hypothesis

To test the significance of the common effect size of all studies, under the FE model, test the null hypothesis $H_0 : \theta = 0$ (that is, $\pi = 0$) against $H_a : \theta \neq 0$ using the test statistic

$$Z = \frac{\hat{\theta}_{FE}}{SE(\hat{\theta}_{FE})} = \frac{p_{FE}}{SE(p_{FE})},$$

where Z follows the standard normal distribution.

Reject H_0 at the α level of significance if the calculated/observed value of the Z statistic (say, z_0) satisfies $|z_0| \geq z_{\alpha/2}$, where $z_{\alpha/2}$ is the $\alpha/2$ level upper cut-off point of the standard normal distribution; otherwise don't reject the null hypothesis. Alternatively, reject H_0 at the α level of significance if the P-value is less than or equal to α; otherwise don't reject the null hypothesis.

Illustration of FE Model for Proportion

Example 6.4 Data on the prevalence of acute schizophrenia in the population with schizophrenia from six independent studies is taken from the Examples of MetaXL Package. Conduct meta-analysis on the appropriate effect size (proportion of acute schizophrenia) for the data in Table 6.1 using fixed effect (FE) model.

Solution:

For the calculation of estimated value of the common effect size and standard error of the estimator, and Q and I^2 statistics we need to find the summary statistics such as p (sample proportion), Var (variance of p), SE (standard error of p), W (study weight), Wp (product of weight and p) and Wp^2 (product of weight and squared p) as in Table 6.2.

The point estimate of the common effect size (proportion) of acute schizophrenia under the FE model is found to be

$$\hat{\theta}_{FE} = \frac{\sum_{i=1}^{k} w_i p_i}{\sum_{i=1}^{k} w_i} = \frac{13244}{22509} = 0.5884 \approx 0.59.$$

Table 6.1 Prevalence data on schizophrenia

Study name	N	Cases
Bondestam et al. (1990)	10	6
Shen et al. (1981)	300	154
Zharikov (1968)	1429	715
Babigian (1980)	3319	2058
Fichter et al. (1996)	7	5
Keith et al. (1991)	305	210

Table 6.2 Calculations of summary statistics for meta-analysis

Study name	N	Cases	p	Var	SE	W	Wp	Wp^2
Bondestam et al. (1990)	10	6	0.6	0.024	0.1549	41.6667	25	15
Shen et al. (1981)	300	154	0.512	0.0008	0.0289	1200.69	614.75	314.75
Zharikov (1968)	1429	715	0.5	0.0002	0.0132	5716	2858	1429
Babigian (1980)	3319	2058	0.62	7E-05	0.0084	14087.4	8734.2	5415.2
Fichter et al. (1996)	7	5	0.75	0.0268	0.1637	37.3333	28	21
Keith et al. (1991)	305	210	0.69	0.0007	0.0265	1425.9	983.87	678.87
						22509	**13244**	**7873.8**

The standard error of the estimator becomes

$$SE(\hat{\theta}_{FE}) = \sqrt{\frac{1}{\sum\limits_{i=1}^{k} w_i}} = \sqrt{\frac{1}{22509}} = 0.006665.$$

So, the 95% confidence interval for the common effect size (proportion) of acute schizophrenia, under the FE model, is provided by the lower limit (LL) and upper limit (UL) as follows:

$$LL = \hat{\theta}_{FE} - z_{\alpha/2} \times SE(\hat{\theta}_{FE}) = 0.5884 - 1.96 \times 0.006665 = 0.57$$
$$UL = \hat{\theta}_{FE} + z_{\alpha/2} \times SE(\hat{\theta}_{FE}) = 0.5884 + 1.96 \times 0.006665 = 0.60.$$

Test of hypothesis
To test the significance of the common effect size of all studies, test the null hypothesis $H_0 : \theta = 0$ (that is, $\pi = 0$) against $H_a : \theta \neq 0$ using the test statistic

$$z = \frac{\hat{\theta}_{FE}}{SE(\hat{\theta}_{FE})} = \frac{0.5884}{0.006665} = 88.27.$$

So, the P-value is $P(|Z| > 88.27) = 0$. Hence the test is significant at the 5% level of significance. Thus the proportion of prevalence of acute schizophrenia is significantly different from 0.

Remark: The 95% confidence interval (0.57, 0.60) does not include 0, and hence the effect size is significant. So, the test of hypothesis and confidence interval lead to the same inference.

Measuring Heterogeneity of between study effects
The heterogeneity of effect size between the studies is measured by Cochran's Q statistic and Higgin's I^2 index.

To test the heterogeneity between study effect sizes, we test the null hypothesis, $H_0 = \theta_1 = \theta_2 = \ldots = \theta_k$ against the alternative hypothesis H_a : not all θ_i's are equal for $i = 1, 2, \ldots, k$ using the Q statistic,

$$Q = \sum_{i=1}^{k} w_i \hat{\theta}_i^2 - \frac{\left(\sum_{i=1}^{k} w_i \hat{\theta}_i\right)^2}{\sum_{i=1}^{k} w_i}.$$

For the data set in Example 6.4, using the summary statistics of Table 6.2, we get

$$Q = \sum_{i=1}^{k} w_i \hat{\theta}_i^2 - \frac{\left(\sum_{i=1}^{k} w_i \hat{\theta}_i\right)^2}{\sum_{i=1}^{k} w_i} = 7873.8 - \frac{(13244)^2}{22509} = 81.4430 \approx 81.44.$$

The Q statistic follows a chi-squared distribution with $(k-1) = 6-1 = 5$ degrees of freedom. Then the P-value of testing equality of population effect sizes becomes

$$p = P\left(\chi_5^2 > 81.44\right) = 0.$$

Using chi-squired distribution table, it is found that the P-value is smaller than 0.001 (exact 0.001 if $Q = 20.515$).

Since the P-value is very small, there is highly significant heterogeneity between the study proportions.

The value of the I^2 statistic is found to be

$$I^2 = \frac{Q - df}{Q} \times 100\% = \left(\frac{81.44 - 5}{81.44}\right) \times 100\% = \left(\frac{76.44}{81.44}\right) \times 100\%$$
$$= 93.86 \times 100\% = 94\%.$$

Hence there is very high heterogeneity between the study proportions.

FE model meta-analysis of proportion using MetaXL
The forest plot under the FE model (indicated by "IV" in the code) is constructed using MetaXL code
=MAInputTable("Schizophrenia Proportion FE","Prev","IV",B9:D14),

where "B9:D14" refers to the data area in Excel Worksheet.

Remark: Explanations of MetaXL Code
For this type of meta-analyses in MetaXL the 'opening' code starts with MA Input Table '= MAInputTable'. This is followed by an open parenthesis inside which the first quote contains the text that appears as the 'title of the output of the forest plot' e.g.

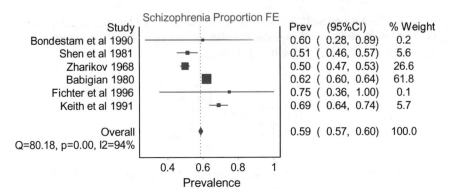

Fig. 6.1 Forest plot of proportion of schizophrenia under fixed effect model

"Schizophrenia Proportion FE" in the above code (user may choose any appropriate title here). Then in the second quote enter the type of effect measure, e.g. "Prev" in the above code tells that the *outcome variable is prevalence and the effect size measure is proportion*. Within the third quote enter the statistical model, e.g. "IV" in the above code stands for the *fixed effect* (inverse variance is abbreviated by (IV) model. Each quotation is followed by a comma, and after the last comma enter the data area in Excel Worksheet, e.g. B9:D14 in the above code tells that the data on the independent studies are taken from the specified cells. The code ends with a closing parenthesis.

The forest plot of the meta-analysis of acute schizophrenic proportion using the above MetaXL code is found to be (Fig. 6.1).

Interpretation
The estimated pooled common effect size (proportion) is 0.59 with the 95% confidence interval (0.57, 0.60). Thus the prevalence of acute schizophrenia in the population is highly significant (as 0 is not included in the confidence interval).

6.5   Random Effects (REs) Model

Under the random effects (REs) model the variance of sample effect size $\hat{\theta}_i$ of the ith study about the population effect size θ is the sum of the within-study and between-study variances, that is, $v_i^* = v_i + \hat{\tau}^2$. Therefore, the modified weight assigned to the ith study becomes

$$w_i^* = \frac{1}{v_i + \hat{\tau}^2}.$$

Then the common effect size estimator of the population proportion (θ) under the random effects (REs) model is given by

$$\hat{\theta}_{RE} = \frac{\sum\limits_{i=1}^{k} w_i^* \hat{\theta}_i}{\sum\limits_{i=1}^{k} w_i^*},$$

with the standard error of the estimator

$$SE(\hat{\theta}_{RE}) = \sqrt{\frac{1}{\sum\limits_{i=1}^{k} w_i^*}}.$$

Estimation of τ^2

The between studies variance is estimated as a scaled excess variation as follows

$$\hat{\tau}^2 = \frac{Q - df}{C},$$

where

$$Q = \sum_{i=1}^{k} w_i \hat{\theta}_i^2 - \frac{\left(\sum\limits_{i=1}^{k} w_i \hat{\theta}_i\right)^2}{\sum\limits_{i=1}^{k} w_i},$$

$$C = \sum_{i=1}^{k} w_i - \frac{\sum\limits_{i=1}^{k} w_i^2}{\sum\limits_{i=1}^{k} w_i}$$

and $df = (k - 1)$ in which k is the number of studies.
Illustration of Random Effects Model for Proportion

Example 6.5 Consider the prevalence of acute schizophrenia data of Example 6.4.

Using the summary statistics in Table 6.2, we get

$$Q = \sum_{i=1}^{k} w_i \hat{\theta}_i^2 - \frac{\left(\sum\limits_{i=1}^{k} w_i \hat{\theta}_i\right)^2}{\sum\limits_{i=1}^{k} w_i} = 7873.8 - \frac{(13244)^2}{22509} = 81.4430 \approx 81.44.$$

Then

Table 6.3 Calculations of summary statistics for meta-analysis under random effects model

Study name	N	Cases	p	Var	τ^2	W*	W* × p
Bondestam et al. (1990)	10	6	0.6	0.024	0.006325	**32.97609**	**19.78566**
Shen et al. (1981)	300	154	0.512	0.0008	0.006325	139.7067	71.52983
Zharikov (1968)	1429	715	0.5	0.0002	0.006325	153.8474	76.9237
Babigian (1980)	3319	2058	0.62	7E-05	0.006325	156.3481	96.93581
Fichter et al. (1996)	7	5	0.75	0.0268	0.006325	30.2017	22.65128
Keith et al. (1991)	305	210	0.69	0.0007	0.006325	142.3222	98.20231
						655.4021	**386.0286**

$$C = \sum_{i=1}^{k} w_i - \frac{\sum_{i=1}^{k} w_i^2}{\sum_{i=1}^{k} w_i} = 22509.028 - \frac{234606499.3}{22509.028} = 12086.25$$

and hence

$$\hat{\tau}^2 = \frac{Q - df}{C} = \frac{81.44304 - 5}{12086.25} = 0.006325.$$

For the calculation of estimated value of the common effect size and standard error of the estimator under the random effects model, we need to find the summary statistics such as τ^2 (between studies variance), W* (the modified weight which is the reciprocal of the sum of within and between studies variances), and W* × p (product of modified weight and p) as in Table 6.3.

From the summary statistics in the above table, the estimated common effect size of population proportion under the random effects model becomes

$$\hat{\theta}_{RE} = \frac{\sum_{i=1}^{6} w_i^* p_i}{\sum_{i=1}^{6} w_i^*} = \frac{\sum_{i=1}^{6} W_i^* \times p_i}{\sum_{i=1}^{6} W_i^*} = \frac{655.4021}{386.0286} = 0.58899 \approx 0.59,$$

with the standard error of the estimator

$$SE(\hat{\theta}_{RE}) = \sqrt{\frac{1}{\sum_{i=1}^{6} w_i^*}} = \sqrt{\frac{1}{\sum_{i=1}^{6} W_i^*}} = \sqrt{\frac{1}{655.4021}} = 0.039061244.$$

The 95% confidence interval for the combined effect size (π) is given by the lower and upper limits:

$$LL = \hat{\theta}_{RE} - 1.96 \times SE(\hat{\theta}_{RE}) = 0.5889 - 1.96 \times 0.0390 = 0.5124 \approx 0.51 \text{ and}$$
$$UL = \hat{\theta}_{RE} + 1.96 \times SE(\hat{\theta}_{RE}) = 0.5889 + 1.96 \times 0.0390 = 0.6653 \approx 0.66.$$

To test the significance of the combined population effect size, θ under the REs model, test $H_0 : \theta = 0$ against $H_a : \theta \neq 0$, based on the observed value of the test statistic Z, $z_0 = \frac{\hat{\theta}_{RE}}{SE(\hat{\theta}_{RE})} = \frac{0.58899}{0.039061} = 15.079 \approx 15.08$ with P-value = P(|Z| > 15.08) = 0.

Hence the test is significant. Therefore, reject the null hypothesis at the 5% level of significance, and conclude that the population prevalence (proportion) is significantly different from 0.

Forest plot of proportion under REs model using MetaXL
The forest plot under the REs model (indicated by "RE" in the code) is constructed using MetaXL code
=MAInputTable("Schizophrenia Proportion RE","Prev","RE",B9:D14),

where "B9:D14" refers to the data area in Excel Worksheet.

Remark: Explanations of MetaXL Code
For this type of meta-analyses in MetaXL the 'opening' code starts with MA Input Table '= MAInputTable'. This is followed by an open parenthesis inside which the first quote contains the text that appears as the 'title of the output of the forest plot' e.g. "Schizophrenia Proportion RE" in the above code (user may choose any appropriate title here). Then in the second quote enter the type of effect measure, e.g. "Prev" in the above code tells that the *outcome variable is prevalence and the effect size measure is proportion*. Within the third quote enter the statistical model, e.g. "RE" in the above code stands for the *random effects* (abbreviated by RE) model. Each quotation is followed by a comma, and after the last comma enter the data area in Excel Worksheet, e.g. B9:D14 in the above code tells that the data on the independent studies are taken from the specified cells. The code ends with a closing parenthesis.

The forest plot of the meta-analysis of prevalence of acute schizophrenia (proportion), under the REs model, using the above MetaXL code is found to be (Fig. 6.2).

Interpretation
The estimated value of the combined effect size, proportion, under the REs model is 0.59 with 95% confidence interval (0.51, 0.66). The 95% confidence interval does not contain 0 (proportion of patients with acute schizophrenia). Hence the prevalence (proportion) of acute schizophrenia is statistically significant.

6.6 Inverse Variance Heterogeneity (IVhet) Model

Under the inverse variance heterogeneity (IVhet) model, the pooled estimate of the common effect size, proportion π ($=\theta$) is given by

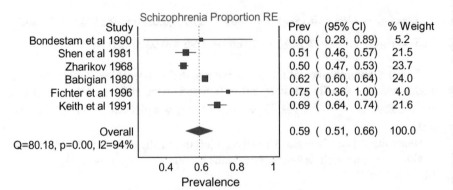

Fig. 6.2 Forest plot of prevalence of schizophrenia (proportion) under random effects model

$$\hat{\theta}_{IVhet} = \frac{\sum\limits_{i=1}^{k} w_i \hat{\theta}_i}{\sum\limits_{i=1}^{k} w_i}.$$

Then the variance of the estimator under the IVhet model is given by

$$Var(\hat{\theta}_{IVhet}) = \sum_{i=1}^{k} \left[\left(\frac{1}{v_i} \Big/ \sum_{i=1}^{k} \frac{1}{v_i} \right)^2 (v_i + \hat{\tau}^2) \right].$$

For the computation of the confidence interval of the common effect size, proportion, based on the IVhet model use the following standard error

$$SE(\hat{\theta}_{IVhet}) = \sqrt{Var(\hat{\theta}_{IVhet})}.$$

Then, the $(1 - \alpha) \times 100\%$ confidence interval for the common effect size θ under the IVhet model is given by the lower limit (LL) and upper limit (UL) as follows:

$$LL = \hat{\theta}_{IVhet} - z_{\alpha/2} \times SE(\hat{\theta}_{IVhet})$$
$$UL = \hat{\theta}_{IVhet} + z_{\alpha/2} \times SE(\hat{\theta}_{IVhet}),$$

where $z_{\alpha/2}$ is the $\frac{\alpha}{2}$th cut-off point of standard normal distribution.

To test the significance of the population proportion, test $H_0 : \theta = 0$, (that is, $\pi = 0$) against $H_a : \theta \neq 0$ using the test statistic $Z = \frac{\hat{\theta}_{IVhet}}{SE(\hat{\theta}_{IVhet})}$ which follows a standard normal distribution under the null hypothesis.

Table 6.4 Calculated summary statistics for meta-analysis of schizophrenia data under IVhet model

Study name	N	Cases	p	Var	W	Wp	Var*	V*
Bondestam et al. (1990)	10	6	0.6	0.024	41.6667	25	0.0303	1.04E-07
Shen et al. (1981)	300	154	0.51	0.0008	1200.69	614.7541	0.0072	2.04E-05
Zharikov (1968)	1429	715	0.5	0.0002	5716	2858	0.0065	0.000419
Babigian (1980)	3319	2058	0.62	7E-05	14087.4	8734.211	0.0064	0.002505
Fichter et al. (1996)	7	5	0.75	0.0268	37.3333	28	0.0331	9.11E-08
Keith et al. (1991)	305	210	0.69	0.0007	1425.9	983.871	0.007	2.82E-05
					22509	**13243.84**	**0.0905**	**0.002973**

Illustration of IVhet Model for Proportion

Example 6.6 Consider the prevalence of acute schizophrenia data in Example 6.4.

Conduct meta-analysis on the appropriate effect size (proportion of acute schizophrenia) under the inverse variance heterogeneity (IVhet) model.

Solution:

For the prevalence of acute schizophrenia data in Table 6.1 the effect size measure of interest, sample proportion (p), variance of estimator (Var), estimated value of modified variance (Var*) by taking into account the between studies variance (τ^2) and modified weight (W*) are provided in Table 6.4.

Illustration of computation in Table 6.4
For the first study (Bondestam et al. 1990):

$W = 1/\text{Var} = 1/0.024 = 41.6667$, the weight,

$\text{Var*} = \text{Var} + \tau^2 = 0.024 + 0.006325 = 0.0303$, the combined variance, and

$V* = \left[\frac{w}{\sum w}\right]^2 \times \text{Var*} = \left[\frac{41.6667}{22509}\right]^2 \times 0.0303 = 0.0000000104$, the modified variance under the IVhet model.

To find the estimated value of the population proportion (θ) under the IVhet model the sums of columns of W and W × p, that is, $\sum W = 22509$ and $\sum W \times p = 13243.84$, of Table 6.4 are required.

The IVhet model estimate of the common effect size, proportion, is given by

$$\hat{\theta}_{IVhet} = \frac{\sum\limits_{i=1}^{k} w_i p_i}{\sum\limits_{i=1}^{k} w_i} = \frac{13243.84}{22509} = 0.5889 \approx 0.59$$

and the variance of the estimator under the IVhet model is given by the sum of the last (W*) column of Table 6.4, that is,

$$Var(\hat{\theta}_{IVhet}) = \sum_{i=1}^{k} \left[\left(\frac{1}{v_i} \bigg/ \sum_{i=1}^{k} \frac{1}{v_i} \right)^2 (v_i + \hat{\tau}^2) \right] = 0.002973.$$

Hence the standard error becomes

$$SE(\hat{\theta}_{IVhet}) = \sqrt{Var(\hat{\theta}_{IVhet})} = \sqrt{0.002973} = 0.054527.$$

Then, the 95% confidence interval for the common effect size proportion under the IVhet model is given by the lower and upper limits:

$$LL = \hat{\theta}_{IVhet} - 1.96 \times SE(\hat{\theta}_{IVhet}) = 0.5884 - 1.96 \times 0.054527 = 0.4815 \approx 0.48 \text{ and}$$

$$UL = \hat{\theta}_{IVhet} + 1.96 \times SE(\hat{\theta}_{IVhet}) = 0.5884 + 1.96 \times 0.054527 = 0.6953 \approx 0.69.$$

Comment: The above point estimate of pooled proportion (0.59) and confidence interval (0.48, 0.69) are reported in the forest plot of Fig. 6.3 in the last row with diamond representing the limits of the 95% confidence interval.

To test the significance of the population proportion, test $H_0 : \theta = 0$, (that is, $\pi = 0$) against $H_a : \theta \neq 0$ the observed value of the test statistic Z is

$$z_0 = \frac{\hat{\theta}_{IVhet}}{SE(\hat{\theta}_{IVhet})} = \frac{0.5884}{0.054527} = 10.79.$$

The two-sided P-value is $P(|Z| > 10.79) = 0$.

Since the P-value is 0, the effect size (proportion of acute schizophrenia) is highly significant (different from 0).

IVhet Meta-analysis of Proportion with MetaXL
The forest plot under the IVhet model (indicated by "IVhet" in the code) is constructed using MetaXL code
=MAInputTable("Schizophrenia Proportion IVhet","Prev","IVhet",B9:D14),

where "B9:D14" refers to the data area in Excel Worksheet.

Remark: Explanations of MetaXL Code
For this type of meta-analyses in MetaXL the 'opening' code starts with MA Input Table '= MAInputTable'. This is followed by an open parenthesis inside which the first quote contains the text that appears as the 'title of the output of the forest plot' e.g. "Schizophrenia Proportion IVhet" in the above code (user may choose any appropriate title here). Then in the second quote enter the type of effect measure, e.g. "Prev" in the above code tells that the *outcome variable is prevalence and the effect size measure is proportion*. Within the third quote enter the statistical model, e.g. "IVhet" in the above code stands for the *inverse variance heterogeneity* (abbreviated by IVhet) model. Each quotation is followed by a comma, and after the last comma enter the data area in Excel Worksheet, e.g. B9:D14 in the above code tells that the

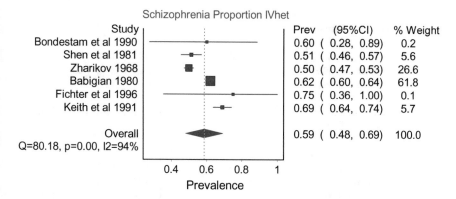

Fig. 6.3 Forest plot of prevalence of schizophrenia (proportion) under IVhet model

data on the independent studies are taken from the specified cells. The code ends with a closing parenthesis.

The forest plot of the meta-analysis of proportion under the IVhet model using the above MetaXL code is found to be (Fig. 6.3).

6.7 Subgroup Analysis

To check if the prevalence of acute schizophrenia differs due to the level of income of the country of study, subgroup analysis of prevalence of acute schizophrenia is required separately for high income and low/medium income countries. In the example, there are three studies (Babigian 1980; Fichter et al. 1996; Keith et al. 1991) from the high income group and another three (Bondestam et al. 1990; Shen et al. 1981; Zharikov 1968) in the low/medium income group. The subgroup analysis conducted by using MetaXL is presented by the forest plot in Fig. 6.4.

Interpretation
For the high income group the estimate of the common effect size (proportion) is 0.63 with 95% confidence interval (0.61, 0.64). This is much higher compared to the estimate of the common effect size in the low/medium income group 0.50 with 95% confidence interval (0.48, 0.53). So, there is much higher prevalence of acute schizophrenia among the people of high income group countries.

The pooled common effect size estimate for all studies is 0.59 with 95% confidence interval (0.57, 0.60). This interval provides compromise figures between the two income groups.

The effect size (proportion) is significant for every subgroup and combined/pooled levels.

For the High income group $Q = 6.29$ with $P = 0.04$ and $I^2 = 68\%$ showing high level of heterogeneity among all the studies.

But for the Low income group there is no heterogeneity among the studies as $Q = 0.48$ with $P = 0.79$ and $I^2 = 0\%$. However, for all the studies, Low and High

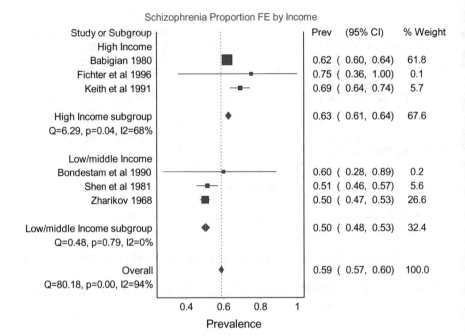

Fig. 6.4 Subgroup analysis of prevalence of acute schizophrenia (proportion) by income group

income combined, $Q = 80.18$ with $P = 0.00$ and $I^2 = 94\%$ indicating very high level of heterogeneity among all the studies.

6.7.1 Discussions and Comparison of Results

The point estimates and 95% confidence intervals of the pooled effect size in Fig. 6.5a–c provide the basis to compare the meta-analysis of acute schizophrenia proportion under the FE, REs and IVhet models.

Interpretations
The point estimate of the population (prevalence) proportion (0.59) is the same under the FE, REs and IVhet model in spite of very high level of heterogeneity among the studies and quite different redistribution of weights under the REs model. Even though the heterogeneity is highly significant in the meta-analysis, the redistributed weights in both FE and IVhet models are the same. However, the 95% confidence interval under FE model (0.57, 0.60) is shorter than that under the RE (0.51, 0.66) and IVhet model (0.48, 0.69).

The 95% confidence interval under the REs model (0.51, 0.66) with width 0.15 is wider than that of the FE model (0.57, 0.60) with width 0.03, but shorter than that of the IVhet model (0.48, 0.69) with width 0.21.

a)

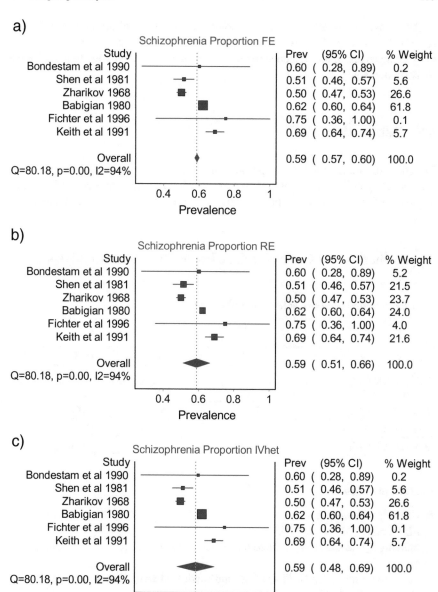

Fig. 6.5 a) Forest plot of Schizophrenia proportion under FE model. **b)** Forest plot of acute Schizophrenia proportion under REs model. **c)** Forest plot of acute Schizophrenia proportion under IVhet model

As always, the point estimates and confidence intervals of all individual studies remain the same in the forest plot regardless of the statistical model of analysis. Only changes are in the pooled estimate and confidence interval due to the different redistributed study weights.

6.8 Publication Bias

The study of publication bias for proportion is very similar to that in Sect. 5.9 of the previous chapter. It is not necessary to re-produce them again here. Readers interested to produce funnel plot or Doi plot and their interpretation are referred that Section.

Appendix 6—Stat Codes for One Proportion Meta-analysis

A6.1 Prevalence of acute schizophrenia data

Study name	N	Cases	p
Bondestam et al. (1990)	10	6	0.6
Shen et al. (1981)	300	154	0.512
Zharikov (1968)	1429	715	0.5
Babigian (1980)	3319	2058	0.62
Fichter et al. (1996)	7	5	0.75
Keith et al. (1991)	305	210	0.69

A6.2 Stata codes

*ssc install metaprop_one
  Fixed effect Meta-analysis
  metaprop_one Cases N, ftt fixed lcols(Studyname)
  or
  metaprop_one Cases N, ftt fixed second(random) lcols(Studyname)
  Random effects Meta-analysis
  metaprop_one Cases N, ftt random lcols(Studyname)
  or
  metaprop_one Cases N, ftt random second(fixed) lcols(Studyname)

References

Borenstein M, Hedges LV, Higgins JP, Rothstein HR (2010) A basic introduction to fixed-effect and random-effects models for meta-analysis. Res Synth Methods 1(2):97–111

Borenstein M, Larry H, Higgins J, Rothstein H (2009) Introduction to meta-analysis. Wiley-Blackwell, Oxford

Doi SA, Barendregt JJ, Khan S, Thalib L, Williams GM (2015a) Advances in the meta-analysis of heterogeneous clinical trials I: the inverse variance heterogeneity model. Contemp Clin Trials 45(Pt A):130–138. https://doi.org/10.1016/j.cct.2015.05.009

Doi SA, Barendregt JJ, Khan S, Thalib L, Williams GM (2015b) Advances in the meta-analysis of heterogeneous clinical trials II: the quality effects model. Contemp Clin Trials 45(Pt A):123–129. https://doi.org/10.1016/j.cct.2015.05.010

Doi SA, Barendregt JJ, Khan S, Thalib L, Williams GM (2015c) Simulation comparison of the quality effects and random effects methods of meta-analysis. Epidemiology 26(4):e42–44

Hartung J, Prof. Dr. Knapp G, Sinha BK (2008) Statistical meta-analysis with applications. Wiley-Blackwell

Chapter 7
Meta-Analysis of Difference of Two Proportions

If the difference of prevalence rates of any specific disease for two different populations/groups is of interest then difference of two proportions is the appropriate effect size measure. The difference between two proportions is often called the risk difference (RD). The meta-analysis of difference between two proportions is covered in this chapter.

7.1 Introduction to Risk Difference

Consider population proportion of treatment population/group to be π_1 and that of the control population/group be π_2. Let the corresponding sample proportions be p_1 and p_2 based on two independent random samples of sizes n_1 and n_2 respectively. Here the statistics p_1 and p_2 are estimators of the unknown population proportions π_1 and π_2 respectively.

Following three different effect size measures (parameters) can be define based on the two population proportions:

(a) Risk difference (RD): $\theta_1 = \pi_1 - \pi_2$.
(b) Odds ratio (OR): $\theta_2 = \frac{\pi_1/(1-\pi_1)}{\pi_2/(1-\pi_2)}$.
(c) Relative risk or risk ratio (RR): $\theta_3 = \frac{\pi_1}{\pi_2}$.

Based on the two sample proportions, the above effect size measures (parameters) are estimated by the following statistics:

$\hat{\theta} = \hat{\theta}_1 = p_1 - p_2$, estimated or sample risk difference (RD),

$\hat{\theta}_2 = \frac{p_1/(1-p_1)}{p_2/(1-p_2)}$, sample odds ratio (OR) or $\hat{\theta}_2^* = \ln\left(\frac{p_1/(1-p_1)}{p_2/(1-p_2)}\right)$, sample ln OR,

and

$\hat{\theta}_3 = \frac{p_1}{p_2}$, sample risk ratio (RR) or $\hat{\theta}_3^* = \ln\left(\frac{p_1}{p_2}\right)$, sample ln RR respectively.

© Springer Nature Singapore Pte Ltd. 2020
S. Khan, *Meta-Analysis*, Statistics for Biology and Health,
https://doi.org/10.1007/978-981-15-5032-4_7

The last two effect size measures (b & c) have been already discussed in Chaps. 4 and 5. In this chapter we concentrate on the meta-analysis of the first effect size, $\theta = \theta_1$, the risk difference (RD).

7.2 Estimation of Effect Size

Based on the two sample proportions, the estimator of the population risk difference, $\theta = \pi_1 - \pi_2$ becomes $\hat{\theta} = p_1 - p_2$.

The variance of the above estimator of the population risk difference is

$$Var(\hat{\theta}) = \frac{p_1(1-p_1)}{n_1} + \frac{p_2(1-p_2)}{n_2}.$$

The standard error of the effect size estimator of the population risk difference is the square root of its variance,

$$SE(\hat{\theta}) = \sqrt{Var(\hat{\theta})} = \sqrt{\frac{p_1(1-p_1)}{n_1} + \frac{p_2(1-p_2)}{n_2}}.$$

Then the $(1 - \alpha) \times 100\%$ confidence interval for the population risk difference $\theta = \pi_1 - \pi_2$ is given by the following lower and upper limits:

$$LL = \hat{\theta} - z_{\alpha/2} \times SE(\hat{\theta})$$
$$UL = \hat{\theta} + z_{\alpha/2} \times SE(\hat{\theta}),$$

where $z_{\alpha/2}$ is $\frac{\alpha}{2}$th cut-off value of the standard normal distribution.

Example 7.1 For a comparative experiment involving two groups of human subjects the sample size for the treatment group is $n_1 = 80$ and that of the control/placebo group is $n_2 = 70$. The observed proportions for the two groups are $p_1 = 0.60$ and $p_2 = 0.80$ respectively. [Adopted from Hartung, Knapp and Sinha, 2008, p. 18].

Find the (i) point estimate of the population effect size (risk difference, θ) and (ii) standard error of its estimator.

Solution:

(i) From the given data, the estimated sample proportions are $p_1 = 0.60$ and $p_2 = 0.80$ with $n_1 = 80$ and $n_2 = 70$. Then the point estimate of the population effect size, θ (risk difference) is

$$\hat{\theta} = p_1 - p_2 = 0.60 - 0.80 = -0.20.$$

The standard error of the effect size estimator is the square root of the variance of the estimator,

$$Var(\hat{\theta}) = \frac{p_1(1 - p_1)}{n_1} + \frac{p_2(1 - p_2)}{n_2} = \frac{0.6 \times 0.4}{80} + \frac{0.8 \times 0.2}{70} = 0.5285, \text{ that is,}$$

$$SE(\hat{\theta})] = \sqrt{Var(\hat{\theta})} = \sqrt{0.5285} = 0.0727.$$

7.2.1 Confidence Interval

Example 7.2 Consider the data in Example 7.1.
Find the 95% confidence interval for the population risk difference, θ.

Solution:
The 95% confidence interval for the population risk difference θ is found by calculating the lower limit (LL) and upper limit (UL) as follows:

$$LL = \hat{\theta} - z_{\alpha/2} \times SE(\hat{\theta})] = -0.20 - 1.96 \times 0.0727 = -0.34 \text{ and}$$
$$UL = \hat{\theta} + z_{\alpha/2} \times SE(\hat{\theta}) = -0.20 + 1.96 \times 0.0727 = -0.06.$$

So the 95% confidence interval for the population risk difference θ is $(-0.34, -0.06)$. Note that the 95% confidence interval does not include 0 (null effect/RD).

7.3 Significance Test on Effect Size, RD

To test the null hypothesis that the population risk difference is 0, we test $H_0 : \theta = 0$ against $H_a : \theta \neq 0$ using the test statistic $Z = \frac{\hat{\theta}}{SE(\hat{\theta})}$, where Z follows the standard normal distribution.

Example 7.3 Consider the data in Example 7.1. Using the data, test the hypothesis that the risk difference is 0.

To test the null hypothesis
$H_0 : \theta = 0$ (risk difference 0) against $H_a : \theta \neq 0$ calculate the observed value of the test statistic Z as

$$z_0 = \frac{\hat{\theta} - 0}{SE(\hat{\theta})} = \frac{-0.2 - 0}{0.0727} = -2.75.$$

The P-value is $P(|Z| > 2.75) = 2 \times P(Z > 2.75) = 0.006$, so we reject the null hypothesis at the 5% level of significance. Since the P-value is too small, there is strong sample evidence to reject the null hypothesis. Thus the risk difference is significantly different from 0.
Conclusion: There is significantly higher risk in the control group compared to the treatment group.

7.4   Fixed Effect (FE) Model

Fixed effect model is used for meta-analysis when the between studies variation is insignificant, that is, the effect size of interest is homogeneous across all studies. For details on the fixed effect and other types of statistical models used for meta-analyses readers may refer to M. Borenstein et al. (2010), Chapter 11 of M. H. Borenstein et al. (2009), Doi et al. (2015a, b, c) for fixed effect and other statistical meta-analytic models.

The estimate of the unknown common effect size, risk difference, θ under the fixed effect model is given by

$$\hat{\theta}_{FE} = \frac{\sum_{i=1}^{k} w_i \hat{\theta}_i}{\sum_{i=1}^{k} w_i},$$

where w_i is the weight and $\hat{\theta}_i$ is the point estimate of the population effect size (RD) of the ith study for i = 1,2, …, k. The standard error of the estimator of the common effect size is $SE(\hat{\theta}_{FE}) = \sqrt{\frac{1}{\sum_{i=1}^{k} w_i}}$.

7.4.1   The Confidence Interval

The $(1 - \alpha) \times 100\%$ confidence interval for the common effect size θ (RD) under the FE model is given by the following lower limit (LL) and upper limit (UL):

$$LL = \hat{\theta}_{FE} - z_{\alpha/2} \times SE(\hat{\theta}_{FE})$$
$$UL = \hat{\theta}_{FE} + z_{\alpha/2} \times SE(\hat{\theta}_{FE}),$$

where $z_{\alpha/2}$ is the $\frac{\alpha}{2}$ th cut-off point of standard normal distribution. For a 95% confidence interval, the z-score becomes $z_{\alpha/2} = z_{0.05/2} = 1.96$.

7.4.2   Test of Significance

To test the significance of the common effect size θ of all studies, under the FE model, test the null hypothesis $H_0 : \theta = 0$ against $H_a : \theta \neq 0$ using the test statistic

$$Z = \frac{\hat{\theta}_{FE}}{SE(\hat{\theta}_{FE})},$$

where Z follows the standard normal distribution.

For a two-tailed test, reject H_0 at the α level of significance if the calculated/observed value of the Z statistic satisfies $|z_0| \geq z_{\alpha/2}$, where $z_{\alpha/2}$ is the $\frac{\alpha}{2}$ level upper cut-off point of the standard normal distribution; otherwise don't reject the null hypothesis. Alternatively, reject H_0 at the α level of significance if the P-value is less than or equal to α; otherwise don't reject the null hypothesis.

7.4.3 Illustration of FE Model for Risk Difference (RD)

Example 7.4 The data in Table 7.1 represent information on seven placebo-controlled randomized trials of the effect of aspirin in preventing death after myocardial infarction (heart attack).

Find the (i) point estimate of the common effect size (risk difference), (ii) standard error of the estimator and (iii) 95% confidence interval for the effect size, RD.

Solution:

For the calculation of the point estimate and confidence interval under the fixed effect model calculations of the summary statistics in Table 7.2 are required.

In Table 7.2, RD is the sample risk difference (RD), Var is the variance of the RD, and W is the study weight. The last row of the table shows the sum of W, sum of W $\times$ RD, sum of W $\times$ RD^2 and sum of W^2.

(i) The estimate of the unknown common effect size, risk difference, θ under the fixed effect model is given by

$$\hat{\theta}_{FE} = \frac{\sum_{i=1}^{k} w_i \hat{\theta}_i}{\sum_{i=1}^{k} w_i} = \frac{-769.624}{57295} = -0.01343 = -0.013,$$

Table 7.1 Count data on death for the aspirin and placebo groups after myocardial infarction

Study	Aspirin			Placebo		
	Patients	Deaths	Alive	Patients	Death	Alive
MRC-1	615	49	566	624	67	557
CDP	758	44	714	771	64	707
MRC-2	832	102	730	850	126	724
GASP	317	32	285	309	38	271
PARIS	810	85	725	406	52	354
AMIS	2267	246	2021	2257	219	2038
ISIS-2	8587	1570	7017	8600	1720	6880

Table 7.2 Calculation of summary statistics for the FE, REs and IVhet Models

Study	p1	p2	RD	Var	W	WRD	WRD^2	W^2
MRC-1	0.0797	0.1074	−0.0277	0.0003	3665.4	−101.519	2.8118	13434800
CDP	0.058	0.083	−0.025	0.0002	5852.7	−146.092	3.6467	34253977
MRC-2	0.1226	0.1482	−0.0256	0.0003	3599.3	−92.2837	2.3661	12955174
GASP	0.1009	0.123	−0.022	0.0006	1574	−34.6759	0.7639	2477359.3
PARIS	0.1049	0.1281	−0.0231	0.0004	2557.4	−59.1801	1.3695	6540400
AMIS	0.1085	0.097	0.0115	8E-05	12271	140.8969	1.6178	150580185
ISIS-2	0.1828	0.2	−0.0172	4E-05	27775	−476.769	8.184	771444238
					57295	**−769.624**	**20.76**	**991686133**

(ii)   The standard error of the estimator of the common effect size is

$$SE(\hat{\theta}_{FE}) = \sqrt{\frac{1}{\sum\limits_{i=1}^{k} w_i}} = \sqrt{0.0000174536} = 0.00418.$$

(iii) The 95% confidence interval for the common effect size θ under the FE model is given by the following lower limit (LL) and upper limit (UL):

$$LL = \hat{\theta}_{FE} - z_{\alpha/2} \times SE(\hat{\theta}_{FE}) = -0.01343 - 1.96 \times 0.00418 = -0.021621 = -0.02$$
$$UL = \hat{\theta}_{FE} + z_{\alpha/2} \times SE(\hat{\theta}_{FE}) = -0.01343 + 1.96 \times 0.00418 = -0.005244 = -0.01.$$

The 95% confidence interval for the common risk difference is $(-0.02, -0.01)$. Since this interval does not contain 0, the effect size is significant at the 5% level of significance.

Example 7.5 Consider the count data on myocardial infarction from seven studies in Example 7.4. Using the data, test the hypothesis that the common risk difference is 0 under the fixed effect model.

Solution:
   To test the null hypothesis
   $H_0 : \theta = 0$ (risk difference 0) against $H_a : \theta \neq 0$ calculate the observed value of the test statistic Z,

$$z_0 = \frac{\hat{\theta}_{FE}}{SE(\hat{\theta}_{FE})} = \frac{-0.01343}{0.00417775} = -3.2153 = -3.22.$$

The P-value is $P(|Z| > 3.22) = 2 \times P(Z > 3.22) = 0.$, so we reject the null hypothesis at the 5% level of significance. Since the P-value is too small, there is strong sample evidence to reject the null hypothesis. Thus the common risk difference is different from 0.

Measuring Heterogeneity between the studies (RD)

The heterogeneity of effect size RD between the studies are measured by Cochran's Q statistic and I^2 statistic.

To test the heterogeneity between study effect sizes, we test the null hypothesis, $H_0 = \theta_1 = \theta_2 = \ldots = \theta_k$ against the alternative hypothesis H_a : not all θ_i's are equal for $i = 1, 2, \ldots, k$ using the Q statistic,

$$Q = \sum_{i=1}^{7} w_i \hat{\theta}_i^2 - \frac{\left(\sum_{i=1}^{7} w_i \hat{\theta}_i\right)^2}{\sum_{i=1}^{7} w_i}.$$

The Q statistic follows a chi-squared distribution with $(k-1) = 7 - 1 = 6$ degrees of freedom.

For the above data set from $k = 7$ studies, using the sums from the bottom row of Table 7.2, we get

$$Q = \sum_{i=1}^{7} w_i \hat{\theta}_i^2 - \frac{\left(\sum_{i=1}^{7} w_i \hat{\theta}_i\right)^2}{\sum_{i=1}^{7} w_i} = 20.7597 - \frac{(-769.624)^2}{57295} = 10.4216 \approx 10.42.$$

Then the P-value of testing equality of population RD becomes

$$p = P\left(\chi_6^2 > 10.42\right) > 0.10$$

(exactly 10% if observed value of chi-squired statistic is 10.6446).

Using chi-squired distribution table, it is found that the P-value is larger than 0.10. Since the P-value is larger than 10%, there is no significant heterogeneity between the study risk differences.

The value of the I^2 statistic is found to be

$$I^2 = \frac{Q - df}{Q} \times 100\% = \left(\frac{10.42 - 6}{10.42}\right) \times 100\% = \left(\frac{4.42}{10.42}\right) \times 100\%$$
$$= 0.424271 \times 100\% = 42\%.$$

Hence there is an indication of some minor heterogeneity, but no real significant heterogeneity between the study risk differences.

7.4.4   FE Model Meta-Analysis of RD Using MetaXL

The forest plot under the FE model (indicated by "IV" in the code) is constructed using MetaXL code
    =MAInputTable("Myocardial RD FE","NumRD","IV",B20:H26),

where "B20:H26" refers to the data area in Excel Worksheet.

Remark: Explanations of MetaXL Code
For this type of meta-analyses in MetaXL the 'opening' code starts with MA Input Table ' = MAInputTable'. This is followed by an open parenthesis inside which the first quote contains the text that appears as the 'title of the output of the forest plot' e.g. "Myocardial RD FE" in the above code (user may choose any appropriate title here). Then in the second quote enter the type of effect measure, e.g. "NumRD" in the above code tells that the *outcome variable is numerical and the effect size measure is risk difference (RD)*. Within the third quote enter the statistical model, e.g. "IV" in the above code stands for the *fixed effect* (inverse variance is abbreviated by IV) model. Each quotation is followed by a comma, and after the last comma enter the data area in Excel Worksheet, e.g. B20:H26 in the above code tells that the data on the independent studies are taken from the specified cells. The code ends with a closing parenthesis (Fig. 7.1).

The forest plot of the meta-analysis of risk difference using the above MetaXL code is in Fig. 7.1.

Interpretation:
Under the FE model the point estimate of the population RD is -0.01 and 95% confidence interval is $(-0.02, -0.01)$. Since the 95% confidence interval does not include 0 (no risk difference) the RD is significant at the 5% level of significance.

Conclusion: The use of aspirin significantly reduce the risk of death after heart attack.

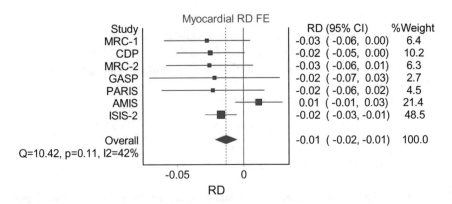

Fig. 7.1 Forest plot of risk difference of aspirin and placebo groups for the myocardial infarction patients under the fixed effect model

Since the value of the Q statistic is 10.42 with P-value 0.11, and $I^2 = 42\%$ there is very small or no real significant heterogeneity among the risk differences of the studies.

7.5   Random Effects (REs) Model

Under the random effects (REs) model the variance of sample risk difference $\hat{\theta}_i$ of the ith study about the population risk difference θ is the sum of the within-study and between-study variances, that is, $v_i^* = v_i + \hat{\tau}^2$. Therefore, the modified weight assigned to the ith study, under the REs model, becomes

$$w_i^* = \frac{1}{v_i + \hat{\tau}^2}.$$

Then the estimator of the population common risk difference (θ) under the random effects (REs) model is given by

$$\hat{\theta}_{RE} = \frac{\sum_{i=1}^{k} w_i^* \hat{\theta}_i}{\sum_{i=1}^{k} w_i^*}, \text{ with the standard error of the estimator } SE(\hat{\theta}_{RE}) = \sqrt{\frac{1}{\sum_{i=1}^{k} w_i^*}}.$$

7.5.1   Estimation of τ^2

The between studies variance is estimated as a scaled excess variation as follows

$$\hat{\tau}^2 = \frac{Q - df}{C},$$

where

$$Q = \sum_{i=1}^{k} w_i \hat{\theta}_i^2 - \frac{\left(\sum_{i=1}^{k} w_i \hat{\theta}_i\right)^2}{\sum_{i=1}^{k} w_i}, C = \sum_{i=1}^{k} w_i - \frac{\sum_{i=1}^{k} w_i^2}{\sum_{i=1}^{k} w_i}$$

and $df = (k - 1)$ in which k is the number of studies.

Table 7.3 Calculations of modified weight and sum of product of modified weight and RD

Study	p1	p2	RD	Var	τ^2	Var*	W*	W*RD
MRC-1	0.0797	0.1074	−0.0277	0.0003	0.0001	0.000384	2605.4	−72.16046
CDP	0.058	0.083	−0.025	0.0002	0.0001	0.000282	3547.8	−88.55972
MRC-2	0.1226	0.1482	−0.0256	0.0003	0.0001	0.000389	2571.8	−65.93929
GASP	0.1009	0.123	−0.022	0.0006	0.0001	0.000746	1339.9	−29.51872
PARIS	0.1049	0.1281	−0.0231	0.0004	0.0001	0.000502	1992	−46.09496
AMIS	0.1085	0.097	0.0115	8E-05	0.0001	0.000192	5195	59.649148
ISIS-2	0.1828	0.2	−0.0172	4E-05	0.0001	0.000147	6802.5	−116.769
							24054	−359.393

7.5.2 Illustration of Random Effects Model for Risk Difference

Example 7.5 Consider the myocardial data in Example 7.4.

Estimate the between-study variance from the data.

Solution:
Using previous calculations in Table 7.3, we find

$$Q = \sum_{i=1}^{k} w_i \hat{\theta}_i^2 - \frac{\left(\sum_{i=1}^{k} w_i \hat{\theta}_i\right)^2}{\sum_{i=1}^{k} w_i} = 20.75971 - \frac{(-769.624)^2}{57295} = 10.4216 \approx 10.42.$$

Now

$$C = \sum_{i=1}^{k} w_i - \frac{\sum_{i=1}^{k} w_i^2}{\sum_{i=1}^{k} w_i} = 57295 - \frac{991686133}{57295} = 39986.25$$

and hence

$$\hat{\tau}^2 = \frac{Q - df}{C} = \frac{10.4216 - 6}{39986.25} = 0.000111.$$

Example 7.6 Under the REs model, find the (i) point estimate (ii) standard error, (iii) 9% confidence interval and (iv) test the significance of the population risk difference.

Solution:

For the calculation of the common risk difference and standard error under the random effects model we need the column sums of W* (modified weight as the reciprocal of the sum of Var and τ^2), and sum of W*RD (modified weight times the RD) as in Table 7.3.

(i)   From the summary statistics in the above table, the estimated common risk difference, under the random effects model becomes

$$\hat{\theta}_{RE} = \frac{\sum\limits_{i=1}^{k} w_i^* \theta_i}{\sum\limits_{i=1}^{k} w_i^*} = \frac{-359.393}{24054} = -0.0149 \approx -0.01.$$

(ii) The standard error of the estimator is

$$SE(\hat{\theta}_{RE}) = \sqrt{\frac{1}{\sum\limits_{i=1}^{k} w_i^*}} = \sqrt{\frac{1}{24054}} = 0.006448.$$

(iii) The 95% confidence interval for the common risk difference, θ, under the random effects model, is given by the lower and upper limits:

$$LL = \hat{\theta}_{RE} - 1.96 \times SE(\hat{\theta}_{RE}) = -0.0149 - 1.96 \times 0.006448 = -0.02758 \approx -0.03 \text{ and}$$
$$UL = \hat{\theta}_{RE} + 1.96 \times SE(\hat{\theta}_{RE}) = -0.0149 + 1.96 \times 0.006448 = -0.0023 \approx -0.00.$$

The 95% confidence interval for the common risk difference is $(-0.03, -0.00)$. This confidence interval does not include 0 (just missed it as the $UL = -0.0023$)

(iv) To test the significance of the population common risk difference, that is, $H_0 : \theta = 0$ against $H_a : \theta \neq 0$, the observed value of the test statistic Z is $z_0 = \frac{\hat{\theta}_{RE}}{SE(\hat{\theta}_{RE})} = \frac{-0.0149}{0.006448} = -2.31725 \approx -2.32$ with P-value $= P(|Z| > 2.32) = 2 \times 0.0102 = 0.0204.$

Since the P-value is small, and hence the test is significant. Therefore, reject the null hypothesis at the 5% level of significance, and conclude that the population risk difference is significantly different from 0.

7.5.3 Forest Plot of RD Under REs Model Using MetaXL

The forest plot under the random effects model (indicated by "RE" in the code) is constructed using MetaXL code

=MAInputTable("Myocardial RD RE","NumRD","RE",B20:H26),

where "B20:H26" refers to the data area in Excel Worksheet.

Remark: Explanations of MetaXL Code
For this type of meta-analyses in MetaXL the 'opening' code starts with MA Input
Table ' = MAInputTable'. This is followed by an open parenthesis inside which the
first quote contains the text that appears as the 'title of the output of the forest plot'
e.g. "Myocardial RD RE" in the above code (user may choose any appropriate title
here). Then in the second quote enter the type of effect measure, e.g. "NUmRD"
in the above code tells that the *outcome variable is numerical and the effect size
measure is risk difference (RD)*. Within the third quote enter the statistical model,
e.g. "RE" in the above code stands for the *random effects* (abbreviated by RE) model.
Each quotation is followed by a comma, and after the last comma enter the data
area in Excel Worksheet, e.g. B20:H26 in the above code tells that the data on the
independent studies are taken from the specified cells. The code ends with a closing
parenthesis.

The forest plot of meta-analysis of risk difference, under the REs model, using
the above MetaXL code is found in Fig. 7.2.

Interpretation:

Under the REs model the point estimate of the population RD is -0.01 and 95%
confidence interval is $(-0.03, 0.00)$. Since the 95% confidence interval does include
0 (no risk difference) the RD is not significant at the 5% level of significance.

Since the value of the Q statistic is 10.42 with P-value 0.11, and $I^2 = 42\%$ there
is very small or no real significant heterogeneity among the risk differences of the
studies.

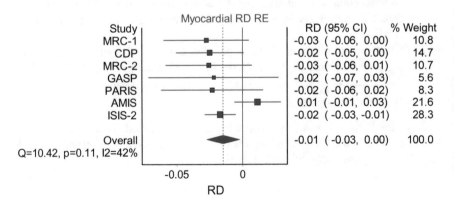

Fig. 7.2 Forest plot of risk difference of aspirin and placebo groups for the myocardial infarction
patients under the random effects model

7.6 Inverse Variance Heterogeneity (IVhet) Model

Under the inverse variance heterogeneity (IVhet) model, the pooled estimate of the common risk difference (θ) is given by

$$\hat{\theta}_{IVhet} = \frac{\sum_{i=1}^{k} w_i \hat{\theta}_i}{\sum_{i=1}^{k} w_i}.$$

Then the variance of the estimator under the IVhet model is given by

$$Var(\hat{\theta}_{IVhet}) = \sum_{i=1}^{k} \left[\left(\frac{1}{v_i} \middle/ \sum_{i=1}^{k} \frac{1}{v_i} \right)^2 (v_i + \hat{\tau}^2) \right].$$

For the computation of the confidence interval of the common risk difference, based on the IVhet model use the following standard error

$$SE(\hat{\theta}_{IVhet}) = \sqrt{Var(\hat{\theta}_{IVhet})}.$$

Then, the $(1 - \alpha) \times 100\%$ confidence interval for the common risk difference θ under the IVhet model is given by the lower limit (LL) and upper limit (UL) as follows:

$$LL = \hat{\theta}_{IVhet} - z_{\alpha/2} \times SE(\hat{\theta}_{IVhet}) \text{ and}$$
$$UL = \hat{\theta}_{IVhet} + z_{\alpha/2} \times SE(\hat{\theta}_{IVhet}),$$

where $z_{\alpha/2}$ is the $\frac{\alpha}{2}$th cut-off point of standard normal distribution.

To test the significance of the population risk difference, test $H_0 : \theta = 0$ against $H_a : \theta \neq 0$ using the test statistic $Z = \frac{\hat{\theta}_{IVhet}}{SE(\hat{\theta}_{IVhet})}$ which follows a standard normal distribution under the null hypothesis.

7.6.1 Illustration of IVhet Model for Risk Difference

Example 7.7 Consider the count data on myocardial infarction from seven studies in Example 7.4.

Under the IVhet model, find the (i) point estimate, (ii) standard error, (iii) 95% confidence interval of the common risk difference, and (iv) test the hypothesis that the common risk difference is 0.

Table 7.4 Calculations of study weights and variance of IVhet model

Study	p1	p2	RD	Var	$\hat{\tau}_2$	w	Var*	W*	W × RD
MRC-1	0.08	0.107	−0.0277	0.0003	0.0001	3665.351	0.0004	1.571E-06	−101.519
CDP	0.058	0.083	−0.025	0.0002	0.0001	5852.69	0.0003	2.941E-06	−146.092
MRC-2	0.123	0.148	−0.0256	0.0003	0.0001	3599.33	0.0004	1.535E-06	−92.2837
GASP	0.101	0.123	−0.022	0.0006	0.0001	1573.963	0.0007	5.632E-07	−34.6759
PARIS	0.105	0.128	−0.0231	0.0004	0.0001	2557.421	0.0005	1E-06	−59.1801
AMIS	0.109	0.097	0.0115	8E-05	0.0001	12271.11	0.0002	8.83E-06	140.8969
ISIS-2	0.183	0.2	−0.0172	4E-05	0.0001	27774.89	0.0001	3.455E-05	−476.769
						57294.75	0.0026	5.099E-05	−769.624

Solution:

First, we need to find the modified weights and variance of the estimator under the IVhet model as in Table 7.4.

In Table 7.4, W is the study weight based on observed variance (Var), Var* is the study level sum of observed variance (Var) and between study variance ($\hat{\tau}_2$) and sum of W* is the variance of the estimator under the IVhet model.

For illustration, consider the first study (MRC-1):

W = 1/Var = 1/0.0003 = 3665.351, the weight based on observed variance (Var), Var* = Var + $\hat{\tau}_2$ = 0.0003 + 0.0001 = 0.0004, the combined variance of the study, and W* = $\left[\frac{w}{\sum w}\right]^2 \times Var^* = \left[\frac{3665.351}{57294.75}\right]^2 \times 0.0004 = 0.00000157$, the modified variance of the study under the IVhet model.

To find the estimated value of the population risk difference (θ) under the IVhet model the sums of columns of W and W × RD, that is, $\sum w_i = 57294.75$ and $\sum w_i \times \hat{\theta}_i = -769.624$, of Table 7.4 are required.

(i)   The IVhet model estimate of the common effect size, RD is given by

$$\hat{\theta}_{IVhet} = \frac{\sum_{i=1}^{k} w_i \hat{\theta}_i}{\sum_{i=1}^{k} w_i} = \frac{\sum_{i=1}^{7} W \times RD}{\sum_{i=1}^{7} W} = \frac{-769.624}{57294.75} = -0.01343 \approx 0 - 0.01.$$

(ii) The variance of the estimator under the IVhet model is given by the sum of the second last column (W*) of the above table, that is,

$$Var(\hat{\theta}_{IVhet}) = \sum_{i=1}^{k}\left[\left(\frac{1}{v_i}\bigg/\sum_{i=1}^{k}\frac{1}{v_i}\right)^2 (v_i + \hat{\tau}^2)\right] = \sum_{i=1}^{7}\left[\left(W\bigg/\sum_{i=1}^{7}W\right)^2 W*\right] = 0.00005099.$$

Hence the standard error becomes

$$SE(\hat{\theta}_{IVhet}) = \sqrt{Var(\hat{\theta}_{IVhet})} = \sqrt{0.00005099} = 0.00714.$$

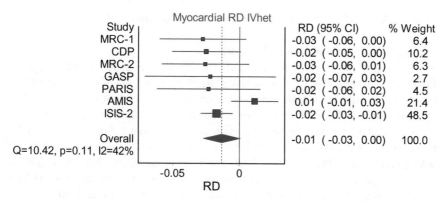

Fig. 7.3 Forest plot of risk difference of aspirin and placebo groups for the myocardial infarction patients under the IVhet model

(iii) Then, the 95% confidence interval for the common risk difference under the IVhet model is given by the lower and upper limits:

$$LL = \hat{\theta}_{IVhet} - 1.96 \times SE(\hat{\theta}_{IVhet}) = -0.01343 - 1.96 \times 0.00714 = -0.02743 \approx -0.03 \text{ and}$$
$$UL = \hat{\theta}_{IVhet} + 1.96 \times SE(\hat{\theta}_{IVhet}) = -0.01343 - 1.96 \times 0.00714 = 0.000563 \approx 0.00.$$

The above point estimate (-0.01) of pooled risk difference and confidence interval $(-0.03, 0.00)$ are reported in the forest plot (See Fig. 7.3) in the last row with the horizontal ends of the diamond representing the limits of the confidence interval.

(iv) To test the significance of the population common risk difference, test H_0 : $\theta = 0$ against $H_a : \theta \neq 0$ the observed value of the test statistic, Z is

$$z_0 = \frac{\hat{\theta}_{IVhet}}{SE(\hat{\theta}_{IVhet})} = \frac{-0.01343}{0.00714} = -1.88121 \approx -1.88.$$

The two-sided P-value is $P(|Z| > 1.88) = 2 \times 0.0301 = 0.0602$.
Since the P-value is greater than 5%, the risk difference is not significant at the 5% level of significance.

7.6.2 Forest Plot of RD Under IVhet Model Using MetaXL

The forest plot under the IVhet model (indicated by "IVhet" in the code) is produced using MetaXL code
=MAInputTable("Myocardial RD IVhet","NumRD","IVhet",B20:H26),

where "B20:H26" refers to the data area in Excel Worksheet.

Remark: Explanations of MetaXL Code

For this type of meta-analyses in MetaXL the 'opening' code starts with MA Input Table ' = MAInputTable'. This is followed by an open parenthesis inside which the first quote contains the text that appears as the 'title of the output of the forest plot' e.g. "Myocardial RD IVhet" in the above code (user may choose any appropriate title here). Then in the second quote enter the type of effect measure, e.g. "NumRD" in the above code tells that the *outcome variable is numerical and the effect size measure is risk difference (RD)*. Within the third quote enter the statistical model, e.g. "IVhet" in the above code stands for the inverse variance heterogeneity (abbreviated by IVhet) model. Each quotation is followed by a comma, and after the last comma enter the data area in Excel Worksheet, e.g. B20:H26 in the above code tells that the data on the independent studies are taken from the specified cells. The code ends with a closing parenthesis.

The forest plot of the meta-analysis of risk difference, under the IVhet model, using the above MetaXL code is found in Fig. 7.3.

Interpretation:

Under the REs model the point estimate of the population RD is -0.01 and 95% confidence interval is $(-0.03, 0.00)$. Since the 95% confidence interval does include 0 (no risk difference) the RD is not significant at the 5% level of significance.

Since the value of the Q statistic is 0.42 with P-value 0.11, and $I^2 = 42\%$ there is very small or no real significant heterogeneity among the risk differences of the studies.

Because the heterogeneity is not significant, the meta-analysis under the IVhet model is very similar to that under the FE model.

7.7   Subgroup Analysis

In the myocardial infarction data there is not enough information to make realistic subgroups of the studies to conduct subgroup analysis. But the procedure to conduct subgroup analysis is very similar to that explained in previous chapters.

7.8   Discussions and Comparison of Results

The meta-analyses of preventing death by using aspirin after myocardial infarction under three different statistical models are presented in this chapter.

Regardless of the model used for meta-analysis, the value of the Q statistic is 10.42 with P-value 0.11, and $I^2 = 42\%$. Therefore, the heterogeneity among the risk differences of the studies is not significant. So, the results of meta-analyses is unlikely to be very different. It is noteworthy to observe that the results of the meta-analysis under the REs model is very similar to that under the IVhet model for this dataset.

The point estimate of the population RD is -0.01 for under all three statistical models. The 95% confidence interval is $(-0.02, -0.01)$ under the FE model, $(-0.03, 0.00)$ under the REs model, and $(-0.03, 0.00)$ under the IVhet model.

The risk difference is significant under the FE model, but not significant under the REs and IVhet models. This is because of including the between study variance in the meta-analysis under the REs and IVhet models.

The redistribution of study weights under the FE and IVhet models are the same. But that under the REs model is very different from the other two models.

7.9 Publication Bias

The study of publication bias for the RD is very similar to that in Sect. 5.9 of the previous chapter. It is not necessary to re-produce them again here. Readers interested to produce funnel plot or Doi plot and their interpretation are referred that Section.

Appendix 7—Stata Codes for Difference of Two Proportions (Risk Difference) Meta-Analysis

A7.1 Myocardial infarction (heat attack) data

Study	AsprPatients	AsprDeath	AsprAlive	PlaceboPatients	PlaceboDeath	PlaceboAlive
MRC-1	615	49	566	624	67	557
CDP	758	44	714	771	64	707
MRC-2	832	102	730	850	126	724
GASP	317	32	285	309	38	271
PARIS	810	85	725	406	52	354
AMIS	2267	246	2021	2257	219	2038
ISIS-2	8587	1570	7017	8600	1720	6880

A7.2 Stata codes for risk difference of heart attack data

Fixed effect model
admetan AsprDeath AsprAlive PlaceboDeath PlaceboAlive, rd **fixed** label(namevar = Study) counts

Random effects model
admetan AsprDeath AsprAlive PlaceboDeath PlaceboAlive, rd random label(namevar = Study) counts

IVhet model
admetan AsprDeath AsprAlive PlaceboDeath PlaceboAlive, rd ivhet label(namevar = Study) counts

Part III
Meta-Analysis for Continuous Outcomes

Chapter 8
Meta-Analysis of Standardized Mean Difference

Meta-analysis of effect sizes for continuous outcome variables are covered in the upcoming three chapters. If the outcome variable is continuous and interest is to compare the effects of two interventions (e.g. treatment and control), standardized mean difference may be the appropriate effects size measure.

Meta-analysis of standardized mean difference (SMD) under different statistical models, subgroup analysis and publication bias are covered in this chapter.

8.1 Introduction

The effect size measure broadly depends on the type of outcome variables involved. There are two major categories of effect measures in meta-analyses based on two kind of outcome variables. There are those based on binary or categorical outcome variables such as the proportion, relative risks or odds ratios. The other category is those effect measures for continuous outcome variables such as the standardised mean difference (SMD), weighted mean difference (WMD), and Pearson's product moment correlation coefficients.

Often interventions or treatments are applied on the experimental units (e.g. patients), called the treatment group, and a placebo is given to another group of patients to measure the size of effect of the intervention through the associated outcome variables. The patients selected to both groups should be randomly chosen to avoid any selection bias. The main objective is to find out if the intervention (e.g. a new drug) is working better than the placebo (control group) or not. So the mean effect measure is assessed for both the treatment and control groups separately for comparison. The difference of the mean effects in treatment group and control group is called the *raw mean difference*, and often used as the effect size measure.

Why Standardise Raw Mean Difference?

The raw mean difference has the same unit of measurement as the outcome variable. However, in some studies outcome variables are measured in difference scales (e.g., cm and inch, or kg and lb). So, direct comparison of means in two different units, using the raw mean difference, is not meaningful. Instead, the raw mean difference is divided by the standard deviation (pooled or not) to find the standardised mean difference (SMD). Any value of SMD is unit free as it is a measure of how many standard deviations the mean of the treatment group is away from the mean of the control group. As such the SMD always produces a unit free number that is unrelated to the unit of measurement of the outcome variable. For this reason, when different study records the same outcome variable in different units of measurement, meta-analysis must use SMD as an appropriate measure of effect size.

In this chapter meta-analytic methods of effect size measure for continuous (numerical) outcome variables, namely the standardised mean difference (SMD) is covered. But first as a precursor to SMD we introduce the raw effect size, the unstandardised/unscaled mean difference, as a measure of effect size. The standardised mean difference is a standardised/scaled version of the raw mean difference (divided by the standard deviation).

Raw Effect Size

The difference between two means may be used to define an effect size. This is called the raw effect size as the raw difference of means is not standardised.

The difference of two means as a measure of effect size may arise in two different contexts (study design), namely from (a) two independent groups and (b) two dependent/matched (paired) groups. The mean difference would differ if the design of the study is independent or matched. Similarly, the variance of the estimator of the population mean difference will depend on the study design.

(a)　Raw Mean Difference for Independent Study Design

Consider a population of patients of the treatment group with mean value of the outcome variable (say Y) to be μ_1 (or μ_T) and that of the patients who received the control/placebo is μ_2 (or μ_P). Then the population mean difference is $\delta = \mu_1 - \mu_2$. This is the raw population effect size expressed as the difference of two independent means. Let the population variance of the patients in the treatment group be σ_1^2 and that of the placebo group be σ_2^2. Assume that the outcome variable of both populations (treatment and placebo) follow the normal distribution.

Based on a random sample of size n_1 from the treatment group, let the sample mean be $\hat{\mu}_1 = \bar{Y}_1$ and sample variance be $\hat{\sigma}_1^2 = S_1^2$. Similarly, for another random sample of size n_2 from the placebo group, let the sample mean be $\hat{\mu}_2 = \bar{Y}_2$ and sample variance be $\hat{\sigma}_2^2 = S_2^2$.

For the purpose of inference, confidence interval and test of significance on $\delta = \mu_1 - \mu_2$, we need to find the point estimate of δ and the standard error (SE) of the estimator of δ.

Table 8.1 Summary data for memory enhancement

Intervention	Count (N)	Mean	Standard deviation
Ginkgo	28	58.4	3.8
Placebo	24	56.8	4.3

The point estimate of the population mean difference is defined as $\hat{\delta} = \bar{Y}_1 - \bar{Y}_2$. However, the SE of the estimator of δ depends on whether the two population variances are equal or not.

(i) SE when $\sigma_1^2 = \sigma_2^2$ (equal variances) assumed

If the two population variances are equal, the variance of $\hat{\delta}$ is $V_{Eq}(\hat{\delta}) = V(\bar{Y}_1 - \bar{Y}_2) = \frac{n_1+n_2}{n_1 n_2} \times S_P^2$, where $S_P^2 = \frac{(n_1-1)S_1^2+(n_2-1)S_2^2}{n_1+n_2-2}$ is the pooled sample variance. Then the standard error of $\hat{\delta}$ is $SE_{Eq}(\hat{\delta}) = \sqrt{V_{Eq}(\hat{\delta})}$.

(ii) SE when $\sigma_1^2 \neq \sigma_2^2$ (unequal variances) assumed

For the case of unequal population variances, the variance of $\hat{\delta}$ is $V_{NEq}(\hat{\delta}) = V(\bar{Y}_1 - \bar{Y}_2) = \frac{S_1^2}{n_1} + \frac{S_2^2}{n_2}$. Then the standard error of $\hat{\delta}$ is $SE_{NEq}(\hat{\delta}) = \sqrt{V_{NEq}(\hat{\delta})}$.

Example 8.1 A researcher wanted to see whether ginkgo biloba enhances memory. In an experiment to find out, subjects were assigned randomly to take ginkgo biloba supplements or a placebo. The memory of both groups of subjects are recoded after the experiment. The summary statistics of the data are noted in Table 8.1.

Let $\mu_1 =$ mean memory score of ginkgo group and $\mu_2 =$ mean memory score of placebo group. Then the population raw mean difference, effect size, is defined as $\delta = \mu_1 - \mu_2$.

Find the (a) point estimate of the population effect size, difference of the means, δ, and (b) the standard error of the estimator of δ assuming the two population variances are (i) equal and (ii) unequal.

Solution:

(a) The point estimate of $\delta = \mu_1 - \mu_2$ is $\hat{\delta} = \hat{\mu}_1 - \hat{\mu}_2 = 58.4 - 56.8 = 1.6$.

(b) To estimate the standard error of the estimator of δ, we have the following two options:

(i) The SE when $\sigma_1^2 = \sigma_2^2$ (equal variances) assumed

First find the pooled sample variance,

$$S_P^2 = \frac{(n_1-1)S_1^2+(n_2-1)S_2^2}{n_1+n_2-2} = \frac{(28-1)\times 3.8^2+(24-1)\times 4.3^2}{28+24-2} = 16.303.$$

Then the variance of the estimator of δ is

$$V_{Eq}(\hat{\delta}) = V(\bar{Y}_1 - \bar{Y}_2) = \frac{n_1+n_2}{n_1 n_2} \times S_P^2 = \frac{28+24}{28\times 24} \times 16.303 = 1.261542,$$ and hence the
standard error becomes

$$SE_{Eq}(\hat{\delta}) = \sqrt{V_{Eq}(\hat{\delta})} = \sqrt{1.261542} = 1.1232.$$

(ii)   The SE when $\sigma_1^2 \neq \sigma_2^2$ (unequal variances) assumed

When the population variances are not equal, the variance of $\hat{\delta}$ is

$$V_{NEq}(\hat{\delta}) = \frac{S_1^2}{n_1} + \frac{S_2^2}{n_2} = \frac{3.8^2}{28} + \frac{4.3^2}{24} = 1.286131.$$

Then the standard error of $\hat{\delta}$ is $SE_{NEq}(\hat{\delta}) = \sqrt{V_{NEq}(\hat{\delta}))} = \sqrt{1.286131} = 1.1341.$

(b)   Raw Mean Difference for Matched Pairs Study Design

Consider a population of pairs of patients or experimental units. The pairs can be pre
and post scores of the same group of patients. It could also be patients at the same stage
of disease or siblings. The idea is to make the experimental units identical or very
similar so that they behave like the same subject. This kind of matched pairs ensures
that the difference in responses of the paired units are only due to the intervention (or
treatment). The main advantage of this design is that the matched pairs ensure internal
control to reduce errors. The numerical data from matched groups are dependent
within the pairs, and hence different from that from the independent groups.

Let the paired values of a variable of interest for a matched paired design experiment be denoted by Y_1 and Y_2 or (Y_1, Y_2). Let the difference of the pair of values of
the variable be denoted by $D = Y_1 - Y_2$. Then D itself is a variable which is assumed
to follow a normal distribution with mean μ_D and variance σ_D^2. Here the mean difference, μ_D is actually the population mean of differences (D) of the matched paired
values of the variable. Similarly, σ_D^2 is the variance of the differences, D. Both μ_D
and σ_D^2 are unknown population parameters, and we need to estimate them from the
sample data.

Consider a random sample of size n from a population of matched pairs (e.g. pre
and post, or before and after) so that the data on the variable appear as n different
pairs (Y_{11}, Y_{21}), $(Y_{12}, Y_{22}), \ldots, (Y_{1n}, Y_{2n})$. Then the differences of the n pairs of
sample values of the variables can be expressed as $D_1 = Y_{11} - Y_{21}$, $D_2 = Y_{12} -
Y_{22}, \ldots, D_n = Y_{1n} - Y_{2n}$. From the sample data, the estimator of the population
mean μ_D and variance σ_D^2 are defined as

$$\hat{\mu}_D = \bar{D} = \frac{\sum D_i}{n},$$ the sample mean of the differences and $\hat{\sigma}_{\bar{D}}^2 = Var(\bar{D}) = \frac{S_D^2}{n},$

the variance of $\bar{D}$, where $S_D^2 = \frac{\sum (D_i - \bar{D})^2}{n-1}$ is the sample variance of the differences.
So, the standard error (SE) of $\bar{D}$ becomes $SE_{\bar{D}} = \sqrt{Var(\bar{D})}.$

The statistic $\bar{D}$ follows a normal distribution. For the confidence interval on the raw population effect size, μ_D and significance test on it, we use the point estimate $\bar{D}$ and the standard error $SE_{\bar{D}}$.

Example 8.2 A new drug is proposed to lower total cholesterol and a study is designed to evaluate the efficacy of the drug in lowering cholesterol. Fifteen patients agreed to participate in the study and each is asked to take the new drug for 6 weeks. However, before starting the treatment, each patient's total cholesterol level is measured. The initial measurement is a pre-treatment or baseline value. After taking the drug for 6 weeks, each patient's total cholesterol level is measured again (post-treatment value). The differences are computed by subtracting the cholesterols measured at 6 weeks from the baseline values, so positive differences indicate reductions and negative differences indicate increases. The summary statistics of the data are shown below:

$$n = 15, \quad \sum_{1}^{15} D_i = 254, \quad \text{and} \quad \sum_{1}^{15} \left(D_i - \bar{D}\right)^2 = 2808.9333.$$

Find the estimated effect size (mean of differences, μ_D) and the standard error of the estimator, $SE_{\bar{D}}$.

Solution:

The estimated value of population mean of differences, μ_D is the sample mean of differences, that is, $\hat{\mu}_D = \bar{D} = \frac{\sum_{1}^{n} D_i}{n} = \frac{254}{15} = 16.9333$.

The sample variance of D is $S_D^2 = \frac{\sum_{1}^{n} (D_i - \bar{D})^2}{n-1} = \frac{2808.9333}{15-1} = 200.6381$. So the variance of the sample mean of differences ($\bar{D}$) is

$$\hat{\sigma}_{\bar{D}}^2 = Var(\bar{D}) = \frac{S_D^2}{n} = \frac{200.6381}{15} = 13.3759.$$

Then the standard error is given by $SE_{\bar{D}} = \sqrt{Var(\bar{D})} = \sqrt{13.3759} = 3.6573$.

8.2 Estimation of Effect Size, SMD

In many meta-analyses when the effect size is measured by the difference between two means some of the popular measures of estimating the unknown population effect size are Cohen's d, Hedges' g and Glass' Δ. All of them are standardized mean difference with the same raw mean difference in the numerator but different denominators. The Cohen's d uses a biased estimator and Hedges' g uses an unbiased estimator of the population standard deviation in the denominator. But Glass' Δ uses the sample standard deviation of the control group as denominator.

The SMD

If the underlying outcome variable of interest is continuous (e.g. systolic blood pressure) the mean of the variable is used to define effect size. Let the mean of the outcome variable in the population of patients who received the treatment be μ_1 (or μ_T) and that of the patients who received the placebo is μ_2 (or μ_P). Again, let the variances of the effect size of the two populations be σ_1^2 and σ_2^2 respectively. Then, assume that the two variances are equal, that is, $\sigma_1^2 = \sigma_2^2 = \sigma^2$, that is, the difference is not significant (cases of unequal variances should be dealt separately in the next chapter). Then the population raw effect size in study i is measured by $\delta_i = \mu_{i1} - \mu_{i2}$ (difference of the two population means), the *mean difference*. Attempt is made to estimate the unknown population effect, δ from the sample data obtained from different independent studies. As an example, an estimate of the effect size of study i is $\hat{\delta}_i = \hat{\mu}_{i1} - \hat{\mu}_{i2}$ (difference of the two sample means), where the 'hat' symbol indicates an estimated value from the observed sample data. Thus, $\hat{\delta}_i$ (calculated from available data) is an estimate of δ_i (unknown parameter) and $\hat{\mu}_{i1}$ is an estimate of μ_{i1} respectively.

The raw mean difference δ can be standardized by dividing the raw mean difference with the standard deviation to get the population effect size, for instance, $\theta = \frac{\mu_1 - \mu_2}{\sigma}$. Then, the unknown population effect size of study i can be defined as the *standardised mean difference* (SMD), $\theta_i = \frac{\mu_{i1} - \mu_{i2}}{\sigma}$ and estimated by $\hat{\theta}_i = \frac{\hat{\mu}_{i1} - \hat{\mu}_{i2}}{\hat{\sigma}}$. This type of effect size expresses the mean difference between two groups in the standard deviation unit.

Let $X_{11}, X_{12}, \ldots, X_{1n_1}$ be a random sample of size n_1 for the treatment group, and $X_{21}, X_{22}, \ldots, X_{2n_2}$ be another random sample of size n_2 for the placebo/control group. Assume that the two samples are independent. The mean of the first sample, $\bar{X}_1$ is an estimate of the population mean μ_1 and that of the second sample, $\bar{X}_2$ is an estimate of μ_2. Similarly, the sample variances S_1^2 and S_2^2 are the estimates of the population variances σ_1^2 and σ_2^2 respectively. Some of the commonly used effect size measures, namely *standardized mean difference*, based on the sample means and standard deviations are discussed below.

(a) **Cohen's d** Cohen (1969, 1987) is an estimate of the population effect size, θ, based on the *standardized mean difference* and is given by

$$d = \frac{\bar{X}_1 - \bar{X}_2}{s},$$

where $s = \sqrt{\frac{n_1 S_1^2 + n_2 S_2^2}{n_1 + n_2}}$ is a **biased** estimator of the common population standard deviation σ. Note that this estimate of σ was defined under the assumption that the two population variances were assumed unequal.

Typically, this is reported as Cohen's d, or simply referred to as "d". The calculated values for effect size, as defined above, are generally low and usually share the range – 3.0 to 3.0. The meaning of effect size varies by context, but the standard interpretation of d offered by Cohen is:

0.8 = large (8/10 of a standard deviation unit)
0.5 = moderate (1/2 of a standard deviation)
0.2 = small (1/5 of a standard deviation)

(b) **Hedges' g** Larry V Hedges (1981, 1982) is another estimate of the population effect size, θ, based on *standardized mean difference* and is given by

$$g = \frac{\bar{X}_1 - \bar{X}_2}{s^*},$$

where $s^* = \sqrt{\frac{(n_1-1)S_1^2+(n_2-1)S_2^2}{n_1+n_2-2}}$, an **unbiased** estimator of the common population standard deviation σ. Note that this pooled estimate of σ was defined under the assumption that two population variances were equal.

If the sample sizes are large, there is no significant difference between the above two effect measures d and g.

(c) **Glass' Δ** Glass et al. (1981) is another estimate of the population effect size θ, based on *standardized mean difference* and is given by

$$\Delta = \frac{\bar{X}_1 - \bar{X}_2}{s_2},$$

where s_2 is the sample standard deviation of the control population.

Although each of the above three effect size estimates has the same numerator, they differ due to the differences in the denominator, different estimators of the population standard deviation σ. Actually, they are scaled differently by using different estimates of σ.

Variances of effect size estimators

The population variance of the above three estimators of the mean difference based effect size are approximated as follows:

$\sigma^2(d) = Var(d) = \left[\frac{n_1+n_2}{n_1 n_2} + \frac{\theta^2}{2(n_1+n_2-2)}\right] \times \left[\frac{n_1+n_2}{n_1+n_2-2}\right]$, where θ represents population counterpart of Cohen's d,

$\sigma^2(g) = Var(g) = \left[\frac{n_1+n_2}{n_1 n_2} + \frac{\theta^2}{2(n_1+n_2-2)}\right]$, where θ represents population counterpart of Hedges' g, and

$\sigma^2(\Delta) = Var(\Delta) = \left[\frac{n_1+n_2}{n_1 n_2} + \frac{\theta^2}{2(n_2-1)}\right]$, where θ represents population counterpart of Glass' Δ.

The corresponding sample/estimated variances of the estimators are given by replacing the unknown parameter θ with its estimate from the sample. Thus

$Var(d) = \left[\frac{n_1+n_2}{n_1 n_2} + \frac{d^2}{2(n_1+n_2-2)}\right] \times \left[\frac{n_1+n_2}{n_1+n_2-2}\right]$, sample variance of Cohen's d,

$$Var(g) = \left[\frac{n_1+n_2}{n_1 n_2} + \frac{g^2}{2(n_1+n_2-2)} \right], \text{ sample variance of Hedges' g and}$$

$$Var(\Delta) = \left[\frac{n_1+n_2}{n_1 n_2} + \frac{\Delta^2}{2(n_2-1)} \right], \text{ sample variance of Glass' } \Delta.$$

Both the point estimate of the effect size, θ and the variance of its estimator from all individual studies are required to perform statistical inference. For the meta-analysis these estimated values from different independent studies are synthesised/pooled to produce a combined estimate for the unknown common effect size θ.

The Standard Error of $\hat{\theta}$

The standard error of the estimator of effect size is calculated from the sample variance of the sample effect sizes. For the Cohen's d statistic, the sample variance is given by

$$Var(d) = \left[\frac{n_1+n_2}{n_1 n_2} + \frac{d^2}{2(n_1+n_2-2)} \right] \times \left[\frac{n_1+n_2}{n_1+n_2-2} \right], \text{ and hence } SE(\hat{\theta}) = \sqrt{Var(d)} \text{ where}$$
$\hat{\theta} = d$.

For the Hedges' g statistic, the sample variance is given by

$$Var(g) = \left[\frac{n_1+n_2}{n_1 n_2} + \frac{g^2}{2(n_1+n_2-2)} \right], \text{ and hence the standard error becomes } SE(\hat{\theta}) =$$
$\sqrt{Var(g)}$, where $\hat{\theta} = g$.

For the Glass' Δ statistic, the sample variance is given by

$$Var(\Delta) = \left[\frac{n_1+n_2}{n_1 n_2} + \frac{\Delta^2}{2(n_2-2)} \right], \text{ so the standard error is } SE(\hat{\theta}) = \sqrt{Var(\Delta)}, \text{ where}$$
$\hat{\theta} = \Delta$.

The above formulae for the standard error are used to find both the confidence interval for θ and the observed value of the test statistic, Z.

Remark The standardised mean difference (SMD) follows a standard normal performing distribution so no transformation is required to define the confidence interval or performing test of hypothesis when the effect size is measured by SMD.

Confidence Interval for θ

In meta-analysis, one of the main interest is to find confidence interval for the population effect size of individual studies as well as for the common effect size by combining summary statistics from selected independent studies.

The generic form of a $(1-\alpha) \times 100\%$ (95% if $\alpha = 0.05$ or 5%) confidence interval for the common effect size θ is

$\hat{\theta} \pm z_{\alpha/2} \times SE(\hat{\theta})$, and that for the ith study θ_i is $\hat{\theta}_i \pm z_{\alpha/2} \times SE(\hat{\theta}_i)$ for $i = 1,2,$ ...,k, where $\hat{\theta}$ is the point estimate of θ, common effect size of all studies, $z_{\alpha/2}$ is the critical value (cut-off point) of the standard normal distribution leaving $\alpha/2$ area to the upper (or lower tail) of the distribution, and SE($\hat{\theta}$) is the standard error of $\hat{\theta}$.

If $\alpha = 0.05$, then from the Normal Table, $z_{\alpha/2} = z_{0.05/2} = 1.96$ and the 95% confidence interval for θ is given by $\hat{\theta} \pm 1.96 \times SE(\hat{\theta})$. The formula for the confidence interval can be simplified by expressing the lower limit (LL) and upper limit (UL) as follows:

$$LL = \hat{\theta} - z_{\alpha/2} \times SE(\hat{\theta}) \text{ and}$$
$$UL = \hat{\theta} + z_{\alpha/2} \times SE(\hat{\theta}).$$

Example 8.3 Consider the data set in Table 8.2 on the quantitative ability of stusents from seven different studies on the sex difference of cognitive abilities (quantitative, verbal, visual-spatial and field articulation) from (Larry V. Hedges 1985), p.17. The data in the following table provide information on the sample size (N), estimated effect size (g) by Hedges and unbiased effect size (g*), both estimating the common effect size θ, difference of mean cognitive ability of the two genders.

Find the standard error, and construct the 95% confidence interval for the population effect size for Study 1. (Similar results are calculated for other studies, if needed).

Solution:

Standard error for Study 1
As an example, consider **Study 1** with N = 76, and Hedges' effect estimate g = 0.72.
Assuming equal sample sizes, we write $N = n_1 + n_2 = 38 + 38 = 76$, and the standard error of g is given by the square root of

$$Var(g) = \left[\frac{n_1+n_2}{n_1 n_2} + \frac{g^2}{2(n_1+n_2-2)}\right] = \left[\frac{38+38}{38\times38} + \frac{0.72^2}{2(38+38-2)}\right] = 0.056134, \quad \text{that is,}$$

$$SE(g) = \sqrt{0.056134} = 0.236927.$$

Confidence interval for Study 1
A 95% confidence interval for the population effect size θ of **Study 1** is computed by working out the lower limit (LL) and upper limit (UL) of the interval as follows:

$$LL = \hat{\theta} - z_{\alpha/2} \times SE(\hat{\theta}) = 0.72 - 1.96 \times 0.236927 = 0.72 - 0.464 = 0.256 \quad \text{and}$$

$$UL = \hat{\theta} + z_{\alpha/2} \times SE(\hat{\theta}) = 0.72 + 1.96 \times 0.236927 = 0.72 + 0.464 = 1.184.$$

So the 95% confidence interval for **Study 1** is (0.256, 1.184). This interval does not include 0 (that is, population effect size 0), the value of θ under the null hypothesis, suggesting significance of the effect size.
Conclusion: The cognitive ability differs between the two genders.

8.3 Tests on Effect Size

Test of significance for θ
To test the significance of the common effect size of all studies (or any individual study effect size), we need to test the hypotheses

Table 8.2 Summary data on gender differences in cognitive (quantitative) ability of students

Study	Sample size (N)	Standardised mean difference (g)	Unbiased standardised mean difference (g*)
Study 1	76	0.72	0.71
Study 2	6167	0.06	0.06
Study 3	355	0.59	0.59
Study 4	1050	0.43	0.43
Study 5	136	0.27	0.27
Study 6	2925	0.89	0.89
Study 7	45222	0.35	0.35

$H_0 : \theta = 0$ against $H_a : \theta \neq 0$
(or $H_0 : \theta_i = 0$ against $H_a : \theta_i \neq 0$ for an individual study i).
The test is based on the standardised normal statistic,
$Z = \frac{\hat{\theta} - 0}{SE(\hat{\theta})}$, $\left(\text{or } Z = \frac{\hat{\theta}_i - 0}{SE(\hat{\theta}_i)} \text{ for any individual study i} \right)$,

where Z follows a standard normal distribution.

For a two-tailed test, reject H_0 at the α level of significance (in favour of the alternative hypothesis) if the observed or calculated value of Z statistic satisfies $|z_0| \geq z_{\alpha/2}$; otherwise don't reject the null hypothesis.

Example 8.4 Using the data in Table 8.2 and the statistics from Example 8.3 test the significance of the population effect size for Study 1. (Similar tests can be performed for other studies, if needed).

Solution:

Test of significance for Study 1
To test the null hypothesis, $H_0 : \theta = 0$ against the two sided alternative $H_0 : \theta \neq 0$ calculate the observed value of the Z statistic,

$$z_o = \frac{\hat{\theta}}{SE(\hat{\theta})} = \frac{g}{SE(g)} = \frac{0.72}{0.236927} = 3.039.$$

The associated (two-sided) P-value is $P(|Z| \geq 3.039) = P(-3.039 < Z) + P(Z > 3.039) = 2 \times 0.0012 = 0.0024$.

Since the P-value is too small (much smaller than even 1%) there is very strong sample evidence against the null hypothesis. So the effect size of this study reveals that the population effect size is significant (that is, significantly different from 0).

Remark The same conclusion is reached if the calculations are based on the value of g* (= 0.71) instead of g for the same study.

8.4 Fixed Effect (FE) Model

Fixed effect model is appropriate for meta-analysis when the between studies variation is insignificant, that is, the effect size of interest is homogeneous across all studies. For details on the fixed effect and other types of statistical models used for meta-analyses readers may refer to Borenstein et al. (2010), Chapter 11 of Borenstein et al. (2009), Doi et al. (2015a, b, c) for fixed effect and other statistical meta-analytic models.

Let us consider k independent primary studies for a meta-analysis of standardised mean difference. Assume that there is an unknown common effect size, θ (SMD) for all the independent studies. Let θ_i be the unknown true (population) study specific effect size of interest which includes systematic bias specific to the study (if no systematic bias then $\theta_i = \theta$) and σ_i^2 be the unknown population variance of the ith study for $i = 1, 2, ..., k$. The sample estimate of the population effect size for the ith primary study based on a random sample of size n_i is denoted by $\hat{\theta}_i$ and the sample variance by v_i. Then the weight of the ith study is estimated by $w_i = \frac{1}{v_i}$.

In meta-analysis, results from all the k independent studies are combined by pooling the summary statistics to a single point estimate and find a confidence interval for the common effect size θ. Under the fixed effect model, the common effect size estimator (SMD) is given by

$$\hat{\theta}_{FE} = \sum_{i=1}^{k} w_i \hat{\theta}_i \bigg/ \sum_{i=1}^{k} w_i$$

which is the weighted mean of the estimated effect sizes of all the independent studies. The variance of the estimator of the common effect size is $Var(\hat{\theta}_{FE}) = 1 \bigg/ \sum_{i=1}^{k} w_i$, and hence the standard error of the estimator of the common effect size is $SE(\hat{\theta}_{FE}) = \sqrt{1 \bigg/ \sum_{i=1}^{k} w_i}$.

The confidence interval

The $(1 - \alpha) \times 100\%$ confidence interval for the effect size θ, based on the sample estimates of θ and SE of its estimator, is given by the lower limit (LL) and upper limit (UL) as follows:

$$LL = \hat{\theta}_{FE} - z_{\alpha/2} \times SE(\hat{\theta}_{FE}) \quad \text{and}$$
$$UL = \hat{\theta}_{FE} + z_{\alpha/2} \times SE(\hat{\theta}_{FE}).$$

Table 8.3 Effect size estimate from six studies of the effect of Open education on Attitude toward School

Study	$n_i^E = n_i^C = n_i$	$\hat{\theta}_i$
Study 1	22	0.563
Study 2	10	0.308
Study 3	10	0.081
Study 4	10	0.598
Study 5	39	-0.178
Study 6	50	-0.24

Here $z_{\alpha/2}$ is the $\frac{\alpha}{2}$ th cut-off point of standard normal distribution and $SE(\hat{\theta}_{FE}) = \sqrt{Var(\hat{\theta}_{FE})}$.

To compute the confidence interval and perform test on the population effect size θ, we need to compute the point estimate and standard error of the estimator for all studies.

Example 8.5 Consider the data on the sample size and estimated effect size from Larry V. Hedges (1985), p. 121 as in Table 8.3. The study is on the effects of Open Education on Attitude toward School for the experimental and control groups.

Find the standard error of the estimator of the population effect size for each of the six studies.

Solution:

From Table 8.3, for the first study (Study 1), we have $n_i^E = n_i^C = n_i = 22$ and estimated effect size $\hat{\theta}_1 = 0.563$ (for $i = 1$).

So, the variance of the effect size estimator is

$Var\left(\hat{\theta}_i\right) = \frac{n^E + n^C}{n^E n^C} + \frac{\hat{\theta}_i^2}{2 \times (n^E + n^C)}$. Then the standard error of the effect size estimator is given by

$$SE(\hat{\theta}_1) = \sqrt{\frac{n^E + n^C}{n^E n^C} + \frac{\hat{\theta}_i^2}{2 \times (n^E + n^C)}} = \sqrt{\frac{22 + 22}{22 \times 22} + \frac{0.563^2}{2 \times (22 + 22)}}$$

$$= \sqrt{0.094511} = 0.307426.$$

Performing the same steps for the other studies we get the following table with the standard errors as in Table 8.4 (at the last column).

Example 8.6 For the data in Table 8.3, find the 95% confidence interval for population effect size of the six studies.

Solution:

The 95% confidence interval for the effect size θ of the first study (Study 1) is obtained by computing the lower limit (LL) and upper limit (UL) as follows:

Table 8.4 Computations of estimated standard deviation of effect estimator

Study	$n_i^E = n_i^C = n_i$	$\hat{\theta}_i$	$SE(\hat{\theta}_i)$
Study 1	22	0.563	0.307426
Study 2	10	0.308	0.449857
Study 3	10	0.081	0.447397
Study 4	10	0.598	0.457100
Study 5	39	−0.178	0.226903
Study 6	50	−0.234	0.200683

$$LL = \hat{\theta}_1 - z_{\alpha/2} \times SE(\hat{\theta}_1) = 0.563 - 1.96 \times 0.3074 = 0.563 - 0.6025 = -0.0395 \text{ and}$$

$$UL = \hat{\theta}_1 + z_{\alpha/2} \times SE(\hat{\theta}_1) = 0.563 + 1.96 \times 0.3074 = 0.563 + 0.6025 = 1.1655.$$

Similar confidence intervals are computed for the other studies and reported in Table 8.5.

Example 8.7 For the data in Table 8.3 find the point estimate and 95% confidence interval for the common effect size θ under the fixed effect model.

Solution:

The estimate of the combined effect size θ under the fixed effect model is based on the sum of the last two columns of Table 8.6.

The point estimate of θ under the FE model is

$$\hat{\theta}_{FE} = \frac{\sum_{i=1}^{k} w_i \hat{\theta}_i}{\sum_{i=1}^{k} w_i} = \frac{1.478124}{69.55727} = 0.02125 \cong 0.021 \text{ and}$$

Table 8.5 The 95% confidence intervals for the population effect size

Study	$n_i^E = n_i^C = n_i$	$\hat{\theta}_i$	$SE(\hat{\theta}_i)$	LL of 95% CI	UL of 95% CI
Study 1	22	0.563	0.307426	−0.0395	1.1655
Study 2	10	0.308	0.449857	−0.5737	1.1897
Study 3	10	0.081	0.447397	−0.7959	0.9578
Study 4	10	0.598	0.457100	−0.2979	1.4939
Study 5	39	−0.178	0.226903	−0.6227	0.2667
Study 6	50	−0.234	0.200683	−0.6273	0.1593

Table 8.6 Computations for combined effect size estimate under FE model

Study	$n_i^E = n_i^C = n_i$	$\hat{\theta}_i$	$Var\left(\hat{\theta}_i\right)$	$w_i = \dfrac{1}{Var\left(\hat{\theta}_i\right)}$	$w_i\hat{\theta}_i$
Study 1	22	0.563	0.094511	10.58078	5.956978
Study 2	10	0.308	0.202372	4.941405	1.521953
Study 3	10	0.081	0.200164	4.995903	0.404668
Study 4	10	0.598	0.20894	4.786061	2.862064
Study 5	39	− 0.178	0.051485	19.42307	− 3.45731
Study 6	50	− 0.234	0.040274	24.83005	− 5.81023
			Sum	69.55727	1.478124

$$Var(\hat{\theta}_{FE}) = \frac{1}{\sum\limits_{i=1}^{k} w_i} = \frac{1}{69.55727} = 0.014377.$$ Therefore, the standard error of the

estimator is $SE(\hat{\theta}_{FE}) = \sqrt{\dfrac{1}{\sum\limits_{i=1}^{k} w_i}} = \sqrt{0.014377} = 0.119903.$

Now the 95% confidence interval for the common effect size θ is computed by obtaining the lower limit (LL) and upper limit (UL) as follows:

$$LL = \hat{\theta}_{FE} - z_{\alpha/2} \times SE(\hat{\theta}_{FE}) = 0.02125 - 1.96 \times 0.1199 = 0.021 - 0.235$$
$$= -0.214 = -0.21 \text{ and}$$

$$UL = \hat{\theta}_{FE} + z_{\alpha/2} \times SE(\hat{\theta}_{FE}) = 0.02125 + 1.96 \times 0.1199 = 0.021 + 0.235$$
$$= 0.256 = 0.26$$

Thus the 95% confidence interval of the common effect size under the fixed effect model is given by (–0.21, 0.26).

The above point estimate (–0.02) and the confidence interval (–0.21, 0.26) for the common effect size are displayed in the forest plot of meta-analysis at the very last row represented by a diamond. See Fig. 8.1.

Significance Test

To test the significance of the mean effect size of any individual study θ_i test the null hypothesis,

$H_0 : \theta_i = 0$ (null) against $H_a : \theta_i \neq 0$ for i = 1,2, ... k, using the test statistic

$$Z_i = \frac{\hat{\theta}_i - 0}{SE(\hat{\theta}_i)},$$

where the statistic Z_i follows the standard normal distribution.

Similarly, to test the significance of the common mean effect size θ of all studies under the FE model, test the null hypothesis

$H_0 : \theta = 0$ against $H_a : \theta \neq 0$ using the test statistic

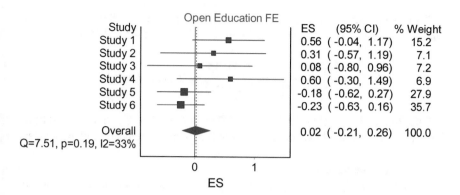

Fig. 8.1 Forest plot of meta-analysis on effects of Open Education on Attitude toward School under FE model

$$Z = \frac{\hat{\theta}_{FE}}{SE(\hat{\theta}_{FE})},$$

where the statistic Z follows the standard normal distribution.

For a two-tailed test, reject H_0 at the α level of significance if the calculated/observed value of the Z statistic (say z_0) satisfies $|z_0| \geq z_{\alpha/2}$, where $z_{\alpha/2}$ is the $\alpha/2$ level upper cut-off point of the standard normal distribution; otherwise don't reject the null hypothesis. Alternatively, reject H_0 at the α level of significance if the P-value is less than or equal to α; otherwise don't reject the null hypothesis.

Example 8.8 Using the data in Table 8.3 test the significance of the (a) mean effect size of the first study, and (b) common mean effect size of all studies under the FE model.

Solution:

(a) From previous calculations, for the first study (Study 1), we have estimated effect size $\hat{\theta}_1 = 0.563$ (for $i = 1$) and the standard error $SE\left(\hat{\theta}_1\right) = 0.307426$.

To test the significance of the population effect size of the first study, test $H_0 : \theta_1 = 0$ against $H_a : \theta_1 \neq 0$ using the observed value of the test statistic Z_1 (say z_{10})

$$z_{10} = \left[\frac{\hat{\theta}_1}{SE(\hat{\theta}_1)}\right] = \frac{0.563}{0.307426} = 1.831335 = 1.83.$$

The P-value is $P(|Z| > 1.83) = 2 \times 0.0336 = 0.0672$. Since the P-value is larger than 5%, we don't reject the null hypothesis at the 5% level of significance.

(b) Similarly, from previous calculations, the estimate of the common effect size under the FE model is $\hat{\theta}_{FE} = 0.02125$ and the standard error is $SE(\hat{\theta}_{FE}) = 0.119903$.

To test the significance of the common effect size, under the FE model, test $H_0 : \theta = 0$ against $H_a : \theta \neq 0$ using the observed value of the test statistic Z is

$$z_0 = \left[\frac{\hat{\theta}_{FE} - 0}{SE(\hat{\theta}_{FE})} \right] = \frac{0.02125}{0.119903} = 0.177227 = 1.77.$$

The P-value is $P(|Z| > 0.177) = 2 \times P(Z > 0.177) = 2 \times 0.4286 = 0.8572$. Since the P-value is too large, there is no sample evidence to reject the null hypothesis.

Measuring Heterogeneity

In many meta-analyses heterogeneity is a real problem and needs to be identified and handled properly for the validity of the results. Heterogeneity means that the variation in the study effect sizes exceeds that is expected due to random error. In practice, the observed variation is often not just random error but includes both true heterogeneity and study biases. Here we cover two the popular methods to identify and measure the extent of heterogeneity among independent studies.

Cochran's Q Statistic (Cochran 1973)

The Cochran's Q statistic is defined as the weighted sum of squares (WSS) of the estimated effect sizes

$$Q = \sum_{i=1}^{k} w_i \left(\hat{\theta}_i - \hat{\theta} \right)^2,$$

where $\hat{\theta}$ is the pooled estimate of the common effect size. The Q statistic can also be written as the sum of standardised differences as

$Q = \sum_{i=1}^{k} \left(\frac{\hat{\theta}_i - \hat{\theta}}{s_i} \right)^2$, where $s_i = \sqrt{v_i}$ is the within-study sample standard deviation of the ith study.

For computations, the following representation of Q is convenient

$$Q = \sum_{i=1}^{k} w_i \hat{\theta}_i^2 - \frac{\left(\sum_{i=1}^{k} w_i \hat{\theta}_i \right)^2}{\sum_{i=1}^{k} w_i}.$$

The above Q statistic follows a chi-squared distribution with $df = (k-1)$, where k is the number of studies included in the meta-analysis. Since the expected (mean) value of a chi-squared variable is its degrees of freedom, the expected value of Q is (k-1), that is, $E(Q) = E(WSS) = (k-1) = df$.

Since Q is the observed WSS (from the sample data) and df is the expected WSS, the difference between the two, $(Q - df)$, is the *excess variation* that represents the extent of heterogeneity in the study effect.

Test of Heterogeneity

To test the null hypothesis of the equality of effect sizes (i.e. equality excluding random error) across all studies, we test

$H_0 : \theta_1 = \theta_2 = \ldots = \theta_k = \theta$ against H_a : not all θ_i's are equal (at least one of them is different), using the following test statistic

$$Q = \sum_{i=1}^{k} w_i \hat{\theta}_i^2 - \frac{\left(\sum_{i=1}^{k} w_i \hat{\theta}_i \right)^2}{\sum_{i=1}^{k} w_i}.$$

Reject the null hypothesis at the α level of significance if the observed value of the Q statistic is larger than or equal to $\chi^2_{k-1,1-\alpha}$, the level α critical value of the chi-squared distribution with (k-1) df, such that $P\left(\chi^2_{k-1} \geq \chi^2_{k-1,1-\alpha}\right) = \alpha$; otherwise don't reject it. Thus higher values of the Q statistic would lead to the rejection of the null hypothesis. Alternatively, find the P-value as $p = P\left(\chi^2_{k-1,0} \geq \chi^2_{k-1}\right)$, where $\chi^2_{k-1,0}$ is the observed value of the chi-squared statistic, and reject H_0 at the α level of significance if the P-value is less than or equal to α; otherwise don't reject the null hypothesis.

The significant P-value leads to the conclusion that there is true difference among the effect sizes. However the non-significant P-value may not mean that the effect sizes are not different as this could happen due to low power of the test. The test should not be used as a sole measure of magnitude of the true differences.

The I^2 Statistic (Higgins et al. 2003)

The value of the Q-statistic increases as the number of studies included in the meta-analysis becomes larger. To dealt with this problem, the I^2 statistic is defined as a ratio of excess variation to the total variation expressed in percentages as follows:

$$I^2 = \left(\frac{Q - df}{Q} \right) \times 100\%,$$

and is viewed as the proportion of between studies variation and total variation (within plus between studies variation).

Table 8.7 Computations for the Q and I^2 statistics

Study	n	d	Var	w	wd	wd^2
Study 1	22	0.563	0.094511	10.58078	0.124609	3.353779
Study 2	10	0.308	0.202372	4.941395	0.009604	0.468761
Study 3	10	0.081	0.200164	4.995903	0.016641	0.032778
Study 4	10	0.598	0.20894	4.786063	0.150544	1.711515
Study 5	39	− 0.178	0.051485	19.42313	0.150544	0.615403
Study 6	50	− 0.234	0.040274	24.82992	0.197136	1.359587
Sum	141	1.138	0.797746	69.55719	0.649078	7.541822

Example 8.9 Using the data in Table 8.3, calculate the value of the Q and I^2 statistics.

Solution:

To answer the question, we need to calculate the weights (w) for each of the six studies and the sum of the products of w and d (wd) and sum of the product of w and d^2 (wd^2) as shown in Table 8.7.

Now, the Q statistic is calculated as

$$Q = \sum_{i=1}^{k} w_i \hat{\theta}_i^2 - \frac{\left(\sum_{i=1}^{k} w_i \hat{\theta}_i\right)^2}{\sum_{i=1}^{k} w_i} = 7.541828 - \frac{1.47814^2}{69.55719} = 7.51041 = 7.51.$$

To test the heterogeneity of effect sizes the P-value is found from the chi-squared Table (with df = 5) as $p = P\left(\chi_5^2 \geq 7.536\right) > 0.10$.

Note if the value of Q was 9.236 then the P-value would be exactly 0.10, since $P\left(\chi_5^2 \geq 9.236\right) = 0.10$. Since the P-value is not small, we can't reject the null hypothesis (of equal effect sizes).

The I^2 statistic is found to be

$$I^2 = \left(\frac{Q - df}{Q}\right) \times 100\% = \left(\frac{7.51041 - (6 - 1)}{7.51041}\right) \times 100\% = 0.334257 \times 100\% = 33\%,$$

where $df = (k - 1) = (6 - 1) = 5$. Note that I^2 represents the percentage of variation across studies that is due to real heterogeneity rather than chance.

Remark The above value of Q statistic, its exact P-value and I^2 statistic are presented in the forest plot produced by MetaXL on the left panel of Fig. 8.1.

Forest plot for SMD under FE model using MetaXL
The forest plot under the FE model (indicated by "IV" in the code) is constructed using MetaXL code

=MAInputTable("Open Education FE","ContSE","IV",B23:D28)

Remark: Explanations of MetaXL Code

For this type of meta-analyses in MetaXL the 'opening' code starts with MA Input Table ' = MAInputTable'. This is followed by an open parenthesis inside which the first quote contains the text that appears as the 'title of the output of the forest plot' e.g. "Open Education FE" in the above code (user may choose any appropriate title here, but FE is chosen to indicate fixed effect model). Then in the second quote enter the type of effect measure, e.g. "ContSE" in the above code which tells that the *outcome variable is continuous and standard error (SE) is used*. Within the third quote enter the statistical model, e.g. "IV" in the above code stands for the *fixed effect* (abbreviated by FE) model. Each quotation is followed by a comma, and after the last comma enter the data area in Excel Worksheet, e.g. B23:D28 in the above code tells that the data on the independent studies are taken from the specified cells of the Excel Worksheet. The code ends with a closing parenthesis.

The forest plot of the meta-analysis using the above MetaXL code is found in Fig. 8.1.

Interpretation

From the above meta-analysis as presented by the forest plot in Fig. 8.1, the estimated common effect size is 0.02, and the 95% confidence interval is (−0.21, 0.20). The effect size is not statistically significant at the 5% level (as 0 is included in the confidence interval).

The value of Q statistic (7.51) with P-value $= 0.19$ and $I^2 = 33\%$ show no significant heterogeneity among the studies.

8.5   Random Effects (RE) Model

For the REs model, there are two sources of errors or variation. The first source of errors is the error in estimating the true common effect size of a specific population (due to random variation within studies). The second source of error is from the variation of the true effect sizes of individual studies that are used to estimate the common true effect size (due to the between studies variation).

The variance of θ_i about θ is τ^2, which is known as the between study variance, and is estimated by the sample variance of $\hat{\theta}_i$ about θ and is denoted by $\hat{\tau}^2$. Thus, under the REs model the variance of the effect size estimator of the ith study is the sum of the within-study and between-study variances, that is, $v_i^* = v_i + \hat{\tau}^2$. Therefore, the weight assigned to each study is modified as follows:

$$w_i^* = \frac{1}{v_i + \hat{\tau}^2}.$$

Note that to make the sum of the weights equal to one, the following modified weight is used $w_i^{**} = \dfrac{\frac{1}{v_i + \hat{\tau}^2}}{\sum\limits_{i=1}^{k} \frac{1}{v_i + \hat{\tau}^2}} = \dfrac{w_i^*}{\sum\limits_{i=1}^{k} w_i^*}$.

The common effect size under the REs model is estimated by

$\hat{\theta}_{RE} = \sum\limits_{i=1}^{k} w_i^* \hat{\theta}_i \Big/ \sum\limits_{i=1}^{k} w_i^*$. The standard error of the estimator of the common effect size under the REs model is

$$ SE(\hat{\theta}_{RE}) = \sqrt{1 \Big/ \sum_{i=1}^{k} w_i^*}. $$

The $(1 - \alpha) \times 100\%$ confidence interval for the effect size θ under the REs model is given by the lower limit (LL) and upper limit (UL) as follows:

$$ LL = \hat{\theta}_{RE} - z_{\alpha/2} \times SE(\hat{\theta}_{RE}) \quad \text{and} $$
$$ UL = \hat{\theta}_{RE} + z_{\alpha/2} \times SE(\hat{\theta}_{RE}), $$

where $z_{\alpha/2}$ is the $\frac{\alpha}{2}$ th cut-off point of standard normal distribution.

Note that the estimator of the common effect size under the REs model is the simple weighted mean of the individual effect sizes, but the weights depend on both the within-study and between-study variances. The weights (w_i^*'s) are also based on the inflated inverse variance such that they add up to 1.

Estimation of τ^2

The between studies variance is estimated as a scaled excess variation as follows
$\hat{\tau}^2 = \frac{Q - df}{C}$,
where

$$ Q = \sum_{i=1}^{k} w_i \hat{\theta}_i^2 - \frac{\left(\sum\limits_{i=1}^{k} w_i \hat{\theta}_i\right)^2}{\sum\limits_{i=1}^{k} w_i}, \quad C = \sum_{i=1}^{k} w_i - \frac{\sum\limits_{i=1}^{k} w_i^2}{\sum\limits_{i=1}^{k} w_i} $$

and $df = (k - 1)$ in which k is the number of studies.

Example 8.10 Consider the data on effect of Open education on the Attitude towards School as in Table 8.3.

Find the (i) estimated value of τ^2 (ii) point estimate of the population effect size and standard error of estimator and (ii) 95% confidence interval of the population effect size under the REs model.

Solution:

To answer this question first we need to compute the summary statistics as in Table 8.8.

Table 8.8 Calculations to find the summary statistics for REs model

Study	d	Var	w	wd	wd^2	w^2	Var*	w*	w*d
Study 1	0.563	0.0945	10.5808	5.957	3.3538	111.9529	0.1422	7.0315	3.9587
Study 2	0.308	0.2024	4.9414	1.5219	0.4688	24.41739	0.2501	3.9987	1.2316
Study 3	0.081	0.2002	4.9959	0.4047	0.0328	24.95905	0.2479	4.0344	0.3268
Study 4	0.598	0.2089	4.78606	2.8621	1.7115	22.9064	0.2566	3.8964	2.33
Study 5	− 0.18	0.0515	19.4231	− 3.457	0.6154	377.2581	0.0992	10.081	− 1.7945
Study 6	− 0.23	0.0403	24.8299	− 5.81	1.3596	616.5247	0.088	11.366	− 2.6597
			69.5572	**1.4781**	**7.5418**	**1178.018**	**1.084**	**40.409**	**3.393**

Here the combined variance (Var*) is the sum of Var and Tau^2, and modified weight (w*) is the weight under the REs model calculated as the reciprocal of Var*.

As an illustration, for **Study 1**, the modified variance for the REs model is found to be $v_1^* = v_1 + \hat{\tau}^2 = 0.0945 + 0.0477 = 0.14222$ and the modified weight becomes $w_1^* = 1/Var_1^* = \frac{1}{0.14222} = 7.0315$.

Similarly for the second study (**Study 2**), the modified variance is $v_2^* = v_2 + \hat{\tau}^2 = 0.2024 + 0.0477 = 0.2501$.

Hence the modified weight becomes

$$w^* = \frac{1}{Var_1^*} = \frac{1}{0.2501} = 3.9987.$$

(i) Using the summary statistics from Table 8.8, we calculate the estimated value of the between studies variance

$$\hat{\tau}^2 = \frac{Q - df}{C},$$

through computing its components as follows:

$$Q = \sum_{i=1}^{k} w_i \hat{\theta}_i^2 - \frac{\left(\sum_{i=1}^{k} w_i \hat{\theta}_i\right)^2}{\sum_{i=1}^{k} w_i} = 1.47814 - \frac{(7.5418)^2}{69.55719} = 7.5104 \approx 7.51,$$

$$C = \sum_{i=1}^{k} w_i - \frac{\sum_{i=1}^{k} w_i^2}{\sum_{i=1}^{k} w_i} = 69.55719 - \frac{1178.0185}{69.55719} = 52.62122$$

and $df = k - 1 = 6 - 1 = 5$.

So the estimated value of the between studies variance becomes

$$\hat{\tau}^2 = \frac{Q - df}{C} = \frac{7.5104 - 5}{52.62122} = 0.047707 \approx 0.05.$$

(ii) The point estimate of the common effect size under the REs model is given by

$$\hat{\theta}_{RE} = \sum_{i=1}^{k} w_i^* \hat{\theta}_i \Bigg/ \sum_{i=1}^{k} w_i^* = \sum_{i=1}^{6} w^* d \Bigg/ \sum_{i=1}^{6} w^* = \frac{3.39399}{40.4085} = 0.083967 \approx 0.08.$$

The standard error of the estimator of the common effect size is

$$SE(\hat{\theta}_{RE}) = \sqrt{1 \Big/ \sum_{i=1}^{k} w_i^*} = \sqrt{1 \Big/ \sum_{i=1}^{k} w^*} = \sqrt{\frac{1}{40.4085}} = 0.157313.$$

(iii) The 95% confidence interval for the population effect size θ under the REs model is given by the lower limit (LL) and upper limit (UL) as follows:

$$LL = \hat{\theta}_{RE} - 1.96 \times SE(\hat{\theta}_{RE}) = 0.083967 - 1.96 \times 0.157313 = -0.2244 \approx -0.22 \text{ and}$$
$$UL = \hat{\theta}_{RE} + 1.96 \times SE(\hat{\theta}_{RE}) = 0.083967 + 1.96 \times 0.157313 = 0.3923 \approx 0.39.$$

Comment The above point estimate (0.08) and the confidence interval (−0.22, 0.39) are presented at the bottom row of the forest plot and represented by a diamond as in Fig. 8.2.

Forest plot for SMD under RE model using MetaXL
The forest plot under the RE model (indicated by "RE" in the code) is constructed using MetaXL code
=MAInputTable("Open Education RE","ContSE","RE",B23:D28)

Remark: Explanations of MetaXL Code
For this type of meta-analyses in MetaXL the 'opening' code starts with MA Input Table '=MAInputTable'. This is followed by an open parenthesis inside which the first quote contains the text that appears as the 'title of the output of the forest plot' e.g. "Open Education RE" in the above code (user may choose any appropriate title here, but RE is chosen to indicate random effects model). Then in the second quote enter the type of effect measure, e.g. "ContSE" in the above code which tells that the *outcome variable is continuous and standard error (SE) is used*. Within the third quote enter the statistical model, e.g. "RE" in the above code stands for the *random*

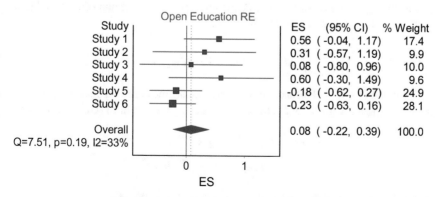

Fig. 8.2 Forest plot of meta-analysis on effects of Open Education on Attitude toward School under REs model

effects (abbreviated by RE) model. Each quotation is followed by a comma, and after the last comma enter the data area in Excel Worksheet, e.g. B23:D28 in the above code tells that the data on the independent studies are taken from the specified cells of the Excel Worksheet. The code ends with a closing parenthesis.

The forest plot of the meta-analysis using the above MetaXL code is found in Fig. 8.2.

Interpretation

From the above meta-analysis as presented by the forest plot, the estimated common effect size is 0.08, and the 95% confidence interval is (–0.22, 0.39). The effect size is not statistically significant (as 0 is included in the confidence interval).

Conclusion: The Open education has not significantly changed Attitude towards School.

8.6   Inverse Variance Heterogeneity (IVhet) Model

Under the inverse variance heterogeneity (IVhet) model estimate of the common effect size θ ($=$ SMD) is given by

$$\hat{\theta}_{IVhet} = \frac{\sum_{i=1}^{k} w_i \hat{\theta}_i}{\sum_{i=1}^{k} w_i}.$$

Then the variance of the estimator under the IVhet model is given by

$$Var(\hat{\theta}_{IVhet}) = \sum_{i=1}^{k} \left[\left(\frac{1}{v_i} \middle/ \sum_{i=1}^{k} \frac{1}{v_i} \right)^2 (v_i + \hat{\tau}^2) \right].$$

For the computation of the confidence interval of the common effect size based on the IVhet model use the following standard error

$$SE(\hat{\theta}_{IVhet}) = \sqrt{Var(\hat{\theta}_{IVhet})}.$$

Then, the $(1 - \alpha) \times 100\%$ confidence interval for the common effect size θ under the IVhet model is given by the lower limit (LL) and upper limit (UL) as follows:

$$LL = \hat{\theta}_{IVhet} - z_{\alpha/2} \times SE(\hat{\theta}_{IVhet})$$
$$UL = \hat{\theta}_{IVhet} + z_{\alpha/2} \times SE(\hat{\theta}_{IVhet}),$$

where $z_{\alpha/2}$ is the $\frac{\alpha}{2}$ th cut-off point of standard normal distribution.

Table 8.9 Calculations of combined variance and modified weights for IVhet model

Study	d	Var	w	Tau^2	Var*	W*	Wd
Study 1	0.563	0.0945	10.581	0.047707	0.14222	0.00329	5.957
Study 2	0.308	0.2024	4.9414	0.047707	0.25008	0.00126	1.5219
Study 3	0.081	0.2002	4.9959	0.047707	0.24787	0.00128	0.4047
Study 4	0.598	0.2089	4.7861	0.047707	0.25665	0.00122	2.8621
Study 5	− 0.178	0.0515	19.423	0.047707	0.09919	0.00773	− 3.4573
Study 6	− 0.234	0.0403	24.83	0.047707	0.08798	0.01121	− 5.8102
			69.557			**0.02599**	**1.4781**

Illustration of IVhet Model for SMD

Example 8.11 Consider the data on the effect of Open education on the Attitude towards School as in Table 8.3.

Find the (i) point estimate of the population effect size and standard error of estimator, and (ii) 95% confidence interval of the population effect size under the IVhet model.

Solution:

To answer this question we need to compute the values in Table 8.9.

Here Var* is the combined variance $\left(Var_i^* = v_i + \hat{\tau}^2\right)$ and W* is the modified weight under the IVhet model calculated as

$$W_i^* = \left[\left(\frac{1}{v_i} \bigg/ \sum_{i=1}^{k} \frac{1}{v_i}\right)^2 (v_i + \hat{\tau}^2)\right] = \left(w_i \bigg/ \sum_{1}^{k} w_i\right) \times Var_i^* \text{ for the ith study.}$$

For example, for **Study 1**,

$Var_1^* = 0.0945 + 0.047707 = 0.14222$, and $W_1^* = \left(\frac{10.581}{69.557}\right) \times 0.14222 = 0.00329$

(i) The point estimate of the common population effect size under the IVhet model is

$$\hat{\theta}_{IVhet} = \frac{\sum_{i=1}^{6} w_i \hat{\theta}_i}{\sum_{i=1}^{6} w_i} = \frac{\sum_{i=1}^{6} wd}{\sum_{i=1}^{6} w} = \frac{1.4781}{69.557} = 0.021251 \approx 0.02,$$

and standard error of estimator is

$$SE(\hat{\theta}_{IVhet}^*) = \sqrt{\sum_{i=1}^{6} W_i^*} = \sqrt{0.02599} = 0.16122.$$

(ii)   The 95% confidence interval of the population effect size under the IVhet model
        is given by the lower limit (LL) and upper limit (UL) as follows:

$$LL = \hat{\theta}_{IVhet} - 1.96 \times SE(\hat{\theta}_{IVhet}) = 0.083967 - 1.96 \times 0.16122 = -0.294744 \approx -0.29$$
$$UL = \hat{\theta}_{IVhet} + z_{\alpha/2} \times SE(\hat{\theta}_{IVhet}) = 0.083967 + 1.96 \times 0.16122 = 0.33725 \approx 0.34.$$

Comment The above point estimate (0.02) and 95% confidence interval (–0.29,
0.34) are presented at the bottom row of the forest plot and represented by a diamond
as in Fig. 8.3.

Forest plot for SMD under IVhet model using MetaXL
The forest plot under the IVhet model (indicated by "IVhet" in the code) is constructed
using MetaXL code
     =MAInputTable("Open Education IVhet","ContSE","IVhet",B23:D28)

Remark: Explanations of MetaXL Code
For this type of meta-analyses in MetaXL the 'opening' code starts with MA Input
Table ' = MAInputTable'. This is followed by an open parenthesis inside which the
first quote contains the text that appears as the 'title of the output of the forest plot'
e.g. "Open Education IVhet" in the above code (user may choose any appropriate title
here, but IVhet is chosen to indicate inverse variance heterogeneity model). Then
in the second quote enter the type of effect measure, e.g. "ContSE" in the above
code which tells that the *outcome variable is continuous and standard error (SE)
is used*. Within the third quote enter the statistical model, e.g. "IVhet" in the above
code stands for the inverse variance heterogeneity (abbreviated by IVhet) model.
Each quotation is followed by a comma, and after the last comma enter the data
area in Excel Worksheet, e.g. B23:D28 in the above code tells that the data on the
independent studies are taken from the specified cells of the Excel Worksheet. The
code ends with a closing parenthesis.

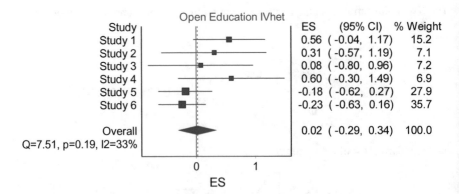

Fig. 8.3 Forest plot of meta-analysis on effects of Open Education on Attitude toward School under
IVhet model

The forest plot of the meta-analysis using the above MetaXL code is found to be

Interpretation
From the above forest plot, the estimated common effect size is 0.02, and the 95% confidence interval is (–0.29, 0.34). The effect size is not statistically significant (as 0 is included in the confidence interval).

8.7 Meta-Analyses of d, g and Δ Under the FE, RE and IVhet Models

Example 8.12 Consider the summary data on operative time for the Laparoscopic-assisted Rectal Resection (LARR) versus Open Rectal Resection (ORR) for Carcinoma from nine independent studies from Memon et al. 2018 (Table 8.10).

The meta-analyses of the data in Table 8.10 using SMD effect size measures of (a) Cohen's d, (b) Hedges' g and (c) Glass' Δ under (i) fixed effect (FE), (ii) random effects (REs), and (iii) inverse variance heterogeneity (IVhet) model are provided below.

(i) Meta-analysis of operative time for LARR and ORR procedures using SMD effect sizes under the fixed effect model

Using the MetaXL Code = MAInputTable("Operative Time Cohen FE","Cohen","RE",B5:H13) the following forest plot is produced for Cohen's d under the fixed effect model (for other methods change the word 'Cohen' by 'Hedges' or 'Glass') (Fig. 8.4).

Comments The common effect size estimate (0.84) and confidence interval (0.77, 0.92) are the same for both Cohen's d and Hedges' g. Because of the large sample

Table 8.10 Summary data on sample size, mean and standard deviation of LARR and ORR groups

Study	LARR			ORR		
	n	Mean	Stdev	n	Mean	Stdev
Bonjer et al. (2015)	699	241	33.6	345	191.5	26.2
Fleshman et al. (2015)	240	266.2	101.9	222	220.6	92.4
Stevenson et al. (2015)	238	210	66.7	235	190	59.2
Jeong et al. (2014)	170	244.9	75.4	170	197	62.9
Ng et al. (2014)	40	211.6	53	40	153	41.1
Liang et al. (2011)	169	138.08	23.79	174	118.53	21.99
Lujan et al. (2009)	101	193.7	45.1	103	172.9	59.4
Ng et al. (2008)	51	213.5	46.2	48	163.7	43.4
Zhou et al. (2004)	82	120	18	89	106	25

(a)

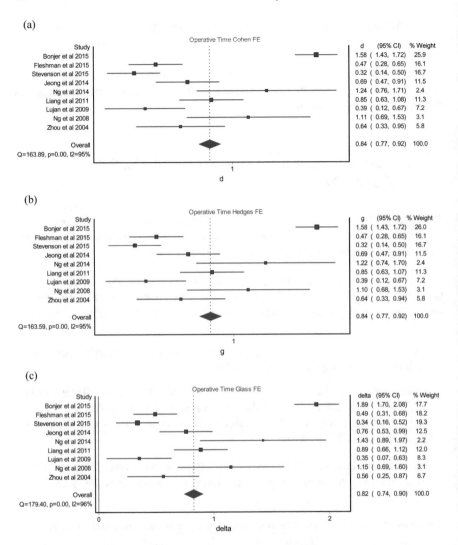

Fig. 8.4 Forest plots under FE model for different SMD measures (**a**) Forest plot of **Cohen's d** under FE model, (**b**) Forest plot of **Hedges' g** under FE model, (**c**) Forest plot of **Glass' Δ** under FE model

sizes there is almost no differences between these two SMDs and confidence intervals. However, the results of Glass' method (estimate 0.82, CI: 0.74, 0.90) are different from the other two methods. Regardless of the method, the effect size is significant as the 95% confidence interval does not include 0 in any of the forest plots. So, there is much longer mean operative time for the LARR procedure compared to the ORR procedure.

(ii) Meta-analysis of operative time for LARR and ORR procedures using SMD effect sizes under the random effects model

Using the MetaXL Code = MAInputTable("Operative Time Cohen RE","Cohen","RE",B5:H13) the following forest plot is produced for Cohen's d under the random effects model (for other methods change the word 'Cohen' by 'Hedges' or 'Glass') (Fig. 8.5).

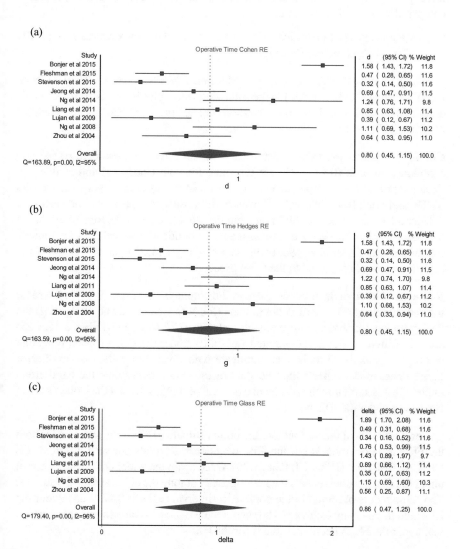

Fig. 8.5 Forest plots under REs model for different SMD measures (**a**) Forest plot of **Cohen's d** under REs model, (**b**) Forest plot of **Hedges' g** under REs model, (**c**) Forest plot of **Glass' Δ** under REs model

Comments Under the REs model the common effect size estimate (0.80) and confidence interval (0.45, 1.15) are the same for both Cohen's d and Hedges' g. Because of the large sample sizes there is almost no differences between the two SMDs and confidence intervals. However, the results of Glass' method (estimate 0.86, and CI: 0.47, 1.25) are different from the other two methods. Regardless of the method, the effect size is significant as the 95% confidence interval does not include 0 in any of the forest plots. So, there is much longer mean operative time for the LARR procedure compared to the ORR procedure.

(iii) Meta-analysis of operative time for LARR and ORR procedures using SMD effect sizes under the IVhet model

Using the MetaXL Code = MAInputTable("Operative Time Cohen IVhet","Cohen","IVhet",B5:H13) the following forest plot is produced for Cohen's d under the IVhet model (for other methods change the word 'Cohen' by 'Hedges' or 'Glass') (Fig. 8.6).

Comments Under the IVhet model the common effect size estimate (0.84) and confidence interval (0.44, 1.25) are the same for both Cohen's d and Hedges' g. Because of the large sample sizes there is almost no differences between the two SMDs and confidence intervals. However, the results of Glass' method (estimate 0.82, and CI: 0.38, 1.26) are different from the other two methods. Regardless of the method, the effect size is significant as the 95% confidence interval does not include 0 in any of the forest plots. So, there is much longer mean operative time for the LARR procedure compared to the ORR procedure.

Remarks Although the point estimate of the common effect size (0.84) is the same for both the fixed effect and IVhet models (for both Cohen's d and Hedges' g) the 95% confidence intervals confidence intervals (FE: 0.77, 0.92) and (IVhet: 0.44, 1.25) are very different. Due to the inflated variability under the IVhet model, reflecting heterogeneity as the Q statistic is significant with P-value = 0, the margin of error in the IVhet model reflects the true state of the nature rather than the fixed effect model. This is similar to the confidence interval of (0.45, 1.15) for the Cohen's d and Hedges' g under the REs model.

For the results of Glass' method, the point estimate (0.82) is the same under both the FE and IVhet models but the 95% confidence intervals are very different (FE CI: 0.74, 0.90) and (IVhet CI: 0.38, 1.26). Once again the wider confidence interval under the IVhet model reflects the heterogeneity among the effect size of the studies. The same fact is observed in the confidence interval (RE CI: 0.47, 1.25) under the REs model. The point estimate (0.86) under the RE model is also slightly higher than that under the FE/IVhet model (0.82) for the Glass' method.

(a) Forest

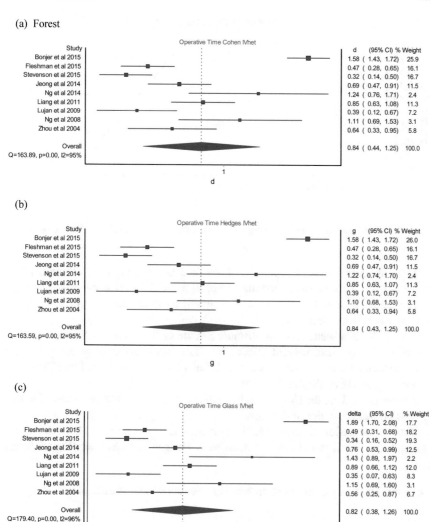

Fig. 8.6 Forest plots under IVhet model for different SMD measures (**a**) Forest plot of **Cohen's d** under IVhet model, (**b**) Forest plot of **Hedges' g** under IVhet model, (**c**) Forest plot of **Glass' Δ** under IVhet model

8.8 Publication Bias

Publication bias is usually detected by using funnel plot or Doi plot. A funnel plot is a scatter plot of standard error of the studies against effect size (or transformed effect size).

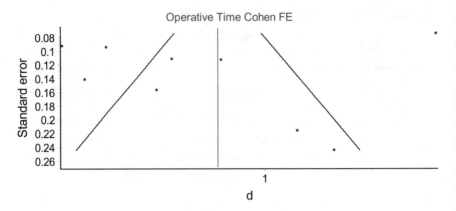

Fig. 8.7 Funnel plot indicating heterogeneity among effect sizes (Cohen's d of Operative Time)

The publication bias of Operative Time data in Example 8.12 (Table 8.10) is studied in this section. The following two plots use Cohen's d as the effect size.

The funnel plot in Fig. 8.7 is roughly symmetrical indicating very low (or no) heterogeneity in the data.

A Doi plot is a scatter plot of absolute z-score of the value of effect size versus the effect size (or transformed effect size). The individual dots on the graph are then connected with a continuous curve. Details are found in A. S. Doi (2018) and Furuya-Kanamori et al. (2018).

For the given data, the Doi plot in Fig. 8.8 indicates no asymmetry indicating that there is no heterogeneity in the data.

Similar conclusion of no heterogeneity in the data is reached from both the funnel plot and Doi plot if the effect size measure is Hedges' g as follows (Figs. 8.9 and 8.10).

Remark The study of publication bias is not based on any statistical models.

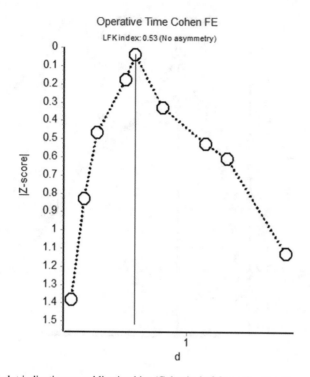

Fig. 8.8 Doi plot indicating no publication bias (Cohen's d of Operative Time)

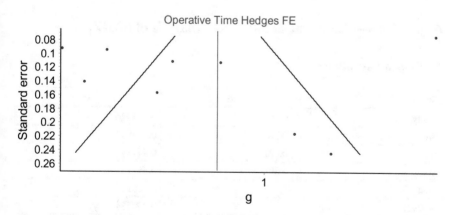

Fig. 8.9 Funnel plot indicating no publication bias (Hedges' g of Operative Time)

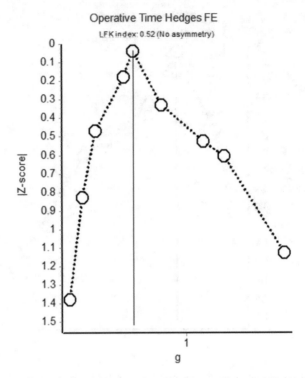

Fig. 8.10 Doi plot indicating no publication bias (Hedges' g of Operative Time)

Appendix 8—Stata Codes for Meta-Analysis of SMD

A8.1 Open Education dataset

Study	d	se
Study 1	0.563	0.307426
Study 2	0.308	0.449858
Study 3	0.081	0.447397
Study 4	0.598	0.4571
Study 5	−0.178	0.226903
Study 6	−0.234	0.200684

A8.2 Stat codes for SMD meta-analysis under different statistical models

```
. ssc install admetan
    Codes for SMD meta-analysis under FE, RRs and Ivhet models
    . admetan d se, iv
    . admetan d se, re
    . admetan d se, ivhet
```

A8.3 Operative Time dataset

study	n_larr	mean_larr	sd_larr	n_orr	mean_orr	sd_orr
Bonjer et al. (2015)	699	241	33.6	345	191.5	26.2
Fleshman et al. (2015)	240	266.2	101.9	222	220.6	92.4
Stevenson et al. (2015)	238	210	66.7	235	190	59.2
Jeong et al. (2014)	170	244.9	75.4	170	197	62.9
Ng et al. (2014)	40	211.6	53	40	153	41.1
Liang et al. (2011)	169	138.08	23.79	174	118.53	21.99
Lujan et al. (2009)	101	193.7	45.1	103	172.9	59.4
Ng et al. (2008)	51	213.5	46.2	48	163.7	43.4
Zhou et al. (2004)	82	120	18	89	106	25

A8.4 Stata codes for SMD meta-analysis of Operation Time dataset

. *ssc install admetan*

Codes for SMD meta-analysis of FE model for different effect sizes

. admetan n_larr mean_larr sd_larr n_orr mean_orr sd_orr, cohen

. admetan n_larr mean_larr sd_larr n_orr mean_orr sd_orr, hedges

. admetan n_larr mean_larr sd_larr n_orr mean_orr sd_orr, glass

Codes for SMD meta-analysis of REs model for different effect sizes

. admetan n_larr mean_larr sd_larr n_orr mean_orr sd_orr, cohen re

. admetan n_larr mean_larr sd_larr n_orr mean_orr sd_orr, hedges re

. admetan n_larr mean_larr sd_larr n_orr mean_orr sd_orr, glass re

Codes for SMD meta-analysis of IVhet model for different effect sizes

. admetan n_larr mean_larr sd_larr n_orr mean_orr sd_orr, cohen ivhet

. admetan n_larr mean_larr sd_larr n_orr mean_orr sd_orr, hedges ivhet

. admetan n_larr mean_larr sd_larr n_orr mean_orr sd_orr, glass ivhet

References

Borenstein M, Hedges LV, Higgins JP, Rothstein HR (2010) A basic introduction to fixed-effect and random-effects models for meta-analysis. Res Synth Methods 1(2):97–111

Borenstein MH, Larry, Higgins J, Rothstein H (2009) Introduction to meta-analysis. Wiley-Blackwell, Oxford

Cochran WG (1973) Experiments for nonlinear functions (R.A. Fisher Memorial Lecture). J Am Stat Assoc 68(344):771–781. https://doi.org/10.1080/01621459.1973.10481423

Cohen J (1969) Statistical power analysis for the behavioral sciences. Academic Press, Nw York

Cohen J (1987) Statistical power analysis for the behavioral sciences. Lawrence Erlbaum Associates, Hillside, NJ

Doi AS (2018) Rendering the Doi plot properly in meta-analysis. Int J Evid-Based Healthc 16(4):242–243. https://doi.org/10.1097/XEB.0000000000000158

Doi SA, Barendregt JJ, Khan S, Thalib L, Williams GM (2015a) Advances in the meta-analysis of heterogeneous clinical trials I: the inverse variance heterogeneity model. Contemp Clin Trials 45(Pt A):130–138. https://doi.org/10.1016/j.cct.2015.05.009

Doi SA, Barendregt JJ, Khan S, Thalib L, Williams GM (2015b) Advances in the meta-analysis of heterogeneous clinical trials II: the quality effects model. Contemp Clin Trials 45(Pt A):123–129. https://doi.org/10.1016/j.cct.2015.05.010

Doi SA, Barendregt JJ, Khan S, Thalib L, Williams GM (2015c) Simulation comparison of the quality effects and random effects methods of meta-analysis. Epidemiology 26(4):e42–44

Furuya-Kanamori JL, Barendregt ARJ, Doi ARS (2018) A new improved graphical and quantitative method for detecting bias in meta-analysis. Int J Evid-Based Healthc 16(4):195–203. https://doi.org/10.1097/XEB.0000000000000141

Glass GV, Smith ML, McGaw B (1981) Meta-analysis in social research. Sage Publications, Incorporated

Hedges LV (1981) Distribution theory for Glass's estimator of effect size and related estimators. J Educ Stat 6(2):107–128

Hedges LV (1982) Estimation of effect size from a series of independent experiments. Psychol Bull 92(2):490–499. https://doi.org/10.1037/0033-2909.92.2.490

Hedges LV (1985) Statistical methods for meta-analysis. Academic Press, Boston

Higgins JP, Thompson SG, Deeks JJ, Altman DG (2003) Measuring inconsistency in meta-analyses. BMJ 327(7414):557–560

Chapter 9
Meta-Analysis of Weighted Mean Difference

Mean difference can be used as an effect size measure if the outcome variable has the same unit of measurement for both the treatment/intervention and placebo/control groups. The raw mean difference can be scaled by the inverse variance weight to define weighted mean difference (WMD). Unlike the SMD, the WMD retains the same unit of measurement as the outcome variable.

Meta-analysis of weighted mean difference (WMD) is covered in this chapter. It provides meta-analysis of WMD under different statistical models along with subgroup analysis with illustrative examples.

9.1 Weighted Mean Difference

For two arms experiments/studies the difference of the two means of an outcome variable is a good starting point to measure the effect size. The raw mean difference is simply the difference of the means of the two arms. It is not essential to standardize the raw mean difference as an effect size measure unless the outcome variable is measured in different units. In many cases the raw mean difference is used as an effect size measure, but it is weighted by the inverse variance. The process produces the weighted mean difference (WMD) as a measure of effect size. This WMD measure retains the same unit of measurement as the outcome variable and is used in many meta-analyses.

9.2 Estimation of Effect Size

Consider an experiment or study with patients randomly divided into two arms, the treatment group with mean of the outcome variable (say Y) to be μ_1 (or μ_T) and control/placebo group having mean μ_2 (or μ_P). Based on a random sample of size

© Springer Nature Singapore Pte Ltd. 2020
S. Khan, *Meta-Analysis*, Statistics for Biology and Health,
https://doi.org/10.1007/978-981-15-5032-4_9

n_1 from the treatment group, let the sample mean be $\hat{\mu}_1 = \bar{Y}_1$ and sample variance be $\hat{\sigma}_1^2 = S_1^2$. Similarly, of another random sample of size n_2 for the placebo group, let the sample mean be $\hat{\mu}_2 = \bar{Y}_2$ and sample variance be $\hat{\sigma}_2^2 = S_2^2$. The sample means and variances are used as estimates of the respective population mean and variance. Assume that both samples are independent the populations are normally distributed.

Then the population raw mean difference $\delta = \mu_1 - \mu_2$ is estimated by the sample mean difference $\hat{\delta} = \bar{Y}_1 - \bar{Y}_2$. As discussed in the previous chapter, the standard error (SE) of the estimator of δ depends on whether the two population standard deviations are equal or not. If the equality of population standard deviations are unknown, we will assume that they are not equal and use appropriate formula to calculate the variance and SE.

For any individual study, let us define population weighted mean difference (WMD) as $\theta = \omega\delta$, where $\omega = 1/\sigma^2$, in which σ^2 is the population variance of δ, is the inverse variance weight of the population mean difference δ. The population WMD, θ is an unknown parameter. An estimator of θ is given by its sample counterpart $\hat{\theta} = w\hat{\delta}$, where $w = 1/v$ is the sample weight, in which $v = \hat{\sigma}^2$ is the sample variance, and $\hat{\delta} = \bar{Y}_1 - \bar{Y}_2$ is the estimate of unknown population mean difference, δ.

In a meta-analysis with $i = 1, 2, \ldots, k$ independent studies, the sample WMD of the ith study is defined as $\hat{\theta}_i = w_i\hat{\delta}_i$ with standard error $SE_i = \sqrt{v_i}$.

So the estimate of the common effect size of all studies is given by $\hat{\theta} = \sum_1^k w_i\hat{\delta}_i \Big/ \sum_1^k w_i$ and the standard error of the estimator of θ becomes $SE(\hat{\theta}) = \sqrt{1 \Big/ \sum_1^k w_i}$.

Then the $(1 - \alpha) \times 100\%$ confidence interval for population WMD, θ is given by the lower limit (LL) and upper limit (UL) as follows:

$$LL = \hat{\theta} - z_{\frac{\alpha}{2}} \times SE(\hat{\theta}) \text{ and}$$

$$LL = \hat{\theta} + z_{\frac{\alpha}{2}} \times SE(\hat{\theta}),$$

where $z_{\frac{\alpha}{2}}$ is the critical value of standard normal distribution leaving $\frac{\alpha}{2}$ area on the upper (or lower) tail of the normal curve.

Example 9.1 Consider the summary data on blood loss for the Laparoscopic-assisted Rectal Resection (LARR) versus Open Rectal Resection (ORR) for Carcinoma from eleven independent studies from Memon et al. 2018.

Table 9.1 Summary statistics of blood loss of eleven studies on sample size, mean and standard deviation of LARR and ORR groups

Study	LARR			ORR		
	n	Mean	Stdev	n	Mean	Stdev
Bonjer et al. (2015)	699	200	222	345	400	370
Fleshman et al. (2015)	240	256.1	305.8	222	318.4	331.7
Stevenson et al. (2015)	238	100	111	235	150	181.5
Jeong et al. (2014)	170	200	148	170	217.5	185
Ng et al. (2014)	40	141.8	500	40	361.1	623
Liu et al. (2011)	98	310	96	88	380	85
Lujan et al. (2009)	101	127.8	113.3	103	234.2	174.3
Ng et al. (2009)	76	280	500	77	337	423
Ng et al. (2008)	51	321.7	750	48	555.6	1188
Braga et al. (2007)	83	213	258	85	396	258
Zhou et al. (2004)	82	20	19	89	92	25

For the above data find the (i) raw mean difference (mean LARR–mean ORR) and standard error of the estimator of population mean difference, (ii) calculate 95% confidence interval for the population mean difference of each of the studies, and (iii) the weight for the first (Bonjer et al. 2015) study.

Solution:
The calculated values of the mean difference (MD), variance of mean difference (Var), standard error of mean difference (SE), weight as inverse variance (W), lower limit (LL) and upper limit (UL) of 95% confidence interval, and sum of W and sum of product of W and MD are shown in Table 9.2.

Explanations of calculations in Table 9.2
To answer the questions in Example 9.1, consider the calculations for the first study (Bonjier et al. 2015):

(i) The raw mean difference is $\hat{\delta}_i = $ MD = difference of mean of LARR and ORR groups $ = 200–400 = -200$.

The variance of the mean difference (assuming population variances are unequal) is

$$\text{Var} = \frac{S_L^2}{n_L} + \frac{S_O^2}{n_O} = \frac{222^2}{699} + \frac{370^2}{345} = 467.318.$$

Then the standard error becomes
$\text{SE} = \sqrt{467.318} = 21.6175$.

Table 9.2 Calculated values of the summary statistics for the mean difference of blood loss

Study	MD	Var	SE	LL	UL	W	WxMD
Bonjer et al. (2015)	−200	467.32	21.618	−242.4	−157.63	0.0021	−0.428
Fleshman et al. (2015)	−62.3	885.25	29.753	−120.6	−3.9839	0.0011	−0.0704
Stevenson et al. (2015)	−50	191.95	13.855	−77.15	−22.845	0.0052	−0.2605
Jeong et al. (2014)	−17.5	330.17	18.171	−53.11	18.114	0.003	−0.053
Ng et al. (2014)	−219	15953	126.31	−466.9	28.26	6E-05	−0.0137
Liu et al. (2011)	−70	176.14	13.272	−96.01	−43.987	0.0057	−0.3974
Lujan et al. (2009)	−106	422.05	20.544	−146.7	−66.134	0.0024	−0.2521
Ng et al. (2009)	−57	5613.2	74.921	−203.8	89.846	0.0002	−0.0102
Ng et al. (2008)	−234	40432	201.08	−628	160.21	2E-05	−0.0058
Braga et al. (2007)	−183	1585.1	39.813	−261	−104.97	0.0006	−0.1155
Zhou et al. (2004)	−72	11.425	3.3801	−78.62	−65.375	0.0875	−6.302
						0.10798	**−7.9085**

(ii) The lower limit of the 95% confidence interval is

LL $= -200 - 1.96 \times 21.6175 = -242.37$ and upper limit is
UL $= -200 + 1.96 \times 21.6175 = -157.63$.

(iii) The weight (for the first study) is $W = \frac{1}{Var} = \frac{1}{467.32} = 0.00214$ and WxMD
$= 0.00214 \times (-200) = -0.428$.

9.3 Tests on Effect Size

To test the significance of the unknown common effect size, θ, test the null hypothesis
$H_0 : \theta = 0$ against $H_A : \theta \neq 0$ using the test statistic
$Z = \frac{\hat{\theta}}{SE(\hat{\theta})}$ which follows a standard normal distribution.
For a two-tailed test, reject H_0 at the α level of significance (in favour of the
alternative hypothesis) if the observed (or calculated) value of Z statistic satisfies
$|z_0| \geq z_{\alpha/2}$; otherwise don't reject the null hypothesis (of a two-sided test).

Example 9.2 Consider the blood loss data from eleven independent studies in
Table 9.1

Test the significance of the common effect size, θ.

Solution:
To test the significance of the unknown common effect size θ, test the null hypothesis
$H_0 : \theta = 0$ against $H_A : \theta \neq 0$ use the test statistic Z as

$$z_0 = \frac{\hat{\theta}}{SE(\hat{\theta})} = \frac{-73.2411}{3.043199} = -24.0671. \text{[see Example 9.3 for details]}$$

The P-value is $P(|Z| > 24.07) = 2 \times P(Z > 24.07) = 0$.

Since the P-value is 0 the test is highly significant. Thus there is strong sample evidence that the mean difference is significantly different from 0. In other words, the mean blood loss in LARR group is significantly different from that of the ORR group.

9.4 Fixed Effect (FE) Model

The fixed effect (FE) model is used if there is no significant heterogeneity of effect size among the independent studies. In this section, the FE model is presented in a general framework for the meta-analysis of RR with example. An introduction to the FE model is found in (Borenstein et al. 2010).

In meta-analysis, results from all the k independent studies are combined by pooling the summary statistics of primary studies to a single point estimate and confidence interval for the common population effect size θ. Under the fixed effect model, the common effect size estimator, WMD ($=\theta$) is given by

$\hat{\theta}_{FE} = \sum_{i=1}^{k} w_i \hat{\delta}_i \Big/ \sum_{i=1}^{k} w_i$ and the variance of the estimator of the common effect

size is $Var(\hat{\theta}_{FE}) = 1 \Big/ \sum_{i=1}^{k} w_i$. Hence the standard error of the estimator of the

common effect size is $SE(\hat{\theta}_{FE}) = \sqrt{1 \Big/ \sum_{i=1}^{k} w_i}$.

The confidence interval

The $(1 - \alpha) \times 100\%$ confidence interval for the common population WMD θ based on the sample estimates is given by the lower limit (LL) and upper limit (UL) as follows:

$$LL = \hat{\theta}_{FE} - z_{\alpha/2} \times SE(\hat{\theta}_{FE}) \text{ and}$$

$$UL = \hat{\theta}_{FE} + z_{\alpha/2} \times SE(\hat{\theta}_{FE}).$$

Here $z_{\alpha/2}$ is the $\frac{\alpha}{2}$ th cut-off point of standard normal distribution and $SE(\hat{\theta}_{FE}) = \sqrt{Var(\hat{\theta}_{FE})}$.

To compute the confidence interval and perform test on the population effect size θ, under the FE model, we need to compute the point estimate and standard error of the estimator for all studies.

Example 9.3 Consider the summary data on blood loss for the Laparoscopic-assisted Rectal Resection (LARR) versus Open Rectal Resection (ORR) for Carcinoma from Table 9.1.

Using the summary statistics at the bottom of Table 9.2 calculate the (i) point estimate of the population WMD, (ii) standard error of estimator and (iii) 95% confidence interval for the population WMD of blood loss under the fixed effect model.

Solution:
To answer the above questions, we use the summary statistics in the last row of Table 9.2 as follows:

(i) The estimate of the population WMD is obtained as the sample WMD as

$$\hat{\theta}_{FE} = \frac{\sum_1^{11} w_i \hat{\delta}_i}{\sum_1^{11} w_i} = \frac{\sum_1^{11} WMD}{\sum_1^{11} W} = \frac{-7.9085}{0.10798} = -73.2411 \approx -73.24.$$

(ii) The standard error is $SE(\hat{\theta}_{FE}) = \sqrt{\frac{1}{\sum_1^{11} w_i}} = \sqrt{\frac{1}{\sum_1^{11} W}} = \sqrt{\frac{1}{0.10798}} = 3.043199.$

(iii) The 95% confidence interval for the common population WMD, θ is given by

$LL = \hat{\theta}_{FE} - 1.96 \times SE(\hat{\theta}_{FE}) = -73.2411 - 1.96 \times 3.043199 = -79.2058 \approx -79.21$ and
$UL = \hat{\theta}_{FE} + 1.96 \times SE(\hat{\theta}_{FE}) = -73.2411 + 1.96 \times 3.043199 = -67.2764 \approx -67.28.$

Comment The above point estimate (-73.24) and confidence limits $(-79.21, -67.28)$ are displayed in the bottom row of forest plot and represented by the diamond as in Fig. 9.1.

Measuring Heterogeneity
Here we consider two popular methods to identify and measure the extent of heterogeneity among the effect sizes of independent studies.

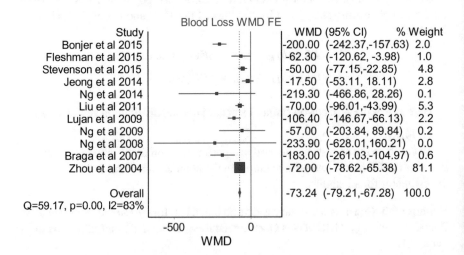

Fig. 9.1 Forest plot of meta-analysis on blood loss for the LARR and ORR groups under FE model

Cochran's Q Statistic (Cochran, 1973)

The Cochran's Q is defined as

$$Q = \sum_{i=1}^{k} w_i \hat{\theta}_i^2 - \frac{\left(\sum_{i=1}^{k} w_i \hat{\theta}_i \right)^2}{\sum_{i=1}^{k} w_i},$$

where w_i is the weight and $\hat{\theta}_i$ is the effect size estimate of the ith study.

The above Q statistic follows a chi-squared distribution with $df = (k-1)$, where k is the number of studies included in the meta-analysis. Since the expected value of a chi-squared variable is its degrees of freedom, the expected value of Q is (k-1), that is, $E(Q) = (k-1) = df$.

Test of Heterogeneity

To test the null hypothesis of the equality of effect sizes (i.e. equality excluding random error) across all studies, test

$H_0 : \theta_1 = \theta_2 = \ldots = \theta_k = \theta$ against H_a : not all θ_i's are equal (at least one of them is different), using the Cochran's Q statistic as defined above.

Reject the null hypothesis at the α level of significance if the observed value of the Q statistic is larger than or equal to $\chi^2_{k-1,1-\alpha}$, the level α critical value of the chi-squared distribution with (k-1) df, such that $P\left(\chi^2_{k-1} \geq \chi^2_{k-1,1-\alpha}\right) = \alpha$; otherwise don't reject it.

The small P-value leads to the conclusion that there is true difference among the effect sizes. However the non-significant P-value may not mean that the effect sizes are not different as this could happen due to low power of the test. The test should not be used to measure the magnitude of the true dispersion.

The I^2 Statistic (Higgins et al. 2003)

The I^2 statistic is a ratio of excess variation to the total variation expressed in percentages as follows:

$$I^2 = \left(\frac{Q - df}{Q} \right) \times 100\%,$$

and is viewed as the proportion of between studies variation and total variation (within plus between studies variation).

Comment

The values of Q and I^2 statistics are calculated from the sample summary data and they are not dependent on any statistical models.

Example 9.4 Consider the summary data on blood loss for the Laparoscopic-assisted Rectal Resection (LARR) versus Open Rectal Resection (ORR) for Carcinoma from Table 9.1.

Find the value of (i) Q statistic and (ii) I^2 statistic for the blood loss data.

Solution:
The following Table 9.3 provides summary calculations for finding Q and I^2 statistics. From the summary statistics in Table 9.3.

(i)   The Q statistic is calculated as

$$Q = \sum_{i=1}^{k} w_i \hat{\delta}_i^2 - \frac{\left(\sum_{i=1}^{k} w_i \hat{\delta}_i\right)^2}{\sum_{i=1}^{k} w_i} = \sum_{i=1}^{k} WMD^2 - \frac{\left(\sum_{i=1}^{k} WMD\right)^2}{\sum_{i=1}^{k} W}$$

$$= 638.3923 - \frac{(-7.9085)^2}{0.10798} = 59.17.$$

To test the heterogeneity of effect sizes the P-value is found from the chi-squared Table (with df $= (11 - 1) = 10$) as
$P\left(\chi_{10}^2 \geq 59.17\right) = 0$. Note there is no area left under the chi-squired density curve to the right of 59.17. Since the P-value is close to 0, we reject the null hypothesis (of equal effect sizes).

The I^2 statistic is found to be

$$I^2 = \left(\frac{Q - df}{Q}\right) \times 100\% = \left(\frac{59.17 - (11 - 1)}{59.17}\right) \times 100\%$$

$$= 0.83098 \times 100\% = 83\%,$$

where $df = (k - 1) = (11 - 1) = 10$.

Table 9.3 Calculated values of the summary statistics for the mean difference of blood loss data

Study	MD	Var	W	WxMD	W^2	WxDM^2
Bonjer et al. (2015)	−200	467.318	0.00214	−0.428	4.6E-06	85.5948
Fleshman et al. (2015)	−62.3	885.2478	0.00113	−0.0704	1.3E-06	4.38441
Stevenson et al. (2015)	−50	191.9487	0.00521	−0.2605	2.7E-05	13.0243
Jeong et al. (2014)	−17.5	330.1706	0.00303	−0.053	9.2E-06	0.92755
Ng et al. (2014)	−219	15953.23	6.3E-05	−0.0137	3.9E-09	3.01459
Liu et al. (2011)	−70	176.1431	0.00568	−0.3974	3.2E-05	27.8183
Lujan et al. (2009)	−106	422.0541	0.00237	−0.2521	5.6E-06	26.8235
Ng et al. (2009)	−57	5613.227	0.00018	−0.0102	3.2E-08	0.57881
Ng et al. (2008)	−234	40432.41	2.5E-05	−0.0058	6.1E-10	1.3531
Braga et al. (2007)	−183	1585.082	0.00063	−0.1155	4E-07	21.1276
Zhou et al. (2004)	−72	11.42491	0.08753	−6.302	0.00766	453.745
			0.10798	**−7.9085**	**0.00774**	**638.392**

The above value of Q = 59.17, its P-value = 0, and $I^2 = 83\%$ are presented in the forest plot produced by MetaXL on the left panel of Fig. 9.1.

Forest plot for WMD under FE model using MetaXL
The forest plot under the FE model (indicated by "IV" in the code) is constructed using MetaXL code
=MAInputTable("Blood Loss WMD FE","WMD","IV",B6:H16)

Remark: Explanations of MetaXL Code
For this type of meta-analyses in MetaXL the 'opening' code starts with MA Input Table ' = MAInputTable'. This is followed by an open parenthesis inside which the first quote contains the text that appears as the 'title of the output of the forest plot' e.g. "Blood Loss WMD FE" in the above code (user may choose any appropriate title here, but FE is chosen to indicate fixed effect model). Then in the second quote enter the type of effect measure, e.g. "WMD" in the above code which tells that the *weighted mean difference is the effect size.* Within the third quote enter the statistical model, e.g. "IV" in the above code stands for the *fixed effect* (abbreviated by FE) model. Each quotation is followed by a comma, and after the last comma enter the data area in Excel Worksheet, e.g. B6:H16 in the above code tells that the data on the independent studies are taken from the specified cells of the Excel Worksheet. The code ends with a closing parenthesis.

The forest plot of the meta-analysis using the above MetaXL code is found in Fig. **9.1**.

Interpretation
From the above forest plot of WMD under the FE model, the estimated common effect size is −73.24, and the 95% confidence interval is (−79.21, −67.28). The effect size is highly statistically significant (as 0 is not included in the 95% confidence interval).

Here Cochran's Q = 59.17 with P-value = 0 indicates highly significant heterogeneity among the mean difference of blood loss between the LARR and ORR groups of independent studies. The $I^2 = 83\%$ also reflects that there is high heterogeneity among the studies.

Remark
The sign of the mean difference (MD = $\hat{\delta}$) and subsequent estimates of the common effect size are all negative because of the way the mean difference is defined here, mean of LARR group minus mean of ORR group. If the order of difference is reversed, that is, if the mean of ORR group is subtracted from that of LARR group then the sign of the MD and other estimates will interchange (negative to positive and vice versa). The results of the meta-analysis on the reversed ordered MD = $\hat{\delta}$ is shown in Fig. 9.2.

Comment The interpretation of the forest plot in Fig. 9.2, significantly different WMD and significant heterogeneity, is the same as that in Fig. 9.1. All the estimates, confidence limits, value of Q statistic and P-value here are the same in magnitude

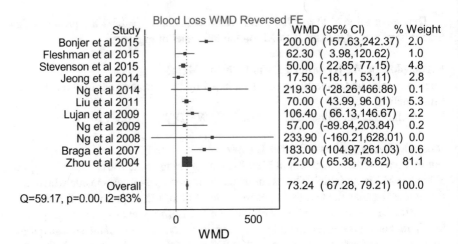

Fig. 9.2 Forest plot of meta-analysis on blood loss for the LARR and ORR groups in reversed order (mean ORR–mean LARR) under FE model

as the previous forest plot but the minus sign is replaced by the plus sign. Thus the order of the raw mean difference does not impact on the final conclusion of the meta-analysis.

9.5   Random Effects (REs) Model

Random effects (REs) model is used when the effect size across the independent studies is significantly heterogeneous. This model was introduced by DerSimonian and Laird, 1986. In spite of its frequent use, some valid criticisms of this model and its poor performance compared with inverse variance heterogeneity (IVhet) and quality effect (QF) models are provided in Doi et al. (2015c, b, c).

Under the random effects model, the population variance of the effect size is the sum of the variance of $\hat{\theta}_i$ about θ (σ^2), the within-study variance, and between-study variances, τ^2. So, for the ith study, the unknown modified variance becomes $\sigma_i^{*2} = \sigma_i^2 + \tau^2$ is estimated by its sample counterpart $v_i^* = v_i + \hat{\tau}^2$, where v_i is the estimate of σ_i^2 and $\hat{\tau}^2$ is the estimate of τ^2. Therefore, the weight assigned to the ith study is defined as

$$w_i^* = \frac{1}{v_i + \hat{\tau}^2} \text{ for i} = 1, 2, ..., k.$$

The common effect size under the REs model is estimated by

$$\hat{\theta}_{RE} = \sum_{i=1}^{k} w_i^* \hat{\delta}_i \left/ \sum_{i=1}^{k} w_i^* \right.$$

The standard error of the estimator of the common effect size is given by

$$SE(\hat{\theta}_{RE}) = \sqrt{1 \left/ \sum_{i=1}^{k} w_i^* \right.}$$

The $(1 - \alpha) \times 100\%$ confidence interval for the effect size θ under the REs model is given by the lower limit (LL) and upper limit (UL) as follows:

$$LL = \hat{\theta}_{RE} - z_{\alpha/2} \times SE(\hat{\theta}_{RE}) \text{ and}$$
$$UL = \hat{\theta}_{RE} + z_{\alpha/2} \times SE(\hat{\theta}_{RE}),$$

where $z_{\alpha/2}$ is the $\frac{\alpha}{2}$ th cut-off point of standard normal distribution.

Estimation of τ^2

The between studies variance is estimated as a scaled excess variation as follows

$$\hat{\tau}^2 = \frac{Q - df}{C},$$

where

$$Q = \sum_{i=1}^{k} w_i \hat{\delta}_i^2 - \frac{\left(\sum_{i=1}^{k} w_i \hat{\delta}_i \right)^2}{\sum_{i=1}^{k} w_i}, \quad C = \sum_{i=1}^{k} w_i - \frac{\sum_{i=1}^{k} w_i^2}{\sum_{i=1}^{k} w_i}$$

and $df = (k - 1)$ in which k is the number of studies.

Example 9.5 Consider the summary data on blood loss for the Laparoscopic-assisted Rectal Resection (LARR) versus Open Rectal Resection (ORR) for Carcinoma from Table 9.1.
Find the estimated value of between studies variance, $\hat{\tau}^2$, for the blood loss data.

Solution:
Using the summary statistics in Table 9.3 of the previous example we calculate the values of Q and C statistics which are required to find the value of $\hat{\tau}^2$. Here

$$Q = \sum_{i=1}^{k} w_i \hat{\delta}_i^2 - \frac{\left(\sum_{i=1}^{k} w_i \hat{\delta}_i\right)^2}{\sum_{i=1}^{k} w_i} = 638.3923 - \frac{(-7.9085)^2}{0.10798} = 59.17,$$

$$C = \sum_{i=1}^{11} w_i - \frac{\sum_{i=1}^{11} w_i^2}{\sum_{i=1}^{11} w_i} = 0.10798 - \frac{0.007742}{0.10798} = 0.0363 \text{ and } df = k-1 = 11-1 = 10.$$

Then, the estimate of the between studies variance becomes
$$\hat{\tau}^2 = \frac{Q-df}{C} = \frac{59.17-10}{0.0363} = 1355.029.$$

Illustration of REs Model for WMD

Example 9.6 Consider the summary data on blood loss for the Laparoscopic-assisted Rectal Resection (LARR) versus Open Rectal Resection (ORR) for Carcinoma from Table 9.1.

Find the (i) point estimate of the combined population WMD, (ii) standard error of the estimator, and (iii) 95% confidence interval of the population effect size, WMD under the random effects model.

In Table 9.4 the combined variance (Var*) is the sum of Var and Tau^2, and modified weight (W*) is the weight under the REs model calculated as the reciprocal of Var*.

As an illustration, for **Study 1** (Bonjer et al. 2015), the modified variance for the REs model is found to be
$$v_1^* = v_1 + \hat{\tau}^2 = 467.318 + 1355.03 = 1822.3 \text{ and the modified weight becomes}$$
$$w_1^* = 1/Var_1^* = \frac{1}{1822.3} = 0.00055.$$
Now using the summary statistics from Table 9.4 we get

Table 9.4 Calculated values of the summary statistics for the REs model

Study	MD	Var	Tau^2	Var*	W*	W*xMD
Bonjer et al. (2015)	−200	467.318	1355.03	1822.3	0.00055	−0.10975
Fleshman et al. (2015)	−62.3	885.2478	1355.03	2240.3	0.00045	−0.02781
Stevenson et al. (2015)	−50	191.9487	1355.03	1547	0.00065	−0.03232
Jeong et al. (2014)	−17.5	330.1706	1355.03	1685.2	0.00059	−0.01038
Ng et al. (2014)	−219	15953.23	1355.03	17308	5.8E-05	−0.01267
Liu et al. (2011)	−70	176.1431	1355.03	1531.2	0.00065	−0.04572
Lujan et al. (2009)	−106	422.0541	1355.03	1777.1	0.00056	−0.05987
Ng et al. (2009)	−57	5613.227	1355.03	6968.3	0.00014	−0.00818
Ng et al. (2008)	−234	40432.41	1355.03	41787	2.4E-05	−0.0056
Braga et al. (2007)	−183	1585.082	1355.03	2940.1	0.00034	−0.06224
Zhou et al. (2004)	−72	11.42491	1355.03	1366.5	0.00073	−0.05269
					0.00475	**−0.42723**

(i) the point estimate of the common effect size, WMD under the REs model to be

$$\hat{\theta}_{RE} = \sum_{i=1}^{11} w_i^* \hat{\delta}_i \bigg/ \sum_{i=1}^{11} w_i^* = \sum_{i=1}^{11} W^* MD \bigg/ \sum_{i=1}^{11} W^* = \frac{-0.42723}{0.00475} = -89.98.$$

(ii) The standard error of the estimator of the common effect size is

$$SE(\hat{\theta}_{RE}) = \sqrt{1 \bigg/ \sum_{i=1}^{11} w_i^*} = \sqrt{1 \bigg/ \sum_{i=1}^{11} W^*} = \sqrt{\frac{1}{0.00475}} = 14.513.$$

(iii) The 95% confidence interval for the population effect size θ under the REs model is given by the lower limit (LL) and upper limit (UL) as follows:

$$LL = \hat{\theta}_{RE} - 1.96 \times SE(\hat{\theta}_{RE}) = -89.98 - 1.96 \times 14.513 = -118.43$$
$$UL = \hat{\theta}_{RE} + 1.96 \times SE(\hat{\theta}_{RE}) = -89.98 + 1.96 \times 14.513 = -61.54.$$

Comment The above point estimate (-89.98) and the 95% confidence interval ($-0118.43, -61.54$) are presented at the bottom row of the forest plot and represented by a diamond as shown in Fig. 9.3.

Forest plot for WMD under REs model using MetaXL
The forest plot under the RE model (indicated by "RE" in the code) is constructed using MetaXL code

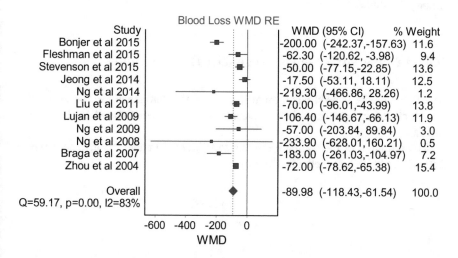

Fig. 9.3 Forest plot of meta-analysis on blood loss for the LARR and ORR groups under REs model

=MAInputTable("Blood Loss WMD RE","WMD","RE",B6:H16)

Remark: Explanations of MetaXL Code
For this type of meta-analyses in MetaXL the 'opening' code starts with MA Input Table ' =MAInputTable'. This is followed by an open parenthesis inside which the first quote contains the text that appears as the 'title of the output of the forest plot' e.g. "Blood Loss WMD RE" in the above code (user may choose any appropriate title here, but RE is chosen to indicate random effects model). Then in the second quote enter the type of effect measure, e.g. "WMD" in the above code which tells that the *weighted mean difference is the effect size*. Within the third quote enter the statistical model, e.g. "RE" in the above code stands for the *random effects* (abbreviated by REs) model. Each quotation is followed by a comma, and after the last comma enter the data area in Excel Worksheet, e.g. B6:D16 in the above code tells that the data on the independent studies are taken from the specified cells of the Excel Worksheet. The code ends with a closing parenthesis.

The forest plot of the meta-analysis using the above MetaXL code is found in Fig. 9.3.

Interpretation
From the above forest plot of WMD of blood loss under the REs model, the estimated common effect size is -89.98, and the 95% confidence interval is $(-118.43, -61.54)$. The effect size is highly statistically significant (as 0 is not included in the confidence interval).

Here Cochran's $Q = 59.17$ with P-value $= 0$ indicates highly significant heterogeneity among the mean difference of blood loss between the LARR and ORR groups of independent studies. The $I^2 = 83\%$ also reflects that there is high heterogeneity among the studies.

9.6   Inverse Variance Heterogeneity (IVhet) Model

The IVhet model is used when there is significant heterogeneity in the effect size across all the independent studies. Details on this model is found in (Doi et al., 2015a).

The estimator of the common effect size WMD ($=\theta$) under the inverse variance heterogeneity (IVhet) model is given by

$$\hat{\theta}_{IVhet} = \frac{\sum_{i=1}^{k} w_i \hat{\delta}_i}{\sum_{i=1}^{k} w_i}.$$

Then the variance of the estimator under the IVhet model is given by

$$Var(\hat{\theta}_{IVhet}) = \sum_{i=1}^{k}\left[\left(\frac{1}{v_i}\bigg/\sum_{i=1}^{k}\frac{1}{v_i}\right)^2 (v_i + \hat{\tau}^2)\right]$$

$$= \sum_{i=1}^{k}\left[\left(w_i\bigg/\sum_{i=1}^{k}w_i\right)^2 \times v_i^*\right].$$

For the computation of the confidence interval of the common effect size based on the IVhet model use the following estimated standard error

$$SE(\hat{\theta}_{IVhet}) = \sqrt{Var(\hat{\theta}_{IVhet})}.$$

Then, the $(1-\alpha) \times 100\%$ confidence interval for the common effect size θ under the IVhet model is given by the lower limit (LL) and upper limit (UL) as follows:

$$LL = \hat{\theta}_{IVhet} - z_{\alpha/2} \times SE(\hat{\theta}_{IVhet})$$
$$UL = \hat{\theta}_{IVhet} + z_{\alpha/2} \times SE(\hat{\theta}_{IVhet}),$$

where $z_{\alpha/2}$ is the $\frac{\alpha}{2}$ th cut-off point of standard normal distribution.

Illustration of IVhet Model for WMD

Example 9.7 Consider the summary data on blood loss for the Laparoscopic-assisted Rectal Resection (LARR) versus Open Rectal Resection (ORR) for Carcinoma from Table 9.1.

Find the (i) point estimate of the population WMD, (ii) standard error of the estimator, and (iii) 95% confidence interval of the population effect size, WMD under the inverse variance heterogeneity model.

Solution:

To answer the questions we need to compute the values in Table 9.5.

In Table 9.5, Var* is the combined variance

$\left(Var_i^* = v_i + \hat{\tau}^2\right)$ and W* is the modified weight under the IVhet model calculated

as $W_i^* = \left[\left(\frac{1}{v_i}\bigg/\sum_{i=1}^{k}\frac{1}{v_i}\right)^2 (v_i + \hat{\tau}^2)\right] = \left(w_i\bigg/\sum_{1}^{k}w_i\right)^2 \times Var_i^*$ for the ith study.

For example, for the first study (Bonjer et al. 2015).

$Var_1^* = 467.318 + 1355.03 = 1822.3$, and

$W_1^* = \left(0.00214\big/0.10798\right)^2 \times 1822.3 = 0.71569.$

Now using the summary statistics in Table 9.5, we answer the questions in Example 9.7.

Table 9.5   Calculated values of the summary statistics for the IVhet model

Study	MD	Var	Tau^2	Var*	W	W*	WxMD
Bonjer et al. (2015)	−200	467.318	1355.03	1822.3	0.00214	0.71569	−0.428
Fleshman et al. (2015)	−62.3	885.2478	1355.03	2240.3	0.00113	0.24518	−0.0704
Stevenson et al. (2015)	−50	191.9487	1355.03	1547	0.00521	3.6011	−0.2605
Jeong et al. (2014)	−17.5	330.1706	1355.03	1685.2	0.00303	1.32585	−0.053
Ng et al. (2014)	−219	15953.23	1355.03	17308	6.3E-05	0.00583	−0.0137
Liu et al. (2011)	−70	176.1431	1355.03	1531.2	0.00568	4.23267	−0.3974
Lujan et al. (2009)	−106	422.0541	1355.03	1777.1	0.00237	0.85564	−0.2521
Ng et al. (2009)	−57	5613.227	1355.03	6968.3	0.00018	0.01897	−0.0102
Ng et al. (2008)	−234	40432.41	1355.03	41787	2.5E-05	0.00219	−0.0058
Braga et al. (2007)	−183	1585.082	1355.03	2940.1	0.00063	0.10036	−0.1155
Zhou et al. (2004)	−72	11.42491	1355.03	1366.5	0.08753	897.864	−6.302
					0.10798	**908.968**	**−7.9085**

(i)   The point estimate of population WMD under the IVhet model is

$$\hat{\theta}^*_{IVhet} = \frac{\sum_{i=1}^{11} w_i \hat{\delta}_i}{\sum_{i=1}^{11} w_i} = \frac{\sum_{i=1}^{11} W \times MD}{\sum_{i=1}^{11} W} = \frac{-7.9085}{0.10798} = -73.24.$$

(ii)   The standard error of the estimator is

$$SE(\hat{\theta}^*_{IVhet}) = \sqrt{\sum_{i=1}^{11} W^*_i} = \sqrt{908.96775} = 30.1491.$$

(iii)   The 95% confidence interval of the effect size under the IVhet model is given by the lower limit (LL) and upper limit (UL) as follows:

$$LL = \hat{\theta}_{IVhet} - 1.96 \times SE(\hat{\theta}_{IVhet}) = -73.24 - 1.96 \times 30.1491 = -132.33 \quad \text{and}$$

$$UL = \hat{\theta}_{IVhet} + z_{\alpha/2} \times SE(\hat{\theta}_{IVhet}) = -73.24 + 1.96 \times 30.1491 = -14.15.$$

Comment   The above point estimate (−73.24) and the 95% confidence interval (−132.33, −14.15) are presented at the bottom row of the forest plot and represented by a diamond as found in Fig. 9.4.

Forest plot for WMD under IVhet model using MetaXL

The forest plot under the IVhet model (indicated by "IVhet" in the code) is constructed using MetaXL code

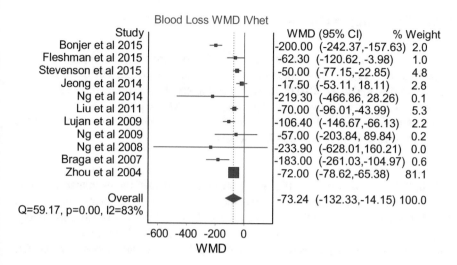

Fig. 9.4 Forest plot of meta-analysis on blood loss for the LARR and ORR groups under IVhet model

=MAInputTable("Blood Loss WMD IVhet","WMD","IVhet",B6:H16)

Remark: Explanations of MetaXL Code
For this type of meta-analyses in MetaXL the 'opening' code starts with MA Input Table ' =MAInputTable'. This is followed by an open parenthesis inside which the first quote contains the text that appears as the 'title of the output of the forest plot' e.g. "Blood Loss WMD IVhet" in the above code (user may choose any appropriate title here, but IVhet is chosen to indicate inverse variance heterogeneity model). Then in the second quote enter the type of effect measure, e.g. "WMD" in the above code which tells that the *weighted mean difference is the effect size*. Within the third quote enter the statistical model, e.g. "IVhet" in the above code stands for the *inverse variance heterogeneity* (abbreviated by IVhet) model. Each quotation is followed by a comma, and after the last comma enter the data area in Excel Worksheet, e.g. B6:D16 in the above code tells that the data on the independent studies are taken from the specified cells of the Excel Worksheet. The code ends with a closing parenthesis.

Interpretation
From the above forest plot, the estimated common effect size is -73.24, and the 95% confidence interval is $(-132.33, -14.15)$. The effect size is highly statistically significant (as 0 is not included in the confidence interval).

Here Cochrane's $Q = 59.17$ with P-value $= 0$ indicates highly significant heterogeneity among the mean difference of blood loss between the LARR and ORR groups of independent studies. The $I^2 = 83\%$ also reflects that there is high heterogeneity among the studies.

9.7 Subgroup Analysis

Consider the Blood loss data in Example 9.5. To illustrate subgroup analysis for
the data, let's divide the studies into two groups: studied published before 2010
(Old Studies) and after 2010 (Recent Studies) to see if there is any difference in the
effect size between the two subgroups. Using MetaXL we produce the forest plot of
subgroup analysis as in Figs. 9.5, 9.6 and 9.7 representing the meta-analyses of the
subgorups under FE, REs and IVhet models.

Interpretation (FE)
From the forest plot (FE) in Fig. 9.5, under the FE model, the estimated common
effect size of Recent Studies is -70.91, and the 95% confidence interval is $(-85.83,$
$-55.98)$, and that for the Old Studies are -73.68 and $(-80.19, -67.18)$ respectively.
The effect size is highly statistically significant (as 0 is not included in the confidence
interval) for both subgroups as well as the pooled results of all studies $(-73,24,$ CI:
$-79.21, 67.28)$.

For the Recent Studies Cochran's $Q = 48.05$ with P-value $= 0$ indicating highly
significant heterogeneity among the mean difference of blood loss between the LARR

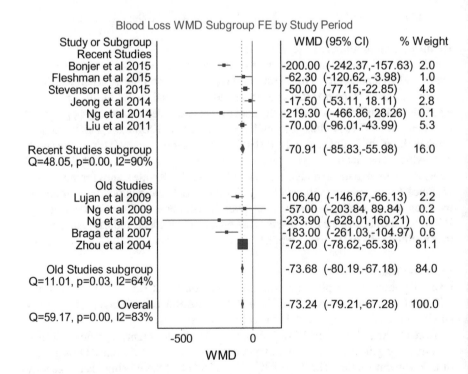

Fig. 9.5 Subgroup analysis by Older and Recent Studies of blood loss after LARR and ORR
procedures under the *FE model*

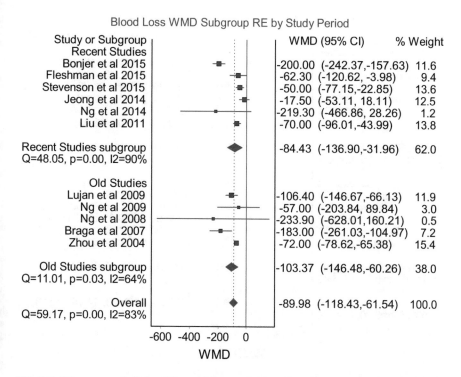

Fig. 9.6 Subgroup analysis by Older and Recent Studies of blood loss after LARR and ORR procedures under the *REs model*

and ORR groups of independent studies. The $I^2 = 90\%$ also reflects that there is high heterogeneity among the studies in this subgroup.

For the Od Studies Cochran's Q = 11.01 with P-value = 0.03 indicating significant heterogeneity among the mean difference of blood loss between the LARR and ORR groups of independent studies. The $I^2 = 64\%$ also reflects that there is high heterogeneity among the studies in this subgroup. But there is more heterogeneity among the Recent Studies than the Old Studies.

Interpretation (REs)

From the forest plot of WMD on blood loss under the REs model, the estimated common effect size of Recent Studies is -84.43, and the 95% confidence interval is $(-136.90, -31.96)$, and that for the Old Studies are -103.37 and $(-146.48, -60.26)$ respectively. The effect size is highly statistically significant (as 0 is not included in the confidence interval) for both subgroups.

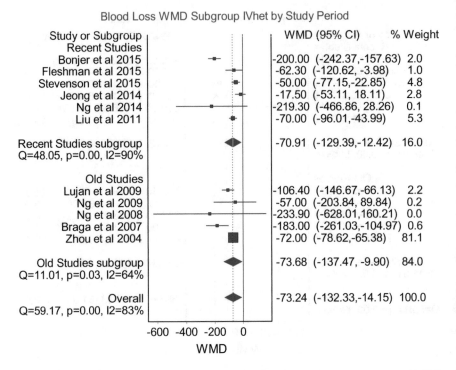

Fig. 9.7 Subgroup analysis by Older and Recent Studies of blood loss after LARR and ORR procedures under the *IVhet model*

The comments on the heterogeneity (Q statistic and P-value) remain the same as that for Fig. 9.5 as these are not dependent on any model.

Interpretation (IVhet)
From the forest plot of WMD on blood loss under the IVhet model, the estimated common effect size of Recent Studies is −70.91, and the 95% confidence interval is (−129.39, −12.42), and that for the Old Studies are −73.68 and (−137.47, −9.90) respectively. The effect size is highly statistically significant (as 0 is not included in the confidence interval) for both subgroups.

9.8   Publication Bias

The study of publication bias for WMD is very similar to that of SMD in Sect. 9.8.8 of the previous chapter. It is not necessary to re-produce thsem again here. Readers interested to produce funnel plot or Doi plot and their interpretation are referred to that Section.

9.9 Conclusions

The weighted mean difference (WMD) method of meta-analysis is covered in this chapter. It is applicable for continuous (numerical) outcome variables for two arms studies. In addition to introducing the WMD method of meta-analysis with step by step illustrations to apply the method on real-life data sets, forest plots are produced under different statistical models by using the MetaXL codes.

The comparison of results for different statistical models show variation in the point estimates and confidence intervals. The heterogeneity among the studies are also studied using Q and I^2 statistics. Subgroup analysis is also provided for the Recent Studies and Old Studies.

Appendix 9—Stata Codes for Meta-Analysis of WMD

A9.1 Blood loss dataset

Study	n_larr	mean_larr	sd_larr	n_orr	mean_orr	sd_orr	study_period
Bonjer et al. (2015)	699	200	222	345	400	370	recent
Fleshman et al. (2015)	240	256.1	305.8	222	318.4	331.7	recent
Stevenson et al. (2015)	238	100	111	235	150	181.5	recent
Jeong et al. (2014)	170	200	148	170	217.5	185	recent
Ng et al. (2014)	40	141.8	500	40	361.1	623	recent
Liu et al. (2011)	98	310	96	88	380	85	recent
Lujan et al. (2009)	101	127.8	113.3	103	234.2	174.3	old
Ng et al. (2009)	76	280	500	77	337	423	old
Ng et al. (2008)	51	321.7	750	48	555.6	1188	old
Braga et al. (2007)	83	213	258	85	396	258	old
Zhou et al. (2004)	82	20	19	89	92	25	old

A9.2 Stata Codes for the Blood loss dataset

```
. ssc install admetan
```
   Codes for WMD meta-analysis of blood loss
```
   . admetan n_larr mean_larr sd_larr n_orr mean_orr sd_orr, wmd
   . admetan n_larr mean_larr sd_larr n_orr mean_orr sd_orr, wmd re
   . admetan n_larr mean_larr sd_larr n_orr mean_orr sd_orr, wmd ivhet
```

A9.3 Codes for WMD Subgroup analysis of blood loss by study period

```
. admetan n_larr mean_larr sd_larr n_orr mean_orr sd_orr, wmd by(study_period)
   . admetan n_larr mean_larr sd_larr n_orr mean_orr sd_orr, wmd re
by(study_period)
   . admetan n_larr mean_larr sd_larr n_orr mean_orr sd_orr, wmd ivhet
by(study_period)
```

References

Borenstein M, Hedges LV, Higgins JP, Rothstein HR (2010) A basic introduction to fixed-effect and random-effects models for meta-analysis. Res Synth Methods 1(2):97–111

Cochran WG (1973) Experiments for nonlinear functions (R.A. Fisher Memorial Lecture). J Am Stat Assoc 68(344):771–781. https://doi.org/10.1080/01621459.1973.10481423

DerSimonian R, Laird N (1986) Meta-analysis in clinical trials. Control Clin Trials 7(3):177–188

Doi SA, Barendregt JJ, Khan S, Thalib L, Williams GM (2015a) Advances in the meta-analysis of heterogeneous clinical trials I: the inverse variance heterogeneity model. Contemp Clin Trials 45(Pt A):130–138. https://doi.org/10.1016/j.cct.2015.05.009

Doi SA, Barendregt JJ, Khan S, Thalib L, Williams GM (2015b) Advances in the meta-analysis of heterogeneous clinical trials II: the quality effects model. Contemp Clin Trials 45(Pt A):123–129. https://doi.org/10.1016/j.cct.2015.05.010

Doi SA, Barendregt JJ, Khan S, Thalib L, Williams GM (2015c) Simulation comparison of the quality effects and random effects methods of meta-analysis. Epidemiology 26(4):e42–44

Higgins JP, Thompson SG, Deeks JJ, Altman DG (2003) Measuring inconsistency in meta-analyses. BMJ 327(7414):557–560

Memon MA, Awaiz A, Yunus RM, Memon B, Khan S (2018) Meta-analysis of histopathological outcomes of laparoscopic assisted rectal resection (LARR) vs open rectal resection (ORR) for carcinoma. Am J Surg 216(5):1004–1015. https://doi.org/10.1016/j.amjsurg.2018.06.012

Chapter 10
Meta-Analysis of Correlation Coefficient

If the linear association/relationship between two continuous/quantitative outcome variables is of interest then the correlation coefficient is the appropriate effect size measure.

Meta-analysis of correlation coefficient is covered in this chapter. It provides meta-analyses of correlation coefficient under different statistical models with illustrative examples.

10.1 Introduction

Correlation arises when the linear association or relationship between two continuous (numerical) outcome variables is of interest. The strength (size) and direction (sign) of linear relationship or association between two numerical variables are measured by the Pearson's correlation coefficient. A common and popular example of correlation would be the linear association between age and systolic blood pressure of adults, or between height and weight of infants. Studies that are interested in the linear association between two continuous variables use correlation coefficient as the effect size measure. The population correlation coefficient is denoted by ρ and its estimate, the sample correlation coefficient, is denoted by r.

By definition the correlation coefficient is a pure number (unit free) and takes value between -1 and 1. If the value of the correlation coefficient is 1 (or -1) there is perfect positive (or negative) linear relationship between the two variables. Closer the value (magnitude) of correlation coefficient to 1 (or -1) stronger the linear relationship between the two numerical variables. There is no linear relationship between the two variables if the value of correlation coefficient is 0 (or very close to 0). Note that this only implies to linear relationship (emphasis on linear) but there may be strong non-linear relationship between the two variables when the correlation coefficient is 0.

Rule of Thumb for interpreting the strength (magnitude) of a correlation coefficient;

© Springer Nature Singapore Pte Ltd. 2020
S. Khan, *Meta-Analysis*, Statistics for Biology and Health,
https://doi.org/10.1007/978-981-15-5032-4_10

Size of correlation	Interpretation
0.90 to 1.00 (-0.90 to -1.00)	Very high positive (negative) correlation
0.70 to 0.90 (-0.70 to -0.90)	High positive (negative) correlation
0.50 to 0.70 (-0.50 to -0.70)	Moderate positive (negative) correlation
0.30 to 0.50 (-0.30 to -0.50)	Low positive (negative) correlation
0.00 to 0.30 (0.00 to -0.30)	negligible correlation

Please see (Hinkle 2003) for further details.

10.2   Estimation of Effect Size

Let ρ be the population correlation coefficient between two continuous/numerical variables. This can be used as the population effect size to measure linear association between two numerical variables. However, often another transformed population effect size measure, $\zeta = \frac{1}{2}\left[\ln\frac{1+\rho}{1-\rho}\right]$ is used. Note here "ln" is the natural logarithm function. The transformation is known as Fisher's variance stabilization. Both ρ and can be used as effect size measure, but the latter is more commonly used because of some advantages.

Let r be the sample correlation coefficient between two sets of sample values of any continuous/(numerical) outcome variable based on two samples of size n each. Then the statistic r is an estimator of the population correlation coefficient, ρ, that is, $\hat{\rho} = r$.

The estimator of the modified/transformed population effect size, ζ is given by $\hat{\zeta} = \frac{1}{2}\left[\ln\frac{1+r}{1-r}\right]$ which is a function of sample correlation coefficient r only.

The exact variance of r and $\hat{\zeta}$ are complicated, but a very good approximation of these are given by $Var(r) = \frac{(1-\rho^2)^2}{n-1}$ which depends on unknown parameter ρ, and $Var(\hat{\zeta}) = \frac{1}{n-3}$ which does not depend on r (or ρ).

The variance of r depends on the value of unknown parameter ρ and also it is not a constant (changes with the change in the value of ρ). However, the variance of the estimator of the modified/transformed population effect size, $\hat{\zeta} = \frac{1}{2}\left[\ln\frac{1+r}{1-r}\right]$ is $Var(\hat{\zeta}) = \frac{1}{n-3}$ which does not depend on r, and is a constant (with respect to r).

The standard error of r is $SE(r) = \sqrt{\frac{(1-r^2)^2}{n-1}} = \frac{(1-r^2)}{\sqrt{n-1}}$, and that of $\hat{\zeta}$ is $SE(\hat{\zeta}) = \sqrt{\frac{1}{n-3}} = \frac{1}{\sqrt{n-3}}$.

Note that $\hat{\zeta} = \frac{1}{2}\left[\ln\frac{1+r}{1-r}\right] = \text{arctanh}(r)$, where "ln" is the natural logarithm function and "arctanh" is the inverse hyperbolic tangent function, and the inverse/back transformation to r is $r = \frac{e^{2\hat{\zeta}}-1}{e^{2\hat{\zeta}}+1} = \tanh(r)$, where "tanh" is the hyperbolic tangent function.

The above transformation of r to $\hat{\zeta}$ is known as the Fisher's Z transformation (cf. (Fisher 1915)) which is an approximate *variance-stabilizing transformation* for r when the two questitative variable, say X and Y, follow a bivariate normal distribution. This means that the variance of $\hat{\zeta}$ is approximately constant for all values of the sample correlation coefficient r.

For statistical inferences, note that both $Z_1 = \frac{r\sqrt{n-1}}{(1-r^2)}$ and $Z_2 = \hat{\zeta}\sqrt{n-3}$ are distributed as standard normal variables (with mean 0 and standard deviation 1), and can be used to find confidence interval and perform statistical tests.

Remark For inference on the population correlation coefficient, ρ we could use either

(i) original sample correlation coefficient, r as the effect size estimate for ρ with
$$SE(r) = \sqrt{\frac{(1-r^2)^2}{n-1}} = \frac{(1-r^2)}{\sqrt{n-1}}, \text{ or}$$

(ii) transformed effect size, $\hat{\zeta} = \frac{1}{2}\left[\ln\frac{1+r}{1-r}\right] = \arctan h(r)$ with $SE(\hat{\zeta}) = \sqrt{\frac{1}{n-3}} = \frac{1}{\sqrt{n-3}}$.

Most of the statistical packages, including MetaXL, use the second method ($\hat{\zeta}$, Fisher's Z transformation of r) for meta-analysis. This is because the variance (and hence the standard deviation) of the estimator of ζ does not change even if the value of r changes from one study to another. In the forthcoming sections we will use the second option, that is, use $\hat{\zeta}$ as the effect size estimate of ρ so that our results are comparable to those produced by popular statistical packages. As a consequence of this choice the lower and upper limits of the confidence interval will initially be computed based on $\hat{\zeta}$ in the transformed (acrcanh) scale and then the limits will be converted into the original scale of r by using the inverse/back (tanh) transformation.

Remarks Readers who are uncomfortable with mathematical explanations may not worry about the above discussions on the transformation of r as the actual meta-analysis will be conducted by MetaXL (or another statistical package) that will automatically use the transformation and produce the final forest plot in r scale.

The confidence interval
A $(1 - \alpha) \times 100\%$ confidence interval for the population effect size ρ, based on the sample correlation coefficient, is given by the lower limit (LL*) and upper limit (UL*) as follows:
$$LL^* = \hat{\zeta} - z_{\alpha/2} \times SE(\hat{\zeta}) \text{ and } UL^* = \hat{\zeta} + z_{\alpha/2} \times SE(\hat{\zeta}) \text{ in the transformed arctanh}$$
scale.

Here $z_{\alpha/2}$ is the $\frac{\alpha}{2}$ cut-off point of standard normal distribution and $SE(\hat{\zeta}) = \sqrt{Var(\hat{\zeta})}$.

Hence the $(1 - \alpha) \times 100\%$ confidence interval for ρ becomes
$$LL = \frac{e^{2 \times LL^*}-1}{e^{2 \times LL^*}+1} = \tanh(LL^*) \text{ and } LU = \frac{e^{2 \times LU^*}-1}{e^{2 \times LU^*}+1} = \tanh(LU^*) \text{ in the original r}$$
scale.

Example 10.1 The following summary statistics on correlation coefficient of 8 independent studies are taken from the MedCalc website.

Table 10.1 Summary data on correlation coefficient of 8 studies

Study	n	r
Moore (2006)	133	0.56
Davis (2008)	149	0.43
Thomas (1999)	131	0.53
Miller (2012)	120	0.51
Williams (2012)	111	0.66
Young (2013)	152	0.46
Baker (2009)	60	0.33
Adams (2006)	122	0.38

For the data in Table 10.1, find the (i) point estimate of ζ and (ii) 95% confidence interval for the population correlation coefficient, ρ for each of the 8 studies.

Solution:

The Table 10.2 provides all relevant calculations and results to answer the above questions.

In Table 10.2, $Z = \hat{\zeta} = \frac{1}{2}\left[\ln \frac{1+r}{1-r}\right] = \text{arctan}h(r)$, Var is the variance of $\hat{\zeta}$ defined as $1/(n-3)$, SE is the standard error of $\hat{\zeta}$ defined as $SE = \sqrt{1/(n-3)}$, LL* and UL* are the lower and upper limits of 95% confidence interval in the $\hat{\zeta}$ scale, and LL and UL are the limits of 95% confidence interval in the r scale using $\tanh(\hat{\zeta})$ back transformation.

Explanation of computations for the first study (Moore 2006)

Note for the first study n $= 133$ and r $= 0.56$.

(i)   From Fisher's transformation, the point estimate of ζ is

Table 10.2 Calculations for the point estimate and confidence interval of correlation coefficient for individual studies

Study	n	r	Z	Var	SE	LL*	UL*	LL	UL
Moore (2006)	133	0.56	0.6328	0.00769	0.08771	0.46093	0.80474	0.4308	0.6667
Davis (2008)	149	0.43	0.4599	0.00685	0.08276	0.29769	0.62211	0.2892	0.5526
Thomas (1999)	131	0.53	0.5901	0.00781	0.08839	0.4169	0.76339	0.3943	0.6431
Miller (2012)	120	0.51	0.5627	0.00855	0.09245	0.38153	0.74393	0.364	0.6315
Williams (2012)	111	0.66	0.7928	0.00926	0.09623	0.60421	0.98141	0.54	0.7537
Young (2013)	152	0.46	0.4973	0.00671	0.08192	0.33674	0.65788	0.3246	0.577
Baker (2009)	60	0.33	0.3428	0.01754	0.13245	0.08322	0.60244	0.083	0.5388
Adams (2006)	122	0.38	0.4001	0.0084	0.09167	0.22039	0.57973	0.2169	0.5225

$$\hat{\zeta} = \tfrac{1}{2}\left[\ln \tfrac{1+r}{1-r}\right] = 0.5 \times ln\left[\frac{1+0.56}{1-0.56}\right] = 0.5 \times \ln(3.54545) = 0.5 \times 1.26567 = 0.6328.$$

Alternatively, directly using the arctanh function, $\hat{\zeta} = arc\tanh(r) = \arctan h(0.56) = 0.6328.$

So the point estimate of $\hat{\zeta}$ is $\zeta = 0.6328$.

(ii) The 95% confidence interval for ρ

First we compute the limits of the 95% confidence interval for ζ and then convert the two limits to find the confidence interval for ρ.

The variance of $\hat{\zeta}$ is $\mathrm{Var} = 1/(n-3) = 1/(133-3) = 1/130 = 0.00769$ and hence the standard error is $SE(\hat{\zeta}) = \sqrt{Var(\hat{\zeta})} = \sqrt{0.00769} = 0.08771$.

Then the lower and upper limits of the 95% confidence interval for ζ are given by

$$LL^* = \hat{\zeta} - 1.96 \times SE(\hat{\zeta}) = 0.6328 - 1.96 \times 0.08771 = 0.46093 \approx 0.46 \text{ and}$$

$$UL^* = \hat{\zeta} + 1.96 \times SE(\hat{\zeta}) = 0.6328 + 1.96 \times 0.08771 = 0.80474 \approx 0.80.$$

Now the lower and upper limits of the 95% confidence interval for ρ become

$$LL = \frac{e^{2 \times LL^*} - 1}{e^{2 \times LL^*} + 1} = \frac{e^{2 \times 0.46093} - 1}{e^{2 \times 0.46093} + 1} = \frac{2.51396 - 1}{2.51396 + 1} = \frac{1.51396}{3.51396} = 0.43084 \approx 0.43 \text{ and}$$

$$LL = \frac{e^{2 \times LL^*} - 1}{e^{2 \times LL^*} + 1} = \frac{e^{2 \times 0.80474} - 1}{e^{2 \times 0.80474} + 1} = \frac{5.00021 - 1}{5.00021 + 1} = \frac{4.00021}{6.00021} = 0.66668 \approx 0.67.$$

Comment The above 95% confidence interval (0.34, 0.67) for ρ along with the value of r (0.56) is reported in the top row (for the first study) of the forest plot in Fig. 10.1.

Similar calculations are done for all other studies to find the 95% confidence interval for the population correlation coefficient ρ for individual studies.

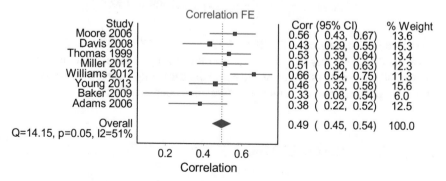

Fig. 10.1 Forest plot of meta-analysis on correlation coefficient under FE model

10.3   Tests on Effect Size, ρ

To test the significance of the population correlation coefficient, test the null hypothesis

$H_0 : \rho = 0$ against $H_a : \rho \neq 0$ using the test statistic

$$Z = \frac{\hat{\zeta}}{SE(\hat{\zeta})} = \frac{\hat{\zeta}}{\sqrt{n-3}},$$

where $\hat{\zeta} = \frac{1}{2}\left[\ln \frac{1+r}{1-r}\right]$, and follows the standard normal distribution.

For a two-tailed test, reject H_0 at the α level of significance if the calculated value of the Z statistic, (say z_o) satisfies $|z_o| \geq z_{\alpha/2}$, otherwise don't reject the null hypothesis.

Example 10.2 Consider the data on correlation coefficient in Table 10.1 of Example 10.1

For the first study (Moore 2006) test the significance of the population correlation coefficient at the 5% level of significance.

Solution:

From the first study (Moore 2006), n $= 133$ and r $= 0.56$.

The appropriate test statistic is $Z = \frac{\hat{\zeta}}{SE(\hat{\zeta})}$.

Here $\hat{\zeta} = \frac{1}{2}\left[\ln \frac{1+r}{1-r}\right] = 0.5 \times ln\left[\frac{1+0.56}{1-0.56}\right] = 0.5 \times \ln(3.54545) = 0.5 \times 1.26567 = 0.6328$. and the standard error of $\hat{\zeta}$ is $SE\left(\hat{\zeta}\right) = \sqrt{Var(\hat{\zeta})} = \sqrt{\frac{1}{n-3}} = \sqrt{\frac{1}{133-3}} = \sqrt{\frac{1}{130}} = \sqrt{0.00769} = 0.08771$.

So the calculated value of the test statistic, Z is

$$z_0 = \frac{\hat{\zeta}}{SE(\hat{\zeta})} = \frac{0.6328}{0.08771} = 7.215408 \approx 7.22.$$

The two-sided P-value is $P(|Z| > 7.22) = 2 \times P(Z > 7.22) = 2 \times 0 = 0$. Since the P-value is less than 5%, we reject the null hypothesis at the 5% level of significance. The test is significant and hence there is strong sample evidence against the null hypothesis that the population correlation coefficient is 0.

10.4   Fixed Effect (FE) Model

In this section, the meta-analysis of correlation coefficient is presented under the fixed effect model. Let the common effect size of population correlation coefficient be denoted by ρ. Then by Fisher transformation define the modified common effect size to be $\theta = \frac{1}{2} \times \ln\left[\frac{1+\rho}{1-\rho}\right] = \text{arctanh}(\rho)$. The point estimate of θ is given by its sample counterpart, $\hat{\theta} = \frac{1}{2} \times \ln\left[\frac{1+r}{1-r}\right] = \text{arctanh}(r)$, where r is the sample correlation coefficient. The standard error becomes, $SE(\hat{\theta}) = \sqrt{Var(\hat{\theta})} = \sqrt{\frac{1}{n-3}}$.

For the ith study, define the point estimate of the modified population effect size, θ_i to be $\hat{\theta}_i = \frac{1}{2} \times \ln\left[\frac{1+r_i}{1-r_i}\right] = \text{arctanh}(r_i)$, and the standard error $SE(\hat{\theta}_i) = \sqrt{\frac{1}{n_i-3}}$ for i $= 1, 2, \dots , k$, where k is the number of studies in the meta-analysis.

Under the fixed effect model, the modified common effect size estimator is given by

$$\hat{\theta}_{FE} = \sum_{i=1}^{k} w_i \hat{\theta}_i \bigg/ \sum_{i=1}^{k} w_i,$$

where $w_i = \frac{1}{v_i}$ is the weight, in which $v_i = Var(\hat{\theta}_i) = \frac{1}{n_i-3}$,

and the variance of the estimator of the modified common effect size is $Var(\hat{\theta}_{FE}) = 1 \bigg/ \sum_{i=1}^{k} w_i$. Hence the standard error of the estimator of the modified common effect size is $SE(\hat{\theta}_{FE}) = \sqrt{1 \bigg/ \sum_{i=1}^{k} w_i}$.

The confidence interval

The confidence interval for the modified common effect size θ based on the sample estimates is given by the lower limit (LL) and upper limit (UL) as follows:

$$LL^* = \hat{\theta}_{FE} - z_{\alpha/2} \times SE(\hat{\theta}_{FE}) \text{ and}$$
$$UL^* = \hat{\theta}_{FE} + z_{\alpha/2} \times SE(\hat{\theta}_{FE}).$$

Here $z_{\alpha/2}$ is the $\frac{\alpha}{2}$ th cut-off point of standard normal distribution and $SE(\hat{\theta}_{FE}) = \sqrt{Var(\hat{\theta}_{FE})}$.

Then the 95% confidence interval for population effect size ρ under the FE model, we transform the above limits using tanh transformation as follows:

$$LL = \frac{e^{2 \times LL^*} - 1}{e^{2 \times LL^*} + 1} \text{ and}$$
$$UL = \frac{e^{2 \times LL^*} - 1}{e^{2 \times LL^*} + 1}.$$

Also, the point estimate of ρ under the FE model is found by transforming that of θ as $\hat{\rho}_{FE} = \tanh(\hat{\theta}_{FE})$.

To compute the confidence interval and perform test on the modified common effect size θ for individual studies, we need to compute the point estimate and standard error of the estimator of θ for all studies.

Example 10.3 Consider the summary data on correlation coefficient from Table 10.1.

Using the sums of W and WZ at the bottom of Table 10.3 calculate the (i) point estimate of θ, (ii) standard error of estimator, and (iii) 95% confidence interval for the population effect size ρ under the fixed effect model.

Solution:

(i) The point estimate of the effect size θ under the FE model is

$$\hat{\theta}_{FE} = \frac{\sum\limits_{1}^{8} w_i \hat{\theta}_i}{\sum\limits_{1}^{8} w_i} = \frac{\sum WZ}{\sum W} = \frac{517.663}{954} = 0.542623 \approx 0.54.$$

(ii) The standard error is $SE(\hat{\theta}_{FE}) = \sqrt{\dfrac{1}{\sum\limits_{1}^{8} w_i}} = \sqrt{\dfrac{1}{\sum W}} = \sqrt{\dfrac{1}{954}} = 0.03238.$

(iii) The 95% confidence interval for the modified common population effect size θ is given by

$$LL^* = \hat{\theta}_{FE} - 1.96 \times SE(\hat{\theta}_{FE}) = 0.542623 - 1.96 \times 0.03238 = 0.47917 \text{ and}$$
$$UL^* = \hat{\theta}_{FE} + 1.96 \times SE(\hat{\theta}_{FE}) = 0.542623 + 1.96 \times 0.03238 = 0.60608.$$

Remark To find the 95% confidence interval for common effect size ρ we transform the above limits using tanh transformation as follows:

$$LL = \frac{e^{2 \times LL^*} - 1}{e^{2 \times LL^*} + 1} = \frac{e^{2 \times 0.47917} - 1}{e^{2 \times 0.47917} + 1} = \frac{2.60736 - 1}{2.60736 + 1} = \frac{1.60736}{3.60736} = 0.44558 \approx 0.44$$

Table 10.3 Summary statistics for the point estimate and confidence interval of correlation coefficient funder fixed effect model

Study	n	r	Z	Var	W	WZ
Moore (2006)	133	0.56	0.6328	0.00769	130	82.2683
Davis (2008)	149	0.43	0.4599	0.00685	146	67.1449
Thomas (1999)	131	0.53	0.5901	0.00781	128	75.5386
Miller (2012)	120	0.51	0.5627	0.00855	117	65.8394
Williams (2012)	111	0.66	0.7928	0.00926	108	85.6239
Young (2013)	152	0.46	0.4973	0.00671	149	74.0994
Baker (2009)	60	0.33	0.3428	0.01754	57	19.5412
Adams (2006)	122	0.38	0.4001	0.0084	119	47.6071
					954	517.663

Note W is the weight calculated as the inverse/reciprocal of variance (Var), and WZ is the product of weight (W) and modified sample effect size (Z)

$$UL = \frac{e^{2 \times LL^*} - 1}{e^{2 \times LL^*} + 1} = \frac{e^{2 \times 0.60608} - 1}{e^{2 \times 0.60608} + 1} = \frac{3.36074 - 1}{3.36074 + 1} = \frac{2.36074}{4.36074} = 0.54236 \approx 0.54.$$

Also, the point estimate of ρ under the FE model is found by transforming that of θ as $\hat{\rho}_{FE} = \tanh(\hat{\theta}_{FE}) = \tanh(0.542623) = 0.494971 \approx 0.49$.

Comment The above point estimate of ρ (0.49) and confidence limits (0.44, 0.54) under the FE model are displayed in the bottom row of forest plot in Fig. 10.1 and represented by the diamond.

Forest plot for correlation under FE model using MetaXL
The forest plot under the FE model (indicated by "IV" in the code) is constructed using MetaXL code
   =MAInputTable("Correlation FE","numcorr","IV",B7:D14)

Remark: Explanations of MetaXL Code
For this type of meta-analyses in MetaXL the 'opening' code starts with MA Input Table ' = MAInputTable'. This is followed by an open parenthesis inside which the first quote contains the text that appears as the 'title of the output of the forest plot' e.g. "Correlation FE" in the above code (user may choose any appropriate title here, but FE is chosen to indicate fixed effect model). Then in the second quote enter the type of effect measure, e.g. "numcorr" in the above code which tells that the variable is numeric and *correlation is the effect size*. Within the third quote enter the statistical model, e.g. "IV" in the above code stands for the *fixed effect* (abbreviated by FE) model. Each quotation is followed by a comma, and after the last comma enter the data area in Excel Worksheet, e.g. B7:D14 in the above code tells that the data on the independent studies are taken from the specified cells of the Excel Worksheet. The code ends with a closing parenthesis.
   The forest plot of the meta-analysis using the above MetaXL code is found in Fig. 10.1.

Interpretation
From the meta-analysis of correlation coefficient under the FE model, the estimated common effect size is 0.49, and the 95% confidence interval is (0.45, 0.54). The effect size is highly statistically significant (as 0 is not included in the confidence interval).
   Here Cochrane's $Q = 14.15$ with P-value slightly less than 0.05 indicates significant heterogeneity among the correlation coefficients among independent studies at the 5% level. The $I^2 = 51\%$ also reflects that there is heterogeneity among the studies.

Measuring Heterogeneity
Heterogeneity is a real concern as it is common in many meta-analyses and makes the analyses much more difficult. It is essential for every meta-analysis to investigate the presence of heterogeneity among the studies so that an appropriate statistical

model could be used to analyse the data properly. Here we cover some of the popular methods to identify and measure the extent of heterogeneity among the effect sizes of independent studies.

Cochran's Q Statistic (Cochran 1973)

The Cochrane's Q is defined as

$$Q = \sum_{i=1}^{k} w_i \hat{\theta}_i^2 - \frac{\left(\sum_{i=1}^{k} w_i \hat{\theta}_i \right)^2}{\sum_{i=1}^{k} w_i},$$

where w_i is the weight and $\hat{\theta}_i$ is the effect size estimate of the ith study.

The above Q statistic follows a chi-squared distribution with $df = (k-1)$, where k is the number of studies included in the meta-analysis. Since the expected value of a chi-squared variable is its degrees of freedom, the expected value of Q is (k-1), that is, $E(Q) = (k-1) = df$.

Test of Heterogeneity

To test the null hypothesis of the equality of effect sizes (i.e. equality excluding random error)

$H_0 : \theta_1 = \theta_2 = \ldots = \theta_k = \theta$ against H_a : not all θ_i's are equal (at least one of them is different), use the Cochrane's Q statistic as defined above.

Any small P-value leads to the conclusion that there is true difference among the effect sizes. However the non-significant P-value may not mean that the effect sizes are not different as this could happen due to low power of the test. The test alone should not be used to measure the magnitude of the true dispersion.

The I^2 Statistic (Higgins et al. 2003)

The value of the Q-statistic increases as the number of studies included in the meta-analysis becomes larger. To dealt with this problem, another statistic that quantifies heterogeneity is the I^2 statistic. It is a ratio of excess variation to the total variation expressed in percentages. This statistic is defined as

$$I^2 = \left(\frac{Q - df}{Q} \right) \times 100\%,$$

and is viewed as the proportion of between studies variation and total variation (within plus between studies variation).

Example 10.4 Consider the summary data on correlation coefficient in Table 8.1.

Find the value of (i) Q statistic and (ii) I^2 statistic for the correlation coefficient data.

Solution:

To answer the above questions, we need to find the summary statistics in Table 10.4 below.

Table 10.4 Calculations for the finding the Q statistic and I^2 statistic of correlation data

Study	n	r	Z	Var	W	WZ	W^2	WZ^2
Moore (2006)	133	0.56	0.6328	0.0077	130	82.2683	16900	52.062
Davis (2008)	149	0.43	0.4599	0.0068	146	67.1449	21316	30.88
Thomas (1999)	131	0.53	0.5901	0.0078	128	75.5386	16384	44.579
Miller (2012)	120	0.51	0.5627	0.0085	117	65.8394	13689	37.05
Williams (2012)	111	0.66	0.7928	0.0093	108	85.6239	11664	67.884
Young (2013)	152	0.46	0.4973	0.0067	149	74.0994	22201	36.85
Baker (2009)	60	0.33	0.3428	0.0175	57	19.5412	3249	6.6993
Adams (2006)	122	0.38	0.4001	0.0084	119	47.6071	14161	19.046
					954	517.663	119564	295.05

Note the squared weight is denoted by W^2 and product of weight (W) and squared modified effect size (Z^2) is denoted by WZ^2

(i)   The Q statistic is calculated as

$$Q = \sum_{i=1}^{8} w_i \hat{\theta}_i^2 - \frac{\left(\sum_{i=1}^{8} w_i \hat{\theta}_i\right)^2}{\sum_{i=1}^{8} w_i} = \sum_{i=1}^{8} WZ^2 - \frac{\left(\sum_{i=1}^{8} WZ\right)^2}{\sum_{i=1}^{8} W}$$

$$= 295.05 - \frac{(517.663)^2}{954} = 14.15.$$

To test the heterogeneity of effect sizes the P-value is found from the chi-squared Table (with df $= (8 - 1) = 7$) as $P\left(\chi_7^2 \geq 14.15\right)$ is slightly less than 5% (between 0.025 and 0.05). Note that the area under the chi-squired density curve to the right of 14.067 is exactly 5%. Since the P-value is smaller than 5%, we may reject the null hypothesis (of equal effect size for all studies) at the 5% level of significance.
   The I^2 statistic is found to be

$$I^2 = \left(\frac{Q - df}{Q}\right) \times 100\% = \left(\frac{14.15 - (8 - 1)}{14.15}\right) \times 100\% = \left(\frac{7.15}{14.15}\right) \times 100\%$$

$$= 0.5054 \times 100\% = 51\%,$$

where $df = (k - 1) = (8 - 1) = 7$.
   The above value of Q statistic, its P-value and I^2 statistic are presented on the left panel of the forest plot produced by MetaXL.

Comment The values of Q and I^2 statistics are calculated from the sample summary data, and they are not dependent on any statistical models.

10.5   Random Effects (REs) Model

The REs model is used when the effect size measure across all the studies is hetero-geneous. There are two sources of variation under the random effects model—the within study variance σ^2 and between-study variances, τ^2. The unknown combined variance $\sigma^{*2} = \sigma^2 + \tau^2$ is estimated by $v^* = v + \hat{\tau}^2$, where v is the estimate of σ^2 and $\hat{\tau}^2$ is the estimate of τ^2. Therefore, the weight assigned to the ith study under the REs model is defined as $w_i^* = \frac{1}{v_i + \hat{\tau}^2}$ for $i = 1, 2, ..., k$.

The common effect size under the REs model is estimated by

$$\hat{\theta}_{RE} = \sum_{i=1}^{k} w_i^* \hat{\theta}_i \left/ \sum_{i=1}^{k} w_i^* \right.$$

The standard error of the estimator of the common effect size is

$$SE(\hat{\theta}_{RE}) = \sqrt{1 \left/ \sum_{i=1}^{k} w_i^* \right.}$$

The $(1 - \alpha) \times 100\%$ confidence interval for the effect size θ under the REs model is given by the lower limit (LL) and upper limit (UL) as follows:

$$LL^* = \hat{\theta}_{RE} - z_{\alpha/2} \times SE(\hat{\theta}_{RE}) \text{ and}$$
$$UL^* = \hat{\theta}_{RE} + z_{\alpha/2} \times SE(\hat{\theta}_{RE}),$$

where $z_{\alpha/2}$ is the $\frac{\alpha}{2}$ th cut-off point of standard normal distribution.

Then the 95% confidence interval for population effect size ρ under the REs model, we transform the above limits using tanh transformation as follows:

$$LL = \frac{e^{2 \times LL^*} - 1}{e^{2 \times LL^*} + 1}$$

$$UL = \frac{e^{2 \times LL^*} - 1}{e^{2 \times LL^*} + 1}.$$

Also, the point estimate of ρ under the REs model is found by transforming that of θ as $\hat{\rho}_{RE} = \tanh(\hat{\theta}_{RE})$.

Estimation of τ^2
The between studies variance is estimated as a scaled excess variation as follows

$$\hat{\tau}^2 = \frac{Q - df}{C},$$

where

$$Q = \sum_{i=1}^{k} w_i \hat{\theta}_i^2 - \frac{\left(\sum_{i=1}^{k} w_i \hat{\theta}_i\right)^2}{\sum_{i=1}^{k} w_i},$$

$$C = \sum_{i=1}^{k} w_i - \frac{\sum_{i=1}^{k} w_i^2}{\sum_{i=1}^{k} w_i}$$

and $df = (k-1)$ in which k is the number of studies.

Example 10.5 Consider the summary data on correlation coefficient from Table 10.1.

Find the estimated value of between studies variance, $\hat{\tau}^2$, for the correlation data.

Solution:

The last row of Table 10.4 provides summary calculations for finding Q and C statistics which are required to find the value of $\hat{\tau}^2$.

From the previous example (or using sums from the bottom row of Table 10.4),

$$Q = \sum_{i=1}^{8} WZ^2 - \frac{\left(\sum_{i=1}^{8} WZ\right)^2}{\sum_{i=1}^{8} W} = 14.15 \text{ (details are in the previous example).}$$

Again, using the summary statistics from Table 10.4,

$$C = \sum_{i=1}^{8} w_i - \frac{\sum_{i=1}^{8} w_i^2}{\sum_{i=1}^{8} w_i} = \sum_{i=1}^{8} W - \frac{\sum_{i=1}^{8} W^2}{\sum_{i=1}^{8} W} = 954 - \frac{119564}{954} = 828.6709 \text{ and}$$

$df = k - 1 = 8 - 1 = 7$.

Then, $\hat{\tau}^2 = \frac{Q-df}{C} = \frac{14.15-7}{828.6709} = 0.008633$.

Illustration of REs Model for correlation coefficient

Example 10.6 Consider the summary data on correlation coefficient of Table 10.1.

Find the (i) point estimate of ζ, (ii) standard error of the estimator, and (iii) 95% confidence interval of the population effect size ζ under the random effects model.

Solution:

In Table 10.5, the estimated between-study variance is presented by Tau^2, the estimate of the combined variance is given by Var*, the modified weight is W* as the reciprocal of Var*, and W*Z represents the product of modified weight (W*) and transformed sample effect size (Z).

As an example, for **Study 1** (Moore 2006), the combined variance for the REs model is found to be

$$v_1^* = v_1 + \hat{\tau}^2 = 0.0077 + 0.0086 = 0.01633$$

Table 10.5 Calculated values of the summary statistics for correlation coefficient under the REs model

Study	n	r	Z	Var	Tau^2	Var*	W*	W*Z
Moore (2006)	133	0.56	0.6328	0.0077	0.0086	0.01633	61.255	38.764
Davis (2008)	149	0.43	0.4599	0.0068	0.0086	0.01548	64.59	29.705
Thomas (1999)	131	0.53	0.5901	0.0078	0.0086	0.01645	60.807	35.885
Miller (2012)	120	0.51	0.5627	0.0085	0.0086	0.01718	58.207	32.755
Williams (2012)	111	0.66	0.7928	0.0093	0.0086	0.01789	55.89	44.31
Young (2013)	152	0.46	0.4973	0.0067	0.0086	0.01534	65.17	32.41
Baker (2009)	60	0.33	0.3428	0.0175	0.0086	0.02618	38.202	13.097
Adams (2006)	122	0.38	0.4001	0.0084	0.0086	0.01704	58.698	23.483
							462.82	**250.41**

and the modified weight becomes

$$W_1^* = \frac{1}{Var_1^*} = \frac{1}{0.01633} = 61.255.$$

Now using the summary statistics from Table 10.5 we get

(i)   the point estimate of the common effect size ζ under the REs model is

$$\hat{\theta}_{RE} = \sum_{i=1}^{8} w_i^* \hat{\theta}_i \bigg/ \sum_{i=1}^{8} w_i^* = \sum_{i=1}^{8} W * Z \bigg/ \sum_{i=1}^{8} W* = \frac{250.41}{462.82} = 0.5411 \approx 0.54.$$

(ii)   The standard error of the estimator of the common effect size ζ is

$$SE(\hat{\theta}_{RE}) = \sqrt{1 \bigg/ \sum_{i=1}^{8} w_i^*} = \sqrt{1 \bigg/ \sum_{i=1}^{8} W*} = \sqrt{\frac{1}{462.82}} = 0.0465.$$

(iii)   The 95% confidence interval for the transformed effect size θ (that is, for ζ) under the REs model is given by the lower limit (LL) and upper limit (UL) as follows:

$LL^* = \hat{\theta}_{RE} - 1.96 \times SE(\hat{\theta}_{RE}) = 0.5411 - 1.96 \times 0.0465 = 0.449943 \approx 0.45$ and

$UL^* = \hat{\theta}_{RE} + 1.96 \times SE(\hat{\theta}_{RE}) = 0.5411 + 1.96 \times 0.0465 = 0.632157 \approx 0.63.$

Remark   To find the 95% confidence interval for population effect size ρ under the REs model, we transform the above limits using tanh transformation as follows:

$$LL = \frac{e^{2 \times LL^*} - 1}{e^{2 \times LL^*} + 1} = \frac{e^{2 \times 0.449943} - 1}{e^{2 \times 0.449943} + 1} = \frac{2.45932 - 1}{2.45932 + 1} = \frac{1.45932}{3.45932}$$

$$= 0.42185 \approx 0.42 \text{ and}$$

$$UL = \frac{e^{2 \times LL^*} - 1}{e^{2 \times LL^*} + 1} = \frac{e^{2 \times 0.632157} - 1}{e^{2 \times 0.632157} + 1} = \frac{3.54066 - 1}{3.54066 + 1} = \frac{2.54066}{4.54066} = 0.55954 \approx 0.56.$$

Also, the point estimate of ρ under the REs model is found by transforming that of θ as $\hat{\rho}_{RE} = \tanh(\hat{\theta}_{RE}) = \tanh(0.5411) = 0.49382 \approx 0.49$.

Comment The above point estimate (0.49) of ρ and the confidence limits (0.42, 0.56) are presented at the bottom row of the forest plot and represented by a diamond as in Fig. 10.2.

Forest plot for correlation under REs model using MetaXL
The forest plot under the REs model (indicated by "RE" in the code) is constructed using MetaXL code
=MAInputTable("Correlation RE","Numcorr","RE",B7:D14)

Remark: Explanations of MetaXL Code
For this type of meta-analyses in MetaXL the 'opening' code starts with MA Input Table ' = MAInputTable'. This is followed by an open parenthesis inside which the first quote contains the text that appears as the 'title of the output of the forest plot' e.g. "Correlation RE" in the above code (user may choose any appropriate title here, but RE is chosen to indicate random effects model). Then in the second quote enter the type of effect measure, e.g. "Numcorr" in the above code which tells that the variable is numeric and *correlation is the effect size*. Within the third quote enter the statistical model, e.g. "RE" in the above code stands for the *random effects* (abbreviated by RE) model. Each quotation is followed by a comma, and after the last comma enter the data area in Excel Worksheet, e.g. B7:D14 in the above code tells that the data on the independent studies are taken from the specified cells of the Excel Worksheet. The code ends with a closing parenthesis.

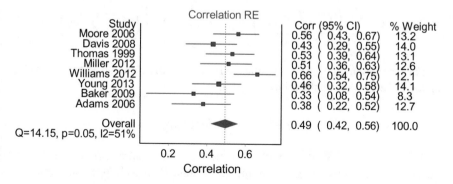

Fig. 10.2 The forest plot of correlation under the REs model

The forest plot of the meta-analysis using the above MetaXL code is found in Fig. 10.2.

Interpretation
From the above forest plot of correlation coefficient under the REs model, the estimated population effect size (common correlation coefficient) is 0.49, and the 95% confidence interval is (0.42, 0.56). The effect size is highly statistically significant (as 0 is not included in the confidence interval). The confidence interval under the REs model is wider than that under the FE model.

The value of the Q statistic (14.15), its P-value (0.05) and I^2 statistic (= 51%) indicate presence of some heterogeneity.

10.6 Inverse Variance Heterogeneity (IVhet) Model

Like the REs model, the IVhet model is appropriate when there is heterogeneity of effect size between the independent studies. But this model does not require some of the unrealistic assumptions of the REs model (cf. (Doi et al. 2015).

The estimator of the transformed common effect size θ (that is, ζ) under the inverse variance heterogeneity (IVhet) model is given by

$$\hat{\theta}^*_{IVhet} = \frac{\sum\limits_{i=1}^{k} w_i \hat{\theta}_i}{\sum\limits_{i=1}^{k} w_i}.$$

Then the variance of the estimator of θ under the IVhet model is given by

$$Var(\hat{\theta}^*_{IVhet}) = \sum_{i=1}^{k}\left[\left(\frac{1}{v_i}\bigg/\sum_{i=1}^{k}\frac{1}{v_i}\right)^2 (v_i + \hat{\tau}^2)\right] = \sum_{i=1}^{k}\left[\left(w_i\bigg/\sum_{i=1}^{k} w_i\right)^2 \times v_i^*\right].$$

For the computation of the confidence interval of the common effect size based on the IVhet model use the following standard error

$$SE(\hat{\theta}^*_{IVhet}) = \sqrt{Var(\hat{\theta}^*_{IVhet})}.$$

Then, the $(1 - \alpha) \times 100\%$ confidence interval for the common effect size $\theta^* = \xi$ under the IVhet model is given by the lower limit (LL) and upper limit (UL) as follows:

$$LL^* = \hat{\theta}^*_{IVhet} - z_{\alpha/2} \times SE(\hat{\theta}^*_{IVhet}) \text{ and}$$
$$UL^* = \hat{\theta}^*_{IVhet} + z_{\alpha/2} \times SE(\hat{\theta}^*_{IVhet}),$$

where $z_{\alpha/2}$ is the $\frac{\alpha}{2}$ th cut-off point of standard normal distribution.

Then the 95% confidence interval for population effect size ρ under the IVhet model, we transform the above limits using tanh transformation as follows:

$$LL = \frac{e^{2 \times LL^*} - 1}{e^{2 \times LL^*} + 1} \text{ and } UL = \frac{e^{2 \times LL^*} - 1}{e^{2 \times LL^*} + 1}.$$

Also, the point estimate of ρ under the IVhet model is found by the following back transformation, $\hat{\rho}_{IVhet} = \tanh(\hat{\theta}^*_{IVhet})$.

Illustration of IVhet Model for correlation coefficient

Example 10.7 Consider the summary data on correlation coefficient in Table 10.1.

Find the (i) point estimate of population effect size ζ, (ii) standard error of the estimator, and (iii) 95% confidence interval of the transformed population effect size ζ under the inverse variance heterogeneity model.

Solution:

To answer the above questions we need to compute the statistics in Table 10.6.

In the above table Var* is the combined variance (Var* = Var + Tau^2) and W* is the modified weight under the IVhet model calculated as $W_i^* =$

$$\left[\left(\frac{1}{v_i} \bigg/ \sum_{i=1}^{8} \frac{1}{v_i} \right)^2 (v_i + \hat{\tau}^2) \right] = \left(W_i \bigg/ \sum_{1}^{8} W_i \right)^2 \times Var_i^* \text{ for the ith study.}$$

For example, for the first study (Moore 2006) $Var_1^* = 0.0077 + 0.0086 = 0.01633$, and $W_1^* = \left(W_1 \bigg/ \sum_{1}^{8} W_i \right)^2 \times Var_1^* = \left(130/954 \right)^2 \times 0.01633 = 0.0003$.

Now, using the summary statistics in the last row of Table 10.6 we answer the questions in Example 10.7 as follows.

(i) The point estimate of ζ under the IVhet model is

Table 10.6 Calculated values of the summary statistics for the IVhet model

Study	n	r	Z	Var	Tau^2	Var*	W	W*	WZ
Moore (2006)	133	0.56	0.6328	0.0077	0.0086	0.01633	130	0.0003	82.268
Davis (2008)	149	0.43	0.4599	0.0068	0.0086	0.01548	146	0.0004	67.145
Thomas (1999)	131	0.53	0.5901	0.0078	0.0086	0.01645	128	0.0003	75.539
Miller (2012)	120	0.51	0.5627	0.0085	0.0086	0.01718	117	0.0003	65.839
Williams (2012)	111	0.66	0.7928	0.0093	0.0086	0.01789	108	0.0002	85.624
Young (2013)	152	0.46	0.4973	0.0067	0.0086	0.01534	149	0.0004	74.099
Baker (2009)	60	0.33	0.3428	0.0175	0.0086	0.02618	57	9E-05	19.541
Adams (2006)	122	0.38	0.4001	0.0084	0.0086	0.01704	119	0.0003	47.607
							954	0.0022	517.66

$$\hat{\theta}^*_{IVhet} = \frac{\sum\limits_{i=1}^{8} w_i \hat{\theta}_i}{\sum\limits_{i=1}^{8} w_i} = \frac{\sum\limits_{i=1}^{8} WZ}{\sum\limits_{i=1}^{8} W} = \frac{517.66}{954} = 0.5426 \approx 0.54.$$

(ii)   The standard error of the estimator is

$$SE(\hat{\theta}^*_{IVhet}) = \sqrt{\sum_{i=1}^{8} W_i^*} = \sqrt{0.0022} = 0.046716.$$

(iii)   The 95% confidence interval of the transformed effect size ζ under the IVhet model is given by the lower limit (LL) and upper limit (UL) as follows:

$$LL^* = \hat{\theta}^*_{IVhet} - 1.96 \times SE(\hat{\theta}^*_{IVhet}) = 0.5426 - 1.96 \times 0.046716$$
$$= 0.451061 \text{ and}$$

$$UL^* = \hat{\theta}^*_{IVhet} + z_{\alpha/2} \times SE(\hat{\theta}^*_{IVhet}) = 0.5426 + 1.96 \times 0.046716 = 0.63419.$$

To find the 95% confidence interval for population effect size ρ under the REs model, we transform the above limits using tanh transformation as follows:

$$LL = \frac{e^{2 \times LL^*} - 1}{e^{2 \times LL^*} + 1} = \frac{e^{2 \times 0.451061} - 1}{e^{2 \times 0.451061} + 1} = \frac{2.46483 - 1}{2.46483 + 1} = \frac{1.46483}{3.46483}$$
$$= 0.422771 \approx 0.42 \text{ and}$$

$$UL = \frac{e^{2 \times LL^*} - 1}{e^{2 \times LL^*} + 1} = \frac{e^{2 \times 0.63419} - 1}{e^{2 \times 0.63419} + 1} = \frac{3.55506 - 1}{3.55506 + 1} = \frac{2.55506}{4.55506} = 0.56093 \approx 0.56.$$

Then, the point estimate of ρ under the IVhet model is found by the following transformation, $\hat{\rho}_{IVhet} = \tanh(\hat{\theta}^*_{IVhet}) = \tanh(0.5426) = 0.495 \approx 0.49$.

Comment The above point estimate (0.49) of ρ and the 95% confidence interval (0.42, 0.56) are presented at the bottom row of the forest plot and represented by the diamond in Fig. 10.3.

Forest plot for correlation under IVhet model using MetaXL
The forest plot under the IVhet model (indicated by "IVhet" in the code) is constructed using MetaXL code
    =MAInputTable("Correlation IVhet","Numcorr","IVhet",B7:D14)

Remark: Explanations of MetaXL Code
For this type of meta-analyses in MetaXL the 'opening' code starts with MA Input Table ' = MAInputTable'. This is followed by an open parenthesis inside which the

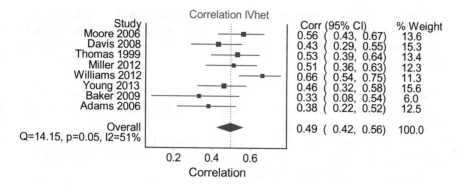

Fig. 10.3   The forest plot of correlation under the IVhet model

first quote contains the text that appears as the 'title of the output of the forest plot' e.g. "Correlation IVhet" in the above code (user may choose any appropriate title here, but IVhet is chosen to indicate inverse variance heterogeneity model). Then in the second quote enter the type of effect measure, e.g. "Numcorr" in the above code tells that the variable is numeric and *correlation is the effect size*. Within the third quote enter the statistical model, e.g. "IVhet" in the above code stands for the *inverse variance heterogeneity* (abbreviated by IVhet) model. Each quotation is followed by a comma, and after the last comma enter the data area in Excel Worksheet, e.g. B7:D14 in the above code tells that the data on the independent studies are taken from the specified cells of the Excel Worksheet. The code ends with a closing parenthesis.

The forest plot of the meta-analysis using the above MetaXL code is found in Fig. 10.3.

Interpretation

From the above forest plot of correlation coefficient under the IVhet model, in Fig. 10.3, the estimated population effect size (common correlation coefficient) is 0.49, and the 95% confidence interval is (0.42, 0.56). The effect size is highly statistically significant (as 0 is not included in the confidence interval).

10.7   Discussions and Comparison of Results

The meta-analyses of the correlation coefficient data in Example 10.3 have been provided in the previous section. The same data has been meta-analysed under the fixed effect, random effects and inverse variance heterogeneity models.

From the calculated value of Cochran's $Q = 14.15$ with its P-value less than 0.05 we find significant heterogeneity in the correlation coefficients among the independent studies. The $I^2 = 51\%$ also reflects that there is heterogeneity among the studies.

Comparison of results

The point estimate of the common population correlation coefficient (0.49) is the same for all three statistical models.

Under the FE model, the 95% confidence interval for the common population correlation coefficient, ρ is (0.45, 0.54) which is highly statistically significant (as 0 is not included in the confidence interval).

The 95% confidence interval under both the REs and IVhet models is (0.42, 0.56) which is also highly significant. So, the confidence interval under the REs and IVhet models is wider than that under the FE model.

Even though the point estimate and 95% confidence interval for the common population correlation coefficient is the same for both REs and IVhet models the re-distributed weights of individual studies are very different.

10.8 Subgroup Analysis

The subgroup analysis for correlation coefficient is very similar to that of WMD in Sect. 9.7. It is not necessary to re-produce them again here. Readers interested to subgroup analysis and their interpretations are referred that Section.

10.9 Publication Bias

The study of publication bias for correlation coefficient is very similar to that of SMD in Sect. 8.8. It is not necessary to re-produce them again here. Readers interested to produce funnel plot or Doi plot and their interpretations are referred that Section.

Appendix 10—Stata Codes for Correlation Coefficient Meta-Analysis

A10.1 Correlation data

Study name	n	r	Z	seZ
Moore (2006)	133	0.56	0.6328	0.0877
Davis (2008)	149	0.43	0.4599	0.0828

(continued)

(continued)

Study name	n	r	Z	seZ
Thomas (1999)	131	0.53	0.5901	0.0884
Miller (2012)	120	0.51	0.5627	0.0925
Williams (2012)	111	0.66	0.7928	0.0962
Young (2013)	152	0.46	0.4973	0.0819
Baker (2009)	60	0.33	0.3428	0.1325
Adams (20067)	122	0.38	0.4001	0.0917

A10.2 Stata codes for meta-analysis

A10.2.1 *metan* function [outputs in terms of $Z = \text{atanh}(r)$]

* Fixed effects meta-analysis
metan Z seZ, fixed lcols(Study) astext(85) xlabels(0(0.25)1) name(forestfixd, replace)
* Random effects meta-analysis
metan Z seZ, random lcols(Study) astext(85) xlabels(0(0.25)1) name(forestrand, replace)
* Combined fixed and random effects forest plots on the same graph
graph combine forestfixd forestrand, ysize(3) xsize(6) name(ROcombined, replace)

A10.2.2 *admetan* function [outputs in terms of $Z = \text{atanh}(r)$]

* **Fixed effects model**
admetan Z seZ, model(fixed) study(Study) or
admetan Z seZ, model(fixed) study(Study) forestplot(effect("Pooled Effect Size")
xlabel(−1 −0.6 −0.3 0 0.3 0.6 1))
* **Random effects model**
admetan Z seZ, model(random) study(Study) or
admetan Z seZ, model(random) study(Study) forestplot(effect("Pooled Effect Size") xlabel(−1 −0.6 −0.3 0 0.3 0.6 1))
* **IVhet model**
admetan Z seZ, model(ivhet) study(Study) or
admetan Z seZ, model(ivhet) study(Study) forestplot(effect("Pooled Effect Size")
xlabel(−1 −0.6 −0.3 0 0.3 0.6 1))
A10.2.2 *admetan* function [outputs in terms of $r = \text{tanh}(Z)$]
** First run any of the above admetan command to generate six new columns (_ES, _seES, _LCI, _UCI, _WT, _rsample) in the dataset
* **Fixed effect model**
clear all
set more off
admetan Z seZ, model(fixed) study(Study)

** _ES is the effect size of each individual studies in z scale, so first transform back Z values to r values

```
generate es = tanh(_ES)
generate lb = tanh(_LCI)
generate ub = tanh(_UCI)
```

** **Create forest plot of r values manually**

* At first prepare data for -forestplot-

```
generate _USE = 1
```

//Generate study labels for -forestplot-

```
generate _LABELS = Study
label var _LABELS "Study"
label var n "Sample size"
```

//Add effect size to data set

```
local new = _N + 1
set obs 'new'
replace _LABELS = "{bf:Overall}" if _n == _N
replace r = tanh(r(eff)) if _LABELS == "{bf:Overall}"
replace lb = tanh(r(eff) - (1.96 * r(se_eff))) if _LABELS == "{bf:Overall}"
replace ub = tanh(r(eff) + (1.96 * r(se_eff))) if _LABELS == "{bf:Overall}"
replace _USE = 5 if _LABELS == "{bf:Overall}"
```

//Forest plot (with weight) under fixed effect model

```
forestplot r lb ub, nonull effect("Correlation") rcol(n) leftjustify
```

* **Random effects model**

```
clear all
set more off
admetan Z seZ, model(random) study(Study)
```

** _ES is the effect size of each individual studies in z scale, so first transform back Z values to r values

```
generate es = tanh(_ES)
generate lb = tanh(_LCI)
generate ub = tanh(_UCI)
```

** **Create forest plot of r values manually**

* At first prepare data for -forestplot-

```
generate _USE = 1
```

//Generate study labels for -forestplot-

```
generate _LABELS = Study
label var _LABELS "Study"
label var n "Sample size"
```

//Add effect size to data set

```
local new = _N + 1
set obs 'new'
replace _LABELS = "{bf:Overall}" if _n == _N
replace r = tanh(r(eff)) if _LABELS == "{bf:Overall}"
replace lb = tanh(r(eff) - (1.96 * r(se_eff))) if _LABELS == "{bf:Overall}"
replace ub = tanh(r(eff) + (1.96 * r(se_eff))) if _LABELS == "{bf:Overall}"
```

```
replace _USE = 5 if _LABELS == "{bf:Overall}"
//Forest plot (with weight) under random effects model
forestplot r lb ub, nonull effect("Correlation") rcol(n) leftjustify
* IVhet model
clear all
set more off
admetan Z seZ, model(ivhet) study(Study)
** _ES is the effect size of each individual studies in z scale, so first transform
back Z values to r values
generate es = tanh(_ES)
generate lb = tanh(_LCI)
generate ub = tanh(_UCI)
** Create forest plot of r values manually
* At first prepare data for -forestplot-
generate _USE = 1
//Generate study labels for -forestplot-
generate _LABELS = Study
label var _LABELS "Study"
label var n "Sample size"
//Add effect size to data set
local new = _N + 1
set obs 'new'
replace _LABELS = "{bf:Overall}" if _n == _N
replace r = tanh(r(eff)) if _LABELS == "{bf:Overall}"
replace lb = tanh(r(eff) - (1.96 * r(se_eff))) if _LABELS == "{bf:Overall}"
replace ub = tanh(r(eff) + (1.96 * r(se_eff))) if _LABELS == "{bf:Overall}"
replace _USE = 5 if _LABELS == "{bf:Overall}"
//Forest plot (with weight) under IVhet model
forestplot r lb ub, nonull effect("Correlation") rcol(n) leftjustify
```

References

Cochran WG (1973) Experiments for nonlinear functions (R.A. Fisher Memorial Lecture). J Am Stat Assoc 68(344):771–781. https://doi.org/10.1080/01621459.1973.10481423

Doi SA, Barendregt JJ, Khan S, Thalib L, Williams GM (2015) Advances in the meta-analysis of heterogeneous clinical trials I: the inverse variance heterogeneity model. Contemp Clin Trials 45(Pt A):130–138. https://doi.org/10.1016/j.cct.2015.05.009

Fisher RA (1915) Frequency distribution of the values of the correlation coefficient in samples from an indefinitely large population. Biometrika 10(4):507–521. https://doi.org/10.2307/2331838

Higgins JP, Thompson SG, Deeks JJ, Altman DG (2003) Measuring inconsistency in meta-analyses. BMJ 327(7414):557–560

Hinkle DE (2003) Applied statistics for the behavioral sciences, 5th edn. Houghton Mifflin, Boston

Part IV
Special Topics in Meta-Analysis

Chapter 11
Meta-Regression

Chang Xu and Suhail A. R. Doi

11.1 Basic Theory

11.1.1 The Classical Meta-Regression Method

Suppose $\hat{\theta}_j$ is the effect estimated in the *jth* study, then under the fixed-effect model,

$$\hat{\theta}_j \sim N(\mu, \sigma_j^2)$$

The fixed-effect model assumes all the studies are from the same population so there is no heterogeneity between these studies (Thompson and Higgins 2002). Now let's consider the random-effect model:

$$\hat{\theta}_j \sim N(\theta_j, \sigma_j^2); \theta_j \sim N(\mu, \tau^2)$$

The heterogeneity term τ^2 is generated under the assumption that the difference between the overall population parameter (μ) and the study population characteristics modified effect (e.g. difference in mean age) is distributed normally with a common variance (Thompson and Sharp 1999). The regression model is then

$$\hat{\theta}_j = \mu + \beta_1 \cdot x_1 + \beta_2 \cdot x_2 + \ldots + \beta_i \cdot x_i + b_j + \varepsilon_j$$

C. Xu (✉) · S. A. R. Doi
Qatar University, Doha, Qatar
e-mail: xuchang2016@runbox.com

S. A. R. Doi
e-mail: sardoi@gmx.net

© Springer Nature Singapore Pte Ltd. 2020
S. Khan, *Meta-Analysis*, Statistics for Biology and Health,
https://doi.org/10.1007/978-981-15-5032-4_11

Here x represents the study-level characteristics and ε_j represents the random error with the variance of σ_j^2 and b the non-random error with the variance of τ^2, both of which share the expectation (mean) of zero. Because all the characteristics (independent variables) are mean or median based on the study-level, each study is independent from another, and these variables are independent from each other. To take account of the variance of error information into the meta-regression, the weighted least square method can be used to get the parameter estimations.

A problem with fixed-effect meta-regression is that most studies are heterogeneous and thus there is overdispersion of the data compared to the model that random-effect meta-regression tries to address (Harbord and Higgins 2008). However, it should be pointed out that with increasing heterogeneity of studies, the random-effect weights become more equal and the regression therefore becomes more and more unweighted and this tends to lead to continued overdispersion with this model as well (Doi et al. 2015). As expected, when variables are added (or dropped) within the regression model, the total weighted variance (Q) will change, while the within study variance (σ_j^2) is known to us and keeps the same. This will result in the change of the between study variance (τ^2) so that when it reduces, this means that the variable can explain part of the heterogeneity and when it increases, this means adding the variable will make the fitting of the model poorer and the variable should not be added and of course is not the source of heterogeneity. The proportion of heterogeneity explained by the added variables is then

$$R^2 = [(\tau_0^2 - \tau_{model}^2)/\tau_0^2, 0]$$

The equation implies that when the heterogeneity is reduced then the $\tau_{model}^2 \leq \tau_0^2$, and when heterogeneity increased that $\tau_{model}^2 > \tau_0^2$, with the proportion tending towards zero (Thompson and Higgins 2009). Here the proportion is actually the same as the R square of the generic regression and is then indexed as R squared.

$$R^2 = \frac{\tau_0^2 - \tau_{model}^2}{\tau_0^2} = 1 - \frac{SS_{res}}{SS_{total}} = \frac{SS_{model}}{SS_{total}}$$

Here τ_0^2 is the heterogeneity when we did not add any variables into the regression and obviously, the result of this model is the pooled effect estimate of the population parameter μ(the constant term).

$$\hat{\theta}_j = \mu + b_j + \varepsilon_j$$

11.1.2   The Robust Error Meta-Regression Method

The classical meta-regression model is based on the random-effect meta-analytic model while this model has the limitation we noted previously. An alternative solution is to use the generic regression with the robust (Huber-Eicker-White-sandwich) error variances to account for the underestimated variance in such analyses under the regression model (Hedges et al. 2010). These standard errors are usually bigger than the ordinary least squares (OLS) standard errors when effect sizes further from the mean are more variable. Weights applied to this model are fixed-effect weights and overdispersion is avoided through use of robust standard errors.

11.2   Application in MetaXL/STATA

11.2.1   The Meta-Regression Dataset

The IHDChol example uses 28 randomized trials of serum cholesterol reduction (by various interventions), and the risk of ischaemic heart disease (IHD) events observed. Both fatal IHD and non-fatal myocardial infarction were included as IHD events, and the analysis is based on the 28 trials reported by Law et al. (Law et al. 1994). In these trials, cholesterol had been reduced by a variety of means, namely dietary intervention, drugs, and, in one case, surgery. The meta-regression looks at if increased benefit in terms of IHD risk reduction is associated with greater reduction in serum cholesterol, in order to lend support to the efficacy of cholesterol reduction and to predict the expected IHD risk reduction consequent upon a specified decrease in serum cholesterol (Table 11.1).

11.2.2   The Robust Error Meta-Regression in STATA

We may first use the inverse-variance weights with the following command to conduct a generic meta-analysis. The reason we use the inverse-variance weights is that with the robust standard errors it mimics the IVhet model (Doi et al. 2015) of meta-analysis which is a robust error fixed-effect model and results can then be compared against the latter. The pooled OR under the IVhet model is 0.83 (95%CI: 0.72, 0.95) and the relative heterogeneity (I^2) is 45.7% and the between-study variance (τ^2) is 0.0188.

Table 11.1 Comparisons on the IDH events of various interventions

Study name	N1	Cases1	Non-cases1	N2	Cases2	Non-cases2	Chol_reduc
T1	5331	173	5158	5296	210	5086	0.55
T2	244	54	190	253	85	168	0.68
T3	350	54	296	367	75	292	0.85
T4	2222	676	1546	2789	936	1853	0.55
T5	145	42	103	284	69	215	0.59
T6	279	73	206	276	101	175	0.84
T7	1906	157	1749	1900	193	1707	0.65
T8	71	6	65	72	11	61	0.85
T9	1149	36	1113	1129	42	1087	0.49
T10	88	2	86	30	2	28	0.68
T11	2051	56	1995	2030	84	1946	0.69
T12	94	1	93	94	5	89	1.35
T13	4541	131	4410	4516	121	4395	0.7
T14	424	52	372	422	65	357	0.87
T15	199	45	154	194	52	142	0.95
T16	229	61	168	229	81	148	1.13
T17	221	37	184	237	24	213	0.31
T18	28	8	20	52	11	41	0.61
T19	130	47	83	134	50	84	0.57
T20	421	82	339	417	125	292	1.43
T21	6582	62	6520	1663	20	1643	1.08
T22	94	2	92	52	0	52	1.48
T23	23	1	22	29	0	29	0.56
T24	60	3	57	30	5	25	1.06
T25	1018	132	886	1015	144	871	0.26
T26	311	35	276	317	24	293	0.76
T27	79	3	76	78	4	74	0.54
T28	76	7	69	79	19	60	0.68

```
. admetan cases1 noncases1 cases2 noncases2, or ivhet summaryonly

Studies included: 28
Participants included: 52350

Meta-analysis pooling of Odds Ratios
using Doi's IVHet model
based on DerSimonian-Laird estimate of tau²
```

	Odds Ratio	[95% Conf. Interval]		% Weight
Overall effect	0.825	0.719	0.946	100.00

```
Test of overall effect = 1:  z =  -2.750  p = 0.006

Heterogeneity Measures
```

	Value	df	p-value
Mantel-Haenszel Q	49.69	27	0.005
I² (%)	45.7%		
Modified H²	0.840		
tau²	0.0294		

From the results, we can see that there is moderate heterogeneity ($I^2 = 45.7\%$, $tau^2 = 0.0294$) between studies. The total variance based on Mantel-Haenszel estimates is 49.69.

Using a robust error meta-regression without covariates, we can reproduce these results as follows:

```
.  regress _ES [aw=1/(_seES^2)], vce(robust) eform(expb)
(sum of wgt is    8.8607e+02)
```

```
Linear regression                    Number of obs   =        28
                                     F(0, 27)        =      0.00
                                     Prob > F        =         .
                                     R-squared       =    0.0000
                                     Root MSE        =    .24116
```

_ES	expb	Robust Std. Err.	t	P>|t|	[95% Conf. Interval]	
_cons	.8245754	.0329994	-4.82	0.000	.7595715	.8951422

We may further investigate whether the amount of cholesterol reduction is associated with the lnORs across studies by the robust error meta-regression analysis with inverse-variance weights and where _ES and _seES are the effect size and standard error of the effect size respectively.

```
. regress _ES chol_reduc [aw=1/(_seES^2)], vce(robust) eform(expb)
(sum of wgt is    8.8607e+02)
```

```
Linear regression                              Number of obs    =          28
                                               F(1, 26)         =       30.23
                                               Prob > F         =      0.0000
                                               R-squared        =      0.2380
                                               Root MSE         =      .21453
```

_ES	expb	Robust Std. Err.	t	P>|t|	[95% Conf. Interval]	
chol_reduc	.6217327	.0537374	-5.50	0.000	.5205299	.7426115
_cons	1.128355	.0764952	1.78	0.087	.9815813	1.297077

The meta-regression analysis suggests there is significant association between amount of cholesterol reduction and lnORs (p < 0.001) and each unit reduction in cholesterol will lead to a 38% reduction of the odds (OR = 0.62, 95%CI: 0.52, 0.74). The proportion of between-study variance explained by cholesterol reduction was 23.8% ($R^2 = \frac{mss}{mss+rss}$, see below). Here mss indicate the model sum of square (SS_{model}) while rss is the residual sum of squares (SS_{res}). The *ereturn list* command allows us to see the total variance when the *chol_reduc* variable was added into the model. The *e(r2_a)* gives the adjusted R^2 (20.9%).

```
. ereturn lis

scalars:
                e(N)   =    28
             e(df_m)   =    1
             e(df_r)   =    26
                e(F)   =    30.23358785102188
               e(r2)   =    .2379548957201425
             e(rmse)   =    .2145287950676138
              e(mss)   =    .3736444210308938
              e(rss)   =    1.196587701742218
             e(r2_a)   =    .2086454686324557
               e(ll)   =    4.407949273183275
             e(ll_0)   =    .6034558100779854
             e(rank)   =    2
```

We may observe that the total variance also reduced (F_{model} = 30.23). And we can use the total variance to calculate the I^2 statistic

$$I^2_{model} = \frac{F_{model} - (df\_r)}{F_{model}} = \frac{30.23 - 26}{30.23} = 13.99\%$$

To depict this relationship we can create a *twoway* plot as follows:

twoway (scatter _ES chol_reduc [w = 1/(_seES²)], msymbol(oh)) (lfit _ES chol_reduc [w = 1/(_seES²)], yline(−0.193) ytitle("Effect size (interval scale)"))

Figure 11.1 presents the regression plot between amount of cholesterol reduction and lnORs. The figure may help us to explain the reason for the reduction on total variance. The dash line is the pooled lnOR by IVhet method [ln(0.825) = −0.193] without adding the chol_reduc variable and the solid line is the linear prediction for

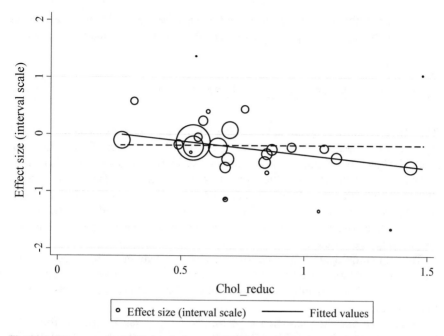

Fig. 11.1 The regression plot between amount of cholesterol reduction and lnORs

cholesterol reduction and lnORs. As we known, the total variance is the sum weighted distance for the observed value to the predicted value ($Q = \sum w_j \cdot \left(\theta - \hat{\theta}\right)^2$). Obviously, the sum weighted distance for the observed value to the dash line is different to the linear prediction and the latter shows better fitting.

As we add the chol_reduc variable into the regression model, the risk of IHD is comparable when the cholesterol reduction is zero (OR = 1.13, 95%CI: 0.98, 1.30).

The meta-regression may also be done using the classic random-effect meta-regression method using the *metareg* command. We then obtain the following results where _seES is the standard error for the effect size (_ES) in each study from the *admetan* command described earlier:

```
. metareg _ES chol_reduc, wsse( _seES ) eform graph mm

Meta-regression                                     Number of obs  =      28
Method of moments estimate of between-study variance  tau2         = .01647
% residual variation due to heterogeneity           I-squared_res  =  31.34%
Proportion of between-study variance explained      Adj R-squared  =  43.97%
With Knapp-Hartung modification
```

_ES	exp(b)	Std. Err.	t	P>|t|	[95% Conf. Interval]	
chol_reduc	.5941587	.113809	-2.72	0.012	.4007817	.8808399
_cons	1.172955	.1707306	1.10	0.283	.8696468	1.582049

The point estimates are similar but in this instance the confidence intervals are slightly different given the Knapp-Hartung modification (Knapp and Hartung 2003).

11.2.3 Meta-Regression in MetaXL

The MetaXL add-in program in Excel also provide solutions for meta-analysis and it allows us to generate data for meta-regression. The MARegresData function in MetaXL allows the creation of a regression dataset that can be directly pasted in Stata and used to run meta-regression analyses under this framework. The dataset appears in a table under the Meta-Regression data tab that will show in the MAInputTable output pop-up window when a MARegresData function is linked to the MAInput-Table function. The MARegresData function creates all the necessary variables and weights required for the analysis.

The regression dataset table consists of nine fixed columns that describe each study's characteristics, and any number of user-defined columns that describe each study's moderator variables. The fixed columns are defined in the table below (Table 11.2).

Please note that the regression is performed on the transformed variables: the transformed effect size called "t_es" as well as a weight under the model of interest called "weight". (The un-transformed variables u_es and its CI are there only for the convenience of the user, useful when back-transformed outputs are cumbersome to obtain, such as with the double arcsine transformation for prevalence). The variable t_es is the outcome variable and this is regressed against the user-defined moderator variables in the dataset.

We open the IHDCholMetaRegres example module and use the MAInputTable and the MARegresData function preparing the meta-regression data by MetaXL. We then see the meta-regression data is presented in the table (Fig. 11.2).

Table 11.2 Definition of variables for meta-regression in cholesterol reduction example

Variable name	Contents
ID	Study name
t_es	Transformed effect size
se_t_es	Standard error of the transformed effect size
var_t_es	Variance of the transformed effect size
u_es	Un-transformed effect size (i.e. natural scale)
lci_u_es	Lower CI of the un-transformed effect size
uci_u_es	Higher CI of the un-transformed effect size
inv_var	Inverse of the variance of the transformed effect size
weight	Weight of the study in the meta-analysis (normalized weights that sum to 1)

Chol_reduc results

Options

Forest plot | Doi plot | Funnel plot | Table | Exclude | Sensitivity | Meta-Regression data

ID	t_es	se_t_es	var_t_es	u_es	lci_u_es	uci_u_es	inv_var	weight	Chol_reduc
T1	-0.207873...	0.1045597...	0.0109327...	0.8123100...	0.6617903...	0.9970645...	91.468350...	0.1032296...	0.55
T2	-0.576727...	0.2037124...	0.0414987...	0.5617337...	0.3768167...	0.8373959...	24.097103...	0.0271955...	0.68
T3	-0.342109...	0.1966084...	0.0386548...	0.7102702...	0.4831369...	1.0441840...	25.869949...	0.0291963...	0.85
T4	-0.144287...	0.0611077...	0.0037341...	0.8656389...	0.7679301...	0.9757797...	267.79770...	0.3022320...	0.55
T5	0.2394721...	0.2294824...	0.0526621...	1.2705783...	0.8103369...	1.9922196...	18.988960...	0.0214306...	0.59
T6	-0.487751...	0.1848466...	0.0341682...	0.6140055...	0.4273961...	0.8820923...	29.266915...	0.0330301...	0.84
T7	-0.230751...	0.1127313...	0.0127083...	0.7939370...	0.6365448...	0.9902460...	78.688407...	0.0888064...	0.65
T8	-0.669649...	0.5379161...	0.2893538...	0.5118881...	0.1783610...	1.4690958...	3.4559765...	0.0039003...	0.85
T9	-0.177788...	0.2310968...	0.0534057...	0.8371197...	0.5322033...	1.3167324...	18.724579...	0.0211322...	0.49
T10	-1.122142...	1.0233973...	1.0473421...	0.3255813...	0.0438068...	2.4197862...	0.9547977...	0.0010775...	0.68
T11	-0.430333...	0.1754338...	0.0307770...	0.6502923...	0.4610830...	0.9171454...	32.491761...	0.0366696...	0.69
T12	-1.653401...	1.1054359...	1.2219886...	0.1913978...	0.0219274...	1.6706514...	0.8183382...	0.0009235...	1.35
T13	0.0759996...	0.1278762...	0.0163523...	1.0789621...	0.8397649...	1.3862919...	61.153330...	0.0690166...	0.7
T14	-0.264301...	0.2002615...	0.0401046...	0.7677419...	0.5185042...	1.1367845...	24.934747...	0.0281409...	0.87
T15	-0.225706...	0.2344968...	0.0549887...	0.7979520...	0.5039329...	1.2635162...	18.185537...	0.0205238...	0.95
T16	-0.410326...	0.2035884...	0.0414482...	0.6634332...	0.4451459...	0.9887626...	24.126465...	0.0272287...	1.13
T17	0.5792204...	0.2807548...	0.0788233...	1.7846467...	1.0293741...	3.0940780...	12.686602...	0.0143178...	0.31
T18	0.3993860...	0.5387943...	0.2902993...	1.4909090...	0.5185953...	4.2862128...	3.4447202...	0.0038876...	0.61
T19	-0.049899...	0.2554007...	0.0652295...	0.9513253...	0.5766755...	1.5693744...	15.330475...	0.0173017...	0.57
T20	-0.570840...	0.1630019...	0.0265696...	0.5650501...	0.4105248...	0.7777401...	37.636953...	0.0424764...	1.43
T21	-0.246948...	0.2586330...	0.0668910...	0.7811809...	0.4705467...	1.2968821...	14.949683...	0.0168719...	1.08
T22	1.0430424...	1.5588003...	2.4298584...	2.8378378...	0.1337009...	60.233876...	0.4115466...	0.0004644...	1.48
T23	1.3694872	1.6568069	2.7450094	3.9333333	0.1529269	101.16666	0.3642974	0.0004111	0.56

Fig. 11.2 The output sheet for meta-regression data prepared for meta-regression

Right-click on the "Meta-regression data" table in the results window and click copy. Then we paste the data into Stata software and run the robust meta-regression.

```
. regress t_es chol_reduc[aw=weight], vce(robust) eform(expb)
(sum of wgt is   1.0000e+00)

Linear regression                               Number of obs     =         28
                                                F(1, 26)          =      30.23
                                                Prob > F          =     0.0000
                                                R-squared         =     0.2380
                                                Root MSE          =     .21453

------------------------------------------------------------------------------
             |               Robust
        t_es |       expb   Std. Err.      t    P>|t|     [95% Conf. Interval]
-------------+----------------------------------------------------------------
  chol_reduc |   .6217327   .0537374    -5.50   0.000       .52053    .7426115
       _cons |   1.128355   .0764952     1.78   0.087     .9815813    1.297077
------------------------------------------------------------------------------
```

11.3 Meta-Regression for Categorical Variables

In the above example we illustrated meta-regression for continues variable, there comes to the question that when the variable is discontinuous how to conduct the meta-regression? Let's use the same dataset to simulate a categorical variable by categorizing the cholesterol reduction into three levels (<0.5, 0.5 ~ 0.99, 1 ~ 1.5) and assign 0, 1, 2 to these three dummy variables.

recode chol_reduc (min/0.499 = 0) (0.5/0.999999 = 1) (1/max = 2), *gen(chol_grp)*

Now we get the dataset as show in the following figure (Fig. 11.3).

Again, we run the meta-regression analysis with indicator variable for group to allow a categorical robust meta-regression.

Data Editor (Edit) - [Untitled]

File   Edit   View   Data   Tools

var10[34]

	studyname	n1	cases1	noncases1	n2	cases2	noncases2	chol
1	T1	5331	173	5158	5296	210	5086	1
2	T2	244	54	190	253	85	168	1
3	T3	350	54	296	367	75	292	1
4	T4	2222	676	1546	2789	936	1853	1
5	T5	145	42	103	284	69	215	1
6	T6	279	73	206	276	101	175	1
7	T7	1906	157	1749	1900	193	1707	1
8	T8	71	6	65	72	11	61	1
9	T9	1149	36	1113	1129	42	1087	0
10	T10	88	2	86	30	2	28	1
11	T11	2051	56	1995	2030	84	1946	1
12	T12	94	1	93	94	5	89	2
13	T13	4541	131	4410	4516	121	4395	1
14	T14	424	52	372	422	65	357	1
15	T15	199	45	154	194	52	142	1
16	T16	229	61	168	229	81	148	2
17	T17	221	37	184	237	24	213	0
18	T18	28	8	20	52	11	41	1
19	T19	130	47	83	134	50	84	1
20	T20	421	82	339	417	125	292	2
21	T21	6582	62	6520	1663	20	1643	2

Length: 3   Vars: 8 Order: Dataset   Obs: 28

Fig. 11.3 Simulated categorical variable for meta-regression

```
. regress t_es i.chol_grp[aw=weight], vce(robust) eform(expb)
(sum of wgt is    1.0000e+00)
```

```
Linear regression                              Number of obs    =          28
                                               F(2, 25)         =        8.32
                                               Prob > F         =      0.0017
                                               R-squared        =      0.1863
                                               Root MSE         =      .22606
```

t_es	expb	Robust Std. Err.	t	P>|t|	[95% Conf. Interval]	
chol_grp						
1	.8534954	.1004852	-1.35	0.191	.6697221	1.087696
2	.6335032	.0836576	-3.46	0.002	.4826499	.8315061
_cons	.9763426	.1075545	-0.22	0.830	.778161	1.224997

We may observe that when using the categorical variable, the proportion of between-study variance explained is much less than the continues one (18.6% versus 23.8%). The constant takes the value of the zero category (reference group).

11.4 Multivariable Meta-Regression

Both classical meta-regression method and the robust error meta-regression method allow us to achieve multivariable meta-regression just like the multivariable regression in individual-level data (Thompson and Higgins 2009). Sometimes multivariable meta-regression is necessary because single covariate generally is only able to explain part of the between-study heterogeneity. In our above example, we know that cholesterol reduction can explain 23.8% of the between-study heterogeneity but not 100%. This means there is still a lot of between-study heterogeneity due to other covariates, which may be the mean age, the region, the mean body mass index and so forth. To address this, we may just add these variables into the meta-regression model. For example, suppose we have another covariate of age in the above example, we may then put both cholesterol and age into the model.

It is notable that more covariates mean we need more studies (one study is a data point) to ensure the statistical power of meta-regression. Then, when we put covariates into the meta-regression model, we should first ensure a sufficient number of studies and note that for every covariate added we need at least 10 additional studies. Therefore, two covariates need at least 20 studies to be present. When the total number of studies is less than 10, it is not appropriate to employ a meta-regression analysis and the subgroup analysis may be employed as an alternative solution to detect the source of heterogeneity. Similarly, when the total number of studies is less than 20, we may only use 1 covariate to fit the meta-regression.

Some characteristics cannot be treated as a covariate for meta-regression, for example, the sample size. This is because sample size in each study is highly correlated with the standard errors of effect estimates. When entered into the meta-regression model, it will break the assumption of orthogonality and make the regression model invalid (Dobson and Barnett 2008).

It might be noted that subgroup analysis is a special case of meta-regression of categorical variables. The difference is that subgroup analysis can only deal with one variable each time and does not have a relative comparison to the reference group within the analysis. The advantage of subgroup analysis to meta-regression is that it does not have the restriction regarding the minimum number of studies. It is notable that for subgroup analysis the interaction test of the potential difference of the effects among sub groups is generally underpowered when there are 3 or more sub groups.

11.5 Summary

In this chapter, we give a detailed introduction to the meta-regression method, including the basic theories, the step-by-step application for meta-regression in Stata and MetaXL as well as the multivariable meta-regression. We suggest that readers read this chapter with Chap. 13 which introduces dose-response meta-analysis, as this may help readers acquire a deeper understanding of both meta-regression and dose-response meta-analysis.

References

Borenstein M, Hedges LV, Higgins JPT et al (2011) Introduction to Meta-Analysis. John Wiley & Sons, New York City

Dobson AJ, Barnett AG (eds) (2008) An introduction to generalized linear models—third edition. Chapman and Hall/CRC Press, Boca Raton

Doi SA, Barendregt JJ, Khan S et al (2015) Advances in the meta-analysis of heterogeneous clinical trials I: the inverse variance heterogeneity model. Contemp Clini Trials 45(Pt A):130–138

Harbord RM, Higgins JPT (2008) Meta-regression in Stata. The Stata J 8(4):493–519

Hedges LV, Tipton E, Johnson MC (2010) Robust variance estimation in meta-regression with dependent effect size estimates. Res Synth Methods 1:39–65

Higgins JP, Thompson SG, Deeks JJ et al (2003) Measuring inconsistency in meta-analyses. BMJ 327(7414):557–560

Knapp G, Hartung J (2003) Improved tests for a random effects meta-regression with a single covariate. Stat Med 22(17):2693–2710

Law MR, Wald NJ, Thompson SG (1994) By how much and how quickly does reduction in serum cholesterol concentration lower risk of ischaemic heart disease? BMJ 308(6925):367–372

Thompson SG, Higgins JP (2002) How should meta-regression analyses be undertaken and interpreted? Stat Med 21(11):1559–1573

Thompson SG, Sharp SJ (1999) Explaining heterogeneity in meta-analysis: a comparison of methods. Stat Med 18(20):2693–2708

Chapter 12
Publication Bias

Luis Furuya-Kanamori and Suhail A.R. Doi

12.1 Introduction

As we have seen in Chap. 1, systematic reviews and meta-analyses of randomised controlled trials generate the highest level of evidence. However, pooled estimates generated from systematic reviews and meta-analyses can be biased due to methodological weakness of the individual trials such as inadequate randomisation, lack of allocation concealment, or incomplete outcome data. Furthermore, meta-analytical pooled estimates can be severely affected if not all existing evidence is included in the analysis. We call this publication bias and is the subject of this Chapter.

For various reasons not all research studies, including randomised controlled trials, are published and hence results or summary statistics on the research question of interest are not always publicly accessible for meta-analysis. One major reason for publication bias is that results that are not statistically significant (p-value > 0.05) are less likely to be published in scientific journals (Koren et al. 1989). Rosenthal described this as the "file drawer problem" where journals are filled with the 5% of studies showing a false-positive result while the remaining non-significant results are being filed in the researcher's drawer (Rosenthal 1979). Another common reason for results not being published are unfavourable findings of trials that contradict funding agency interests. Other reasons that may also lead to publication bias include language bias (i.e. including only studies published in English), time-lag bias (i.e. results of negative trials take longer to get published than positive trials), and outcome reporting bias (i.e. selective reporting of pre-specified outcomes in a trial) (Thornton and Lee 2000).

L. Furuya-Kanamori (✉)
Research School of Population Health, Australian National University, Canberra, Australia
e-mail: luis.furuya-kanamori@anu.edu.au

S. A.R. Doi
Qatar University, Doha, Qatar
e-mail: sardoi@gmx.net

© Springer Nature Singapore Pte Ltd. 2020
S. Khan, *Meta-Analysis*, Statistics for Biology and Health,
https://doi.org/10.1007/978-981-15-5032-4_12

12.2   Detection Methods

When conducting a meta-analysis, the presence of publication bias can be examined either through direct or indirect evidence. Direct evidence is available from trial registries (e.g. ClinicalTrials.gov) generally for interventional and cohort studies which are required to register the research protocol before the study can be conducted. Researchers can then search these registries for studies that have been conducted, yet have not been published or the results not been made available.

Several graphical and statistical methods have been developed to gather indirect evidence of publication bias. Large trials are expected to be of better quality, more precise, and usually get published even if the results are not statistically significant; while smaller trials, are less precise and require a larger effect size (either positive or negative) to be statistically significant in order to be considered for publication. Therefore, most of these indirect methods operate under the assumption that if there is no publication bias, there should not be an association between the treatment effect and the study size (measured through its precision) of the studies included in a meta-analysis. If there is an association between treatment effect size and study size, it is likely that publication bias is present due to the lack of inclusion of small negative trials in the meta-analysis. However, an association between treatment effect and study size can be due to reasons other than publication bias, such as true heterogeneity between studies included in the meta-analysis and chance (Sterne et al. 2011).

12.2.1   Graphical Methods

Two datasets (provided in the Appendices A12.1 and A12.2) were used for the examples in this Chapter. The *Fibrinolysis* dataset contains data from a meta-analysis of randomised controlled trials that examined the effect of fibrinolytic therapy on reduction of mortality after a myocardial infarction (Yusuf et al. 1985). The *Magnesium* dataset contains information from randomised controlled trials that assessed the effect of intravenous magnesium sulphate on mortality in patients with acute myocardial infarction (Nüesch and Jüni 2008). In both cases, the effect measure was the natural log of the relative risk (Ln RR).

Funnel Plot
Funnel plots are the most commonly used graphical methods to detect publication bias. Funnel plots are scatter plots of the effect size (or Ln transformed effect size for RR and OR) against a measure of precision (usually the standard error). In the absence of publication bias, it is expected that these plots will resemble an inverted funnel where smaller studies will scatter widely at the bottom of the plot (due to random variation), with the spread narrowing with increasing size of the study and thus its precision. The funnel plots are not recommended to be used when the number of studies in a meta-analysis is small (less than 10) (The Cochrane Collaboration 2011) as well as in proportion meta-analysis (Hunter et al. 2014).

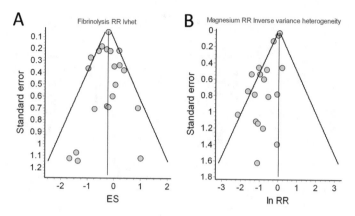

Fig. 12.1 Funnel plots with ES = Ln RR depicting the fibrinolysis (left) and magnesium (right) meta-analyses

The funnel plot is not dependent on the meta-analytical model because it uses the fixed effect pooled estimate as the centre of the funnel, regardless of model of meta-analysis in use. In this example, the meta-analysis used the IVhet model but the funnel plots (Fig. 12.1) were generated using the fixed effect model in MetaXL. Funnel plots can also be generated in Stata (the codes are provided in the Appendix A12.3).

From the funnel plots in Fig. 12.1 it likely that there is no publication bias in the fibrinolysis meta-analysis (left panel) as the plot is symmetrical. A symmetrical plot indicates that there is no association between effect size and study size.

The funnel plot for the magnesium meta-analysis (right panel) is asymmetrical. The majority of the studies included in this meta-analysis indicate that magnesium reduces the risk of mortality after myocardial infarction. A medium sized study and two large ones are on the right side of the vertical line indicating a null or harmful effect of magnesium, while there are no negative small studies. This finding is highly suggestive of publication bias.

Contour-Enhanced Funnel Plot

The contour-enhanced funnel plot is a variation of the standard funnel plot, where levels of statistical significance (e.g., < 0.01, < 0.05, < 0.1) are added to funnel plots (Peters et al. 2008). The addition of areas with different levels of statistical significance assist with the interpretation of the funnel plot, particularly if studies are missing from areas of statistical non-significance, which suggests publication bias. Contour-enhanced funnel plots (Fig. 12.2) were generated in Stata (codes are provided in the Appendix A12.4).

The contour-enhanced funnel plot in the left panel shows studies of different sizes on both sides of the statistical non-significance area (white area) suggesting that publication bias is not present. The plot on the right panel does not contain small and medium sized studies on the right side of statistical non-significance area, and

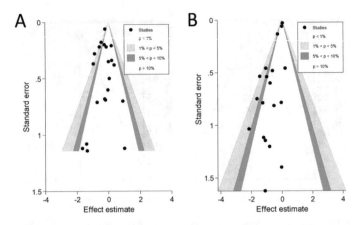

Fig. 12.2 Contour-enhanced funnel plot where effect estimate = Ln RR depicting the fibrinolysis (left) and magnesium (right) meta-analyses

is thus indicative that the results of the meta-analysis may be affected by publication bias.

Doi Plot

Another graphical method that is increasingly being used to assess publication bias is the Doi plot (Furuya-Kanamori et al. 2018; Barendregt 2016). Like the funnel plot, the Doi plot is a graph of effect size versus a measure of precision; however, in this plot the measure of precision is the absolute Z-score. The individual dots on the graph are then connected and the tip of the Doi plot is formed by the most precise study, the one with the Z-score closer to zero. Smaller and less precise studies will produce an effect size that scatters increasingly widely, and the absolute Z-score will gradually increase for both smaller and larger effect sizes on either side of the effect size of the most precise study. If studies are homogeneously spread on both sides of the most precise study this indicates that they are not affected by publication bias. The plot will resemble a symmetrical mountain with similar number of studies and equal spread on each side. Like the funnel plot, the Doi plot is used to alert researchers of possible publication bias affecting the pooled estimate; however, the Doi plots have some significant advantages—they are more sensitive than the funnel plots, can be used for proportion meta-analysis, and the number of studies in a meta-analysis does not impact its visual interpretation (Furuya-Kanamori et al. 2018).

Similar to the funnel plot, the Doi plot does not depend on any meta-analytical models, hence it can be generated from MetaXL regardless of the model selected. The Doi plots in Fig. 12.3 were produced from meta-analyses using the IVhet model in MetaXL. For the appropriate way to render the Doi plots, please follow the instructions provided by Suhail AR Doi in *International Journal of Evidence-Based Healthcare* (Doi 2018). A Stata package has been developed to produce Doi plots, the instructions for its installation and Stata codes are provided in the Appendix A12.5.

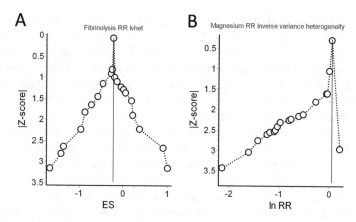

Fig. 12.3 Doi plots where ES = Ln RR depicting the fibrinolysis (left) and magnesium (right) meta-analyses

The interpretation is much like that of the funnel plot, a symmetrical Doi plot like in Fig. 12.3 (left panel) is suggestive of no publication bias. The Doi plot of the magnesium meta-analysis depicted in the right panel is clearly asymmetric suggestive of presence of publication bias towards publications favouring the use of magnesium.

12.2.2 Quantifying Asymmetry

We have described commonly used graphical methods to visually assess publication bias through the asymmetry of the plots. There are several quantitative methods to formally examine the (a)symmetry of the plots. There are two main approaches for such quantitative methods, one that relies on statistical tests (i.e. p-value) and one that creates an effect measure to quantify asymmetry depicted by either the funnel or Doi plots.

Statistical Tests
In 1994, Begg and Mazumdar (1994) proposed a rank correlation test to assess the association of treatment effect size and study size in funnel plots. However, it was noticed that the test has moderate to little power to detect funnel plot asymmetry when the number of studies in the meta-analysis was less than 25.

The most commonly used test to detect funnel plot asymmetry is the Egger's regression. This test was developed by Egger et al. (1997) and consists of a simple linear regression of normalised effect size (effect size divided by its standard error) against precision (reciprocal of the standard error). If the funnel plot is symmetrical (suggestive of no publication bias), the intercept of the regression model should not be significantly different from zero.

In 2006, Harbord et al. (2006) proposed a modified version of the Egger's regression. The components of the simple linear regression were replaced with a Z score over the square root of its variance. Like the Egger's test, the funnel plot was considered symmetrical if the intercept of the modified regression model was not significantly different from zero. A simulation study revealed that the modified Harbord's regression has a lower false-positive rate than the Egger's regression when there is little or no between study heterogeneity.

Another popular alternative to the Egger's regression was proposed by Peters et al. (2006). The Peters' tests is a simple weighted linear regression model of the LnOR against the inverse of the total sample size. The interpretation of the Peters' regression test is similar to the Egger's and Harbord's regression.

Given that these tests examine the asymmetry of the funnel plot, they are constrained by the limitations of the funnel plot such as the minimum number of studies in a meta-analysis (at least 10 studies) and are not recommended for proportion meta-analysis. Furthermore, it has been demonstrated that these tests have little to moderate power to detect asymmetry and their power is dependent on the number of studies included in a meta-analysis (Furuya-Kanamori et al. 2020).

Effect Measure Based Index

To overcome the drawbacks with the statistical tests to detect publication bias, in 2016 an effect measure of asymmetry (i.e. LFK index) was proposed. Rather than a test of association, this index compares the two halves of the Doi plot to detect asymmetry (Furuya-Kanamori et al. 2018; Barendregt 2016). The Doi plot is divided into two areas using a vertical line from the study with the absolute Z-score closest to zero. The LFK index quantifies the difference between these two areas (weighted by the number of studies in each half). If the areas are similar, the Doi plot is considered symmetrical and thus unlikely to be affected by publication bias. The Doi plot and the LFK index are increasingly being used by the research community(Negoi et al. 2018; Kaesmacher et al. 2018; Lee et al. 2019; Murphy et al. 2018). Simulation studies have shown that the LFK index has better operating characteristics than the Egger's regression and is not dependent on the number of studies in the meta-analysis (Furuya-Kanamori et al. 2018).

Examples

The p-values of Begg's, Egger's, Harbord's, and Peters' tests and the LFK index were estimated for the fibrinolysis and magnesium meta-analyses and are presented in Table 12.1. The p-values of Begg's, Egger's, Harbord's, and Peters' tests were estimated using Stata (codes provided in Appendix 12.6). The LFK index are automatically calculated when the Doi plots are generated in MetaXL as well as in Stata (Appendix A12.5).

A p-value of 0.1 is used in these tests is used as the threshold to define asymmetry. An LFK index value between -1 and 1 indicates symmetry, values between -2 to -1 and 1 to 2 indicate minor asymmetry, and values less than -2 and more than 2 indicate major asymmetry of the Doi plot.

Table 12.1 Results of the different statistical methods using the Fibrinolysis and Magnesium datasets

	Fibrinolysis	Magnesium
Begg's test	0.63	0.51
Egger's regression	0.77	<0.001
Harbord's regression	–	<0.001
Peters' regression	–	0.001
LFK index	−0.67	−10.09

The Begg's test and the Egger's regression p-values of 0.63 and 0.77 indicate that the funnel plot for the fibrinolysis is symmetrical. The LFK index of −0.67 indicates that the Doi plot is symmetrical. Therefore, there is no evidence to suggest that the fibrinolysis meta-analysis is affected by publication bias. The p-values of Harbord's and Peter's regression could not be estimated because Stata requires the raw data (i.e. *event_treat noevent_treat event_ctrl noevent_ctrl*) for each individual study.

In the magnesium meta-analysis, the Egger's, Harbord's, and Peters' regression indicate that the funnel plots are asymmetrical, while the Begg's test failed to detect asymmetry. The LFK index of −10.09 is a clear indication of major asymmetry of the Doi plot.

Appendix

A12.1. Fibrinolysis meta-analysis dataset

Study	es	se
Fletcher	−1.66	1.12
Schreiber	−1.40	1.08
Lasierra	−1.35	1.14
Second Frankfurt	−0.96	0.37
Third European	−0.87	0.28
Dewar	−0.73	0.71
Austrian	−0.57	0.22
Second European	−0.45	0.18
Australian	−0.26	0.20
Witchitz	−0.25	0.68
GISSI	−0.21	0.06
Olson	−0.19	0.69
UK Collaborative	−0.13	0.22
Frank	−0.04	0.60

(continued)

(continued)

Study	es	se
Italian	0.01	0.35
Valcre	0.06	0.50
N. German Collab	0.19	0.21
Heikenheimo	0.22	0.34
First European	0.37	0.38
NHLBISMIT	0.91	0.70
Klein	1.01	1.12

A12.2. Magnesium meta-analysis dataset

Study_name	total_treat	event_treat	noevent_treat	total_ctrl	event_ctrl	noevent_ctrl
Abraham (1987)	48	1	47	46	1	45
Bhargava (1995)	40	3	37	38	3	35
Ceremuzynski (1989)	25	1	24	23	3	20
Feldstedt (1991)	150	10	140	148	8	140
Gyamlani (2000)	50	2	48	50	10	40
ISIS-4 (1995)	29011	2216	26795	29039	2103	26936
Shechter (1990)	50	1	49	53	9	44
Morton (1984)	40	1	39	36	2	34
Nakashima (2004)	89	1	88	91	3	88
Raghu (1999)	169	6	163	181	18	163
Rasmussen (1986)	56	4	52	74	14	60
Santoro (2000)	75	0	75	75	1	74
MAGIC (2000)	3113	475	2638	3100	472	2628
Shechter (1991)	21	2	19	25	4	21
Shechter (1995)	96	4	92	98	17	81
Singh (1990)	81	6	75	81	11	70
Smith (1986)	92	2	90	93	7	86
Thogersen (1995)	130	4	126	122	8	114
Woods (1992)	1150	90	1060	1150	118	1032

A12.3. Stata codes for the funnel plots

. *For the fibrinolysis meta-analysis
. ssc install metafunnel
. metafunnel es se
. *For the magnesium meta-analysis
. ssc install metafunnel
. ssc install admetan

. admetan event_treat noevent_treat event_ctrl noevent_ctrl
. metafunnel _ES _SE

A12.4. Stata codes for the contour-enhanced funnel plots

. *For the fibrinolysis meta-analysis
. ssc install confunnel
. confunnel es se
. *For the magnesium meta-analysis
. ssc install confunnel
. ssc install admetan
. admetan event_treat noevent_treat event_ctrl noevent_ctrl
. confunnel _ES _SE

A12.5. Stata codes for the Doi plots
The LFK package for Stata is available from the Boston College Statistical Software Components.

. *For the fibrinolysis meta-analysis
. ssc install lfk
. lfk es se
. *For the magnesium meta-analysis
. lfk admetan event_treat noevent_treat event_ctrl noevent_ctrl

A12.6. Stata codes for the Begg's, Egger's, Harbord's, and Peters' tests

. *For the fibrinolysis meta-analysis
. ssc install metabias
. metabias es se, begg
. metabias es se, egger
. metabias es se, harbord
. metabias es se, peters
. *For the magnesium meta-analysis
. ssc install metabias
. metabias event_treat noevent_treat event_ctrl noevent_ctrl, begg
. metabias event_treat noevent_treat event_ctrl noevent_ctrl, egger
. metabias event_treat noevent_treat event_ctrl noevent_ctrl, harbord
. metabias event_treat noevent_treat event_ctrl noevent_ctrl, peters

References

Barendregt JJ, Doi SA (2016) MetaXL User Guide version 5.3

Begg CB, Mazumdar M (1994) Operating characteristics of a rank correlation test for publication Bias. Biometrics 50:1088–1101

Doi SA (2018) Rendering the Doi plot properly in meta-analysis. Int J Evid Based Healthcare 16:242–243

Egger M, Davey Smith G, Schneider M, Minder C (1997) Bias in meta-analysis detected by a simple, graphical test. BMJ 315:629–634

Furuya-Kanamori L, Barendregt JJ, Doi SAR (2018) A new improved graphical and quantitative method for detecting bias in meta-analysis. Int J Evid Based Healthcare 16:195–203

Furuya-Kanamori L, Xu C, Lin L, Doan T, Chu H, Thalib L, et al. (2020) P-value driven methods were underpowered to detect publication bias: analysis of Cochrane review meta-analyses. J Clin Epidemiol 118:86–92

Harbord RM, Egger M, Sterne JA (2006) A modified test for small-study effects in meta-analyses of controlled trials with binary endpoints. Stat Med 25:3443–3457

Hunter JP, Saratzis A, Sutton AJ, Boucher RH, Sayers RD, Bown MJ (2014) In meta-analyses of proportion studies, funnel plots were found to be an inaccurate method of assessing publication bias. J Clin Epidemiol 67:897–903

Kaesmacher J, Dobrocky T, Heldner MR, Bellwald S, Mosimann PJ, Mordasini P et al (2018) Systematic review and meta-analysis on outcome differences among patients with TICI2b versus TICI3 reperfusions: success revisited. J Neurol Neurosurg Psychiatry 89:910

Koren G, Shear H, Graham K, Einarson T (1989) Bias against the null hypothesis: the reproductive hazards of cocaine. Lancet 334:1440–1442

Lee YY, Stockings EA, Harris MG, Doi SAR, Page IS, Davidson SK, et al. (2019) The risk of developing major depression among individuals with subthreshold depression: a systematic review and meta-analysis of longitudinal cohort studies. Psychol Med 49:92–102

Murphy P, Bentall RP, Freeman D, O'Rourke S, Hutton P (2018) The paranoia as defence model of persecutory delusions: a systematic review and meta-analysis. Lancet Psychiatry 5:913–929

Negoi I, Beuran M, Hostiuc S, Negoi RI, Inoue Y (2018) Surgical anatomy of the superior mesenteric vessels related to pancreaticoduodenectomy: a systematic review and meta-analysis. J Gastrointest Surg 22:802–817

Nüesch E, Jüni P (2008) Commentary: which meta-analyses are conclusive? Int J Epidemiol 38:298–303

Peters JL, Sutton AJ, Jones DR, Abrams KR, Rushton L (2008) Contour-enhanced meta-analysis funnel plots help distinguish publication bias from other causes of asymmetry. J Clin Epidemiol 61:991–996

Peters JL, Sutton AJ, Jones DR, Abrams KR, Rushton L (2006) Comparison of two methods to detect publication bias in meta-analysis. JAMA 295:676–680

Recommendations on testing for funnel plot asymmetry. In: Higgins JPT, Green S, editors. Cochrane Handbook for Systematic Reviews of Interventions Version 510 [updated March 2011]: The Cochrane Collaboration; 2011

Rosenthal R (1979) The file drawer problem and tolerance for null results. Psychol Bull 86:638–641

Sterne JAC, Sutton AJ, Ioannidis JPA, Terrin N, Jones DR, Lau J et al (2011) Recommendations for examining and interpreting funnel plot asymmetry in meta-analyses of randomised controlled trials. BMJ 343:d4002

Thornton A, Lee P (2000) Publication bias in meta-analysis: its causes and consequences. J Clin Epidemiol 53:207–216

Yusuf S, Collins R, Peto R, Furberg C, Stampfer MJ, Goldhaber SZ et al (1985) Intravenous and intracoronary fibrinolytic therapy in acute myocardial infarction: overview of results on mortality, reinfarction and side-effects from 33 randomized controlled trials. Eur Heart J 6:556–585

Chapter 13
Dose-Response Meta-Analysis

Chang Xu and Suhail A. R. Doi

This chapter deals witth the Dose-Response meta analysis.

13.1 Basic Theory

We define dose-response meta-analysis (DRMA) as a type of meta-analytic method that combines dose-specific effects of various doses of exposure on outcome from conceptually similar research in order to establish the potential dose-response relationship between them. There are three key questions to be considered for a dose-response meta-analysis: (1) how to conceptualize the unknown dose-response relationship? (2) how to pool the dose-response relationship from multiple studies? (3) how to deal with the correlations among dose-specific effects (effect estimates) when there are multiple estimates per study?

13.1.1 Dose-Response Relationship

To answer the first question, we need to understand the concept of dose-response relationship. A dose-response relationship describes the changes on the association between exposure and outcome at different levels of exposure (Steenland and Deddens 2004). If a higher dose of exposure leads to a higher or lower effect size, then we may assume that there is a dose-response relationship. The dose-response

C. Xu (✉) · S. A. R. Doi
Qatar University, Doha, Qatar
e-mail: xuchang2016@runbox.com

S. A. R. Doi
e-mail: sardoi@gmx.net

© Springer Nature Singapore Pte Ltd. 2020
S. Khan, *Meta-Analysis*, Statistics for Biology and Health,
https://doi.org/10.1007/978-981-15-5032-4_13

Table 13.1 Categorical data for dose-response relationship

ID	Exposure level	Events	Total number	Effect sizes	Confidence interval
1	$\leq L_1$	r_0	n_0	Reference	Reference
1	L_1-L_2	r_1	n_1	RR_1	$\ln RR_1 \pm Z_{a/2} * SE_1$
1	L_2-L_3	r_2	n_2	RR_2	$\ln RR_2 \pm Z_{a/2} * SE_2$
1	$\geq L_4$	r_3	n_3	RR_3	$\ln RR_3 \pm Z_{a/2} * SE_3$

RR indicates relative risk, including risk ratio, odds ratio, and hazard ratio; Za/2 is the z-score at alpha/2 level, and SE is the standard error

relationship can be presented in a categorical form and a continuous form. The categorical dose-response relationship means that the exposure variable was categorized into several intervals with each interval as a category and there are real differences in effect (not by chance) as the categorical dose increases (Table 13.1). The continuous dose-response relationship means that the exposure variable was treated as continuous and that the relationship between exposure and effect size can be smoothed as a simple linear, piecewise linear, or nonlinear curve.

The problem usually faced is that the majority of studies present their data in a categorical form rather than a dose-response curve. This will make it easier for the reader (physicians and patients) to follow, while it is difficult then to meta-analyze because the categories in each study are mostly different. In very few cases where the categories are the same in included studies we can combine the effect estimates category by category. For the more usual case, a practical and valid approach is to smooth the categories by assigning a dose (e.g. the middle, the median, or the mean value) for each category to represent the interval and these doses allow us to create a dose-response curve using the effect estimates from each study and the curves in each study can then be pooled using the regression coefficients. The method for assigning a dose for each category is generally based on nonparametric assumption as there are usually only two point values, say, lower boundary and upper boundary, which is insufficient to establish a parametric model (Bekkering et al. 2008; Takahashi and Tango 2010). The most commonly used method is to use the middle value of the interval. Sometimes, authors may also provide the median or the mean value for each category. We put more weight on the establishment of the dose-response curve then on defining a dose from the interval.

13.1.2 Synthesis of the Dose-Response Relationship

In the dose-response data, there is correlations when the effect estimates are relative effects (*RR, OR, HR*) or absolute difference (*RD, MD, SMD*) for the non-reference categories. One valid solution to take account of the correlation is the generalized least squares (*GLS*) estimation (Dobson and Barnett 2008). Since there is usually a reference category that is common to all effect estimates per study, there is covariance between effects within study and the condition for applying *GLS* estimation is that the covariance is known to us.

The estimator for the variance of effect estimates is given in relevant chapters. Here we give the estimator for the variance of the reference group. In Table 13.1, we've indexed r_i and n_i as the number of events and totals in each category. For cohort studies or randomized controlled trials, the reference variance is calculated as:

$$var(\theta_0) = \frac{1}{r_0} - \frac{1}{n_0}.$$

For case-control studies

$$var(\theta_0) = \frac{1}{r_0} + \frac{1}{n_0 - r_0}$$

It may be noted that if the relative risks have been adjusted for confounding variables then ideally we require the variance of these adjusted risks. We can obtain the variance of adjusted risks of the non-reference groups while there is no information necessary to estimate the variance of adjusted risk of the reference. Therefore, for observational studies, the estimation of the covariance between effect estimates is somewhat biased.

With the estimates of the regression coefficients and variances we can pool them by either a two-stage regression or a one-stage regression model. The two-stage approach was first introduced by Greenland et al. (1992) and further developed by Orsini et al. (2006, 2012) and is known as generalized least squares for trend (*GLST*). This method uses the *GLS* estimation to get the regression coefficients and variances within each study in the first stage and then combines the estimates by a fixed-effect or random-effect meta-analytic model in the second stage. As the process consists of two stages, we call it a "two-stage" approach. *GLST* forces the regression through the origin as it is based on the mathematical expectation that the intercept is zero (Liu et al. 2009).

An alternative approach to pool the dose-response relationship is the inverse variance weighted least squares (*WLS*) regression with cluster robust error variances (*REMR* model) based on the one-stage framework (Xu and Doi 2018). This method has a particular advantage in addressing the correlations between regression coefficients because it treats each study as a cluster and fits these studies into a cluster robust log-linear model without generating regression coefficients study-by-study. While for the correlations between effect estimates within each study (before the regression is done), a cluster robust error variance is employed to address this. This is a special case of the generalized linear mixed model where only one stage is required and covariance need not be imputed from the data. In addition, by applying the maximum within-study weights to the reference, we need not force the intercept through zero thus minimizing potential bias.

13.2   Application in Stata

13.2.1   Binary Outcome

Let's use alcohol consumption and risk of lung cancer as the first example to illustrate the application of dose-response meta-analysis using the Stata software. The relationship between alcohol consumption and lung cancer has been investigated in several epidemiological studies. We collected the data from a published meta-analysis, which is a commonly used example. The data-set covers 4 cohort studies with the dose range for alcohol from 0 to 45.6 g/day and the reference dose of each study being zero. Table 13.2 gives the layout of the data for analysis.

In this table, the first column "id" indexes the four studies, RR, LCI and UCI index the relative risks, lower boundary of the confidence interval, and upper boundary of the confidence interval respectively. The consumption of alcohol was measured in g/day and is the "dose". The events of lung cancer in each category were labeled as "cases" and the "person-years" indicates the total follow-up years for the subjects. These two variables (person-years and cases) are required for covariance computation

Table 13.2   Alcohol consumption (dose in g/day) and risk of lung cancer

Id	Author	rr	lci	uci	dose	Cases	Person_years	Studytype
1	at	1.00	1.00	1.00	0.00	45.00	5931.51	2
1	at	0.82	0.56	1.22	1.85	61.00	12143.00	2
1	at	0.87	0.60	1.27	9.09	79.00	14671.50	2
1	at	0.81	0.54	1.20	22.86	60.00	12854.30	2
1	at	0.83	0.55	1.26	45.60	53.00	10925.80	2
2	hp	1.00	1.00	1.00	0.00	51.00	96659.20	2
2	hp	0.80	0.53	1.21	2.10	41.00	99390.70	2
2	hp	0.97	0.67	1.40	9.50	67.00	111752.00	2
2	hp	0.51	0.29	0.87	18.80	18.00	53704.70	2
2	hp	1.26	0.86	1.84	40.30	67.00	47657.00	2
3	nt	1.00	1.00	1.00	0.00	111.00	1356.69	2
3	nt	1.11	0.78	1.57	2.20	136.00	1782.74	2
3	nt	1.20	0.86	1.66	9.30	200.00	2456.36	2
3	nt	1.10	0.79	1.54	22.50	193.00	2069.80	2
3	nt	1.69	1.18	2.44	41.30	188.00	1266.80	2
4	ny	1.00	1.00	1.00	0.00	47.00	20756.50	2
4	ny	0.73	0.52	1.02	0.97	135.00	90930.20	2
4	ny	0.95	0.66	1.36	11.40	86.00	42534.00	2
4	ny	0.85	0.57	1.26	22.80	53.00	25430.00	2
4	ny	1.16	0.80	1.70	45.60	71.00	19493.40	2

in this study type which uses incidence rate (ir). Parallel to incidence rate for cohort studies, there could also be cumulative incidence (ci) reported where person-years is replaced with number of non-cases. For case-control (cc) studies, the person-years is replaced with number of controls. The variable *studytype* must take value 1 for case–control, 2 for cohort with incidence-rate, and 3 for cohort with cumulative incidence. These details are important as they are used to calculate the correlations between lnRRs or lnORs when the *GLS* estimation based method (GLST) is employed.

GLST approach

Before we start the dose-response meta-analysis in Stata, the following two commands should be installed in advance: *glst* and *xblc*. To install type into the command window in Stata:

. *ssc install glst*

. *net install st0215_1*

The reference of each study is the same in this data-set and all equal zero so there is good homogeneity among them and no further process is needed to make them more homogeneous. The following commands allow us to transform *RR* from the natural to the log scale and for each study, the reference effects are relative to 1 (zero when log transformed).

. *gen logrr = log(rr)*

. *gen loglci = log(lci)*

. *gen loguci = log(uci)*

. *gen se = (loguci-loglci)/(2*invnormal(0.975))*

A restricted cubic spline can be created with 3 knots across the reported dose distribution, which generates two splines (*n-1*) named *doses1* and doses2 and these will then be employed for potential non-linear dose-specific modelling.

. *mkspline doses = dose, cubic nk(3) disp*

The *glst* commend then can be used to run the spline regression within each study and pool the regression coefficients across studies. It provides fixed-effect and random-effect models.

. *glst logrr doses*, cov(person_years cases) se(se) pfirst(id studytype) r*

We can use the *xblc* commend to convert the coefficients to RRs for the pre-defined doses and plot the summarized dose-response curve. *GLST* requires a reference dose as the regression has no constant. The dose-response relationship is plotted as follows:

. *quietly levelsof dose, local(levels)*

. *xblc doses*, covname (dose) at('r(levels)') ref (0) eform line*

The *pfirst* option requires variable *id* which is a numeric indicator variable that takes the same value across correlated log relative risks within a study. The *pfirst* option also requires the variable *studytype,* which as mentioned above takes the value 1 for case–control, 2 for cohort with incidence-rate, and 3 for cohort with cumulative incidence. Within each group of log relative risks, the first observation is assumed to be the reference and data must be ordered by dose within study. The *pfirst* option specifies the pooling method with multiple summarized studies. The fixed effect (*f*) or random effects model (*r*) can be assigned with the *pfirst* option. To understand the meaning of *pfirst*, we may use the following command (without "*pfirst*") to fit

Table 13.3 The regression coefficients of each study by fitting a restricted cubic spline function

Study ID	Beta 1	Standard error	Beta 2	Standard error
1	−0.00819	0.017	0.00717	0.018
2	−0.02091	0.020	0.03158	0.023
3	−0.00037	0.016	0.01137	0.017
4	0.01011	0.014	−0.00313	0.016

regression to the first study and we can find that when do not use the "*pfirst*" option it works when only one study is present while it fails to work when two or more studies are present. Therefore, the *pfirst* option is used to specify the pooling of multiple summarized studies while removing this option would allow *glst* to fit a regression for effect estimates against the dose in one study (requires study type to be indicated as *ir, ci or cc*).

. *glst logrr doses* if id ==1, cov(person_years cases) se(se) ir*

The regression coefficients of each study are listed in Table 13.3. These regression coefficients can then be pooled by the multivariate meta-analytic method.

REMR approach

This is our preferred approach and the code for the *REMR* approach is similar to that for the *GLST* approach. One difference however is that before fitting the pooled dose-response relationship, we need to first compute weights and also assign a maximum weight to the reference dose.

. *gen wt = 1/(se^2)*

. *bysort id: egen maxwt = max(wt)*

. *replace wt = maxwt if wt ==.*

Again, we create a restricted cubic spline across the reported dose distribution.

. *mkspline doses = dose, cubic nk(3) disp*

Then the *regress* commend allows us to establish an inverse-variance weighted robust error regression across studies.

. *regress logrr doses* [aweight = wt], vce(cluster id)*

A Wald-type test for non-linearity can be obtained by testing the regression coefficient of the second spline equal to zero.

. *test doses2*

A Wald-type test for the hypothesis of no exposure-disease association can be obtained by testing simultaneously both regression coefficients equal to zero.

test doses1 doses2

We can use the *xblc* commend to convert the coefficients to RRs for the pre-defined doses and plot the summarized dose-response curve. Unlike *GLST* that requires a reference dose as the regression has no constant, REMR does not require this reference dose as there is a constant term.

. *quietly levelsof dose, local(levels)*

Table 13.4 Pooled regression parameters and standard errors by different models

Alcohol and lung cancer	Estimating models		
	REMR	GLST-fixed	GLST-random
$\beta_1(se)$	−0.00561 (0.008)	−0.00065 (0.008)	−0.00232 (0.040)
$\beta_2(se)$	0.01223 (0.009)	0.00702 (0.009)	0.00878 (0.009)
P for non-linearity	0.861	0.438	0.335

. xblc doses*, covname (dose) at('r(levels)') eform line

Explanation of the results

The entire code for the two methods can be found in Xu and Doi (2018). Table 13.4 presents the pooled estimates of regression parameters and standard errors by the two models. With the *GLST* random-effect we get regression estimates of $\beta_1(-0.002)$, $\beta_2(0.009)$; with the *GLST* fixed-effect we get regression estimates of $\beta_1(-0.001)$, $\beta_2(0.007)$; and with the *REMR* model, we get regression estimates of $\beta_1(-0.006)$ and $\beta_2(0.01)$.

Let's look at Fig. 13.1 of the dose-specific relationship between alcohol consumption and risk of lung cancer based on the REMR model. There is a more-or-less linear trend between alcohol consumption and risk of lung cancer (P for non-linear test = 0.261). The two dashed lines present the confidence interval and the solid line is the linear prediction of the dose-specific effects. The hollow circle is the weighted effect estimates from each study and a larger circle indicates larger weight. The confidence interval line covers horizontal line at 1 (RR) and indicates no significant association by current studies. The dose-specific effects are listed below:

Dose	RR	(95% CI)
0.00	0.95	(0.86−1.04)
0.97	0.94	(0.85−1.04)
1.85	0.94	(0.85−1.04)
2.10	0.94	(0.84−1.04)
2.20	0.94	(0.84−1.04)
9.09	0.91	(0.77−1.09)
9.30	0.91	(0.76−1.09)
9.50	0.91	(0.76−1.09)
11.40	0.92	(0.75−1.11)
18.80	0.95	(0.77−1.18)
22.50	0.98	(0.79−1.23)
22.80	0.98	(0.79−1.23)
22.86	0.99	(0.79−1.23)
40.30	1.14	(0.86−1.52)
41.30	1.15	(0.86−1.54)

(continued)

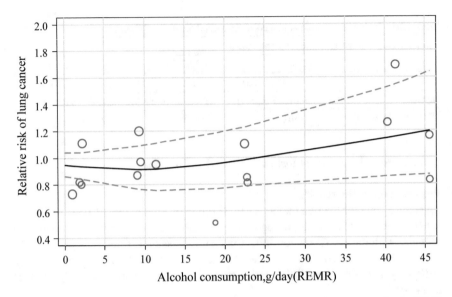

Fig. 13.1 Dose-response curve between alcohol consumption and risk of lung cancer (by the *REMR* approach)

(continued)

Dose	RR	(95% CI)
45.60	1.20	(0.87–1.64)

13.2.2 Continuous Outcome

In meta-analysis of continuous outcomes, the effect estimates include means, mean difference, standardized mean difference etc. Let's use the data of a meta-analysis used by Crippa as an example to show the dose-response meta-analysis of continuous outcomes (Crippa and Orsini 2016). Aripiprazole is an antipsychotic drug for schizoaffective disorder, and the improvement in the condition of patients is measured by a score on the Positive and Negative Symptoms Scale (PANSS). Five clinical trials have investigated the potential dose-response effect of aripiprazole on the improvement of the PANSS score (Table 13.5). The mean score of PANSS, standard deviation of the mean and number of patients refers to the category and are listed in Table 13.5. The data can be downloaded using the following command.

.*use* http://www.stats4life.se/data/aripanss, *clear*

We may first construct a dose-response relationship for aripiprazole and the mean score. This process is the same as the dose-response meta-analysis for binary outcomes that just uses the lnRRs instead of the mean score. Then we can construct a one-stage dose-response meta-analysis for the mean score against the doses using the *REMR* approach. It is important to note that when we use absolute mean (not mean difference) as an outcome measurement, the *GLST* method is not applicable as it requires the effects and variance at the reference to be at zero (or 1).

gen sterr = sd/sqrt(n)
gen wt = 1/(sterr ^2)
bysort id: egen maxwt = max(wt)
replace wt = maxwt if wt ==.
mkspline doses = dose, cubic nk(3) disp
regress mean doses* [aweight = wt], vce(cluster id)
test doses1 = doses2
quietly levelsof dose, local(levels)
xblc doses*, covname (dose) at('r(levels)') line

We get the following pooled regression estimates with β_1 as 1.017204 and β_2 as -0.7326656. The non-linear test ($P = 0.0011$) suggests an obvious non-linear relationship between the different doses of aripiprazole and the mean scores.

Table 13.5 Aripiprazole for the improvement on the PANSS score of shizoaffective patients

ID	Author and Year	Dose	Mean score	sd (Standard deviation)	n (number. of patients)
1	Cutler (2006)	0	5.30	18.31	85
1		2	8.23	18.32	92
1		5	10.60	18.31	89
1		10	11.30	18.32	94
2	McEvoy (2007)	0	2.33	26.10	107
2		10	15.04	27.60	103
2		15	11.73	26.20	103
2		20	14.44	25.90	97
3	Kane (2002)	0	2.90	24.28	102
3		15	15.50	26.49	99
3		30	11.40	22.90	100
4	Potkin (2003)	0	5.00	21	103
4		20	14.50	20.16	98
4		30	13.90	20.88	96
5	Study 94202	0	1.40	25.73	57
5		2	11.00	25.00	51
5		10	11.50	25.20	51
5		30	15.80	28.51	54

```
Linear regression                                       Number of obs     =         18
                                                        F(2, 4)           =      58.21
                                                        Prob > F          =     0.0011
                                                        R-squared         =     0.8500
                                                        Root MSE          =     1.8333
```

(Std. Err. adjusted for 5 clusters in id)

mean	Coef.	Robust Std. Err.	t	P>|t|	[95% Conf. Interval]	
doses1	1.017204	.1580657	6.44	0.003	.5783437	1.456065
doses2	-.7326656	.1557566	-4.70	0.009	-1.165115	-.3002159
_cons	4.664162	.8159043	5.72	0.005	2.398849	6.929475

The dose-response trend for different doses of aripiprazole and mean scores can be established (Fig. 13.2). The pooled baseline mean score of PANSS is 4.66 (95%CI: 2.39–6.93, and as the dose of aripiprazole increases, the mean score increases and at the dose of 15 mg/day the effects reached the best (Mean = 14.20, 95%CI: 13.39–15.01).

Physicians may further want to know the absolute improvement on the mean score for aripiprazole therapy to the pre-drug score. For this purpose, we need to use the mean difference as effect estimate instead of the mean score. Let's generate the mean difference (indexed as d) for non-reference groups to the reference group (dose = 0) in each study and the next step is to calculate the variance and the covariance matrix of d. In the reference group, the variance of d is regarded as missing. For the non-reference groups, the variances are calculated as:

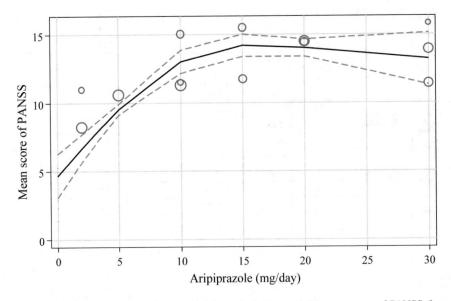

Fig. 13.2 Dose-response curve between aripiprazole therapy and the mean score of PANSS (by REMR approach)

$$Var(dij) = \sqrt{\frac{sd_{ij}^2}{n_{ij}} + \frac{sd_{0j}^2}{n_{0j}}}$$

Here the subscript 0 indexes the reference group. The following commends allow us to generate d as well as the variance for each d. Please note that these commends are based on the fact that the "sterr" variable has been generated earlier as "gen sterr = sd/sqrt(n)".

. drop wt maxwt doses1 doses2
. bysort id:gen cat = _n-1
. bysort id: gen d = mean - mean[1]
. bysort id: gen var = sterr[_n]^2
. bysort id: gen sumvar = var[_n] + var[1]
. replace sumvar = . if cat ==0
. bysort id: gen s_pooled = sqrt(sumvar)
. drop var sumvar

As a result, we get the effect estimators and the variance of the non-reference categories and can then establish the dose-response relationship between them. If we want to use standard mean difference as effect estimators, we can calculate standard mean difference and its variance based on Hedge's g (Hedges 1981) and Cohen's d (Cohen 1988) two methods. Let's continue to use the *REMR* approach to establish the absolute improvement of the score for aripiprazole therapy. Again, we first generate the weights.

. gen wt = 1/(s_pooled ^2)
. bysort id: egen maxwt = max(wt)
. replace wt = maxwt if wt ==.

Again, we create a restricted cubic spline across the reported dose distribution.

. mkspline doses = dose, cubic nk(3) disp

Finally, we get the pooled regression estimates and the dose-specific mean difference from the following command.

. regress d doses* [aweight = wt], vce(cluster id)
. quietly levelsof dose, local(levels)
. xblc doses*, covname (dose) at('r(levels)') line

From the results, we know that as the dose for aripiprazole increased to 15 mg/day, the improvements reached the maximum effect with the mean difference of 10.55 (95%CI: 8.28−12.82). This means the best dose for aripiprazole therapy is about 15 mg/day and on average an improvement of 10.55 points on the score will be achieved under this dose. The dose-response curve is presented in Fig. 13.3.

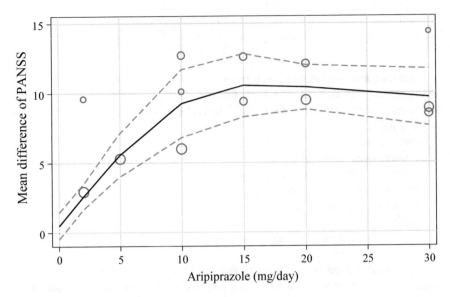

Fig. 13.3 Dose-response curve between aripiprazole therapy and the improvement (mean difference) on the mean score compared to no therapy (by *REMR* approach)

13.3 Additional Issues and Guidance

13.3.1 Heterogeneous Reference Doses

From the above examples we may notice that all the reference dose are zero. This is obviously important that it ensures all the studies have the same control. While in some situations the reference doses are different across studies which would bring large amount of heterogeneity and uncertainty for the pooled evidence. An extreme example is that in some studies the reference dose is larger than the non-reference dose in other studies. This is the same situation that in intervention meta-analysis, if we treat the intervention as different treatments, the controls are different and the interventions is also different. It is not suitable to conduct a dose-response meta-analysis when the reference doses are substantially heterogeneous. Let's consider another situation that several studies with the reference doses are of great difference, while the rest of them are relatively homogeneous, we may exclude those studies with substantial heterogeneous on the reference dose and use the rest of the studies to conduct the dose-response meta-analysis. Even when the differences among the reference doses are not substantial a further procedure is necessary to make them more harmonious. This procedure is the concept of centering, a method that subtracts the reference dose from all other doses thus in effect moving from dose to "dose increment".

```
.sort id dose
.bysort id: gen dosec = dose – dose[1]
```

This centering procedure creates a common reference dose of zero but also makes the results more difficult to explain in terms of its clinical value. We may use a two-stage centering procedure to deal with this problem. The first stage is the same while in the second stage, we add the median value of the reference doses (original value) to the centered reference. For example, suppose the range of reference doses is between 1 and 3 and the median value of the reference doses across studies is 2, then this value is added to the centered reference. We then use the centered doses instead of the original dose to establish the dose-response relationship.

.sort id dose
.bysort id: gen dosec = dose – dose[1] + 2

The above issue is based on the assumption that all the studies the reference dose is located in the lowest category or the highest category of the exposure spectrum. Think about the situation where some studies have the reference doses located in the lowest category while some others have it located in the middle category. Although the doses at the lowest category may be the same across studies, but some studies did not set the lowest category as reference. This is another case of heterogeneity on reference doses. For such a situation, a transformation of the reference is needed and there is an Excel macro add-in program (RREst_trend) that may facilitate the transformation and this can be downloaded from http://www.pnlee.co.uk/software. htm. Readers can get the manual for the program from the web page.

13.3.2 Missing Data

Missing data represents a tough challenge in meta-analysis. Some missing information can be obtained by contacting authors while most of which cannot be obtained. For dose-response meta-analysis missing data mainly includes missing on the "dose", missing on confidence interval of effect estimates, and missing on the group size information. In the original study, the "dose" is always presented as interval rather than a point value, for such types of missing the most commonly used method is to use the mean value, median value, or middle value of the interval. Some studies may stratify exposure dose as a qualitative interval (e.g. low, moderate, high), but even more crude than this is to map the qualitative interval to another study with a similar population. When the confidence interval is missing that the weight of each effect estimate cannot be obtained, due to the nature of dose-response meta-analysis, we may use sample size in each category to generate the frequency weight. But this may lead to the biased variance estimation. The missing on group size information means that the *GLST* approach is not possible as it needs this information to estimate the within study variance-covariance matrix while missing on group size has no problem in the *REMR* approach, Therefore, when such information is missing, the optimal method is to use the *REMR* approach to conduct the dose-response meta-analysis.

Table 13.6 Summarized characters for GLST and REMR

Characters for compare	GLST	REMR
Framework	Two-stage and One-stage	One-stage
Regression	Generalized least squares	Cluster robust variance
Weighting scheme (Effect models)	Fixed-effect and Random-effect	Inverse variance heterogeneity (IVhet)
Information required	Effect estimates, variance, doses, group sizes, study type	Effect estimates, variance, doses
Dose-specific effects	2 categories for one-stage and 3 categories for two-stage	2 categories
Binary outcomes	Yes	Yes
Continuous outcomes	Yes	Yes
Absolute effect estimators (Mean, prevalence)	No. Relevant risk or absolute difference is needed	Yes
Software	Stata, R, SAS	Stata, Mlwin
IPD dose-response meta-analysis	Yes	Yes

13.3.3 GLST Versus REMR

The summarized characteristics of the GLST approach and the REMR approach are presented in Table 13.6. The main features (which may not really be advantages) of the GLST approach include: (1) it supports both one-stage and two-stage frameworks; (2) it supports both fixed-effect and random effects models; and (3) there is software available to implement it. The main advantages of *REMR* approach include: (1) the information required is much less than *GLST* while it can achieve a similar estimation on the dose-response relationship; (2) it support the dose-response meta-analysis of absolute effect estimators such as mean, prevalence; (3) it drops the use of the classic and fixed effect and random effects models of meta-analysis in favour of the IVhet model (Doi et al. 2015) that avoids the problem of overdispersion.

13.4 Practical Guidance for DRMA

What types of exposure are to be considered?

In DRMA, both a *continuous variable* and a *discontinuous variable* are potential exposures that may be considered. The nature of these two types of exposures determines which regression function are appropriate to be fitted. For exposure of a continuous variable, the simple linear, piecewise linear, and non-linear regression functions are reasonable since all the data points are continuous. The non-linear function is the optimal choice when there is no evidence of linear relationship. Piecewise linear is seldom utilized when exposure is continuous since the non-linear function fits better than the piecewise linear. However, for U-shaped or J-shaped dose-response relationship, a piecewise linear may be used to predict the "average trend" (effects refer to each unit increase) in each segment of the curve instead of the simple linear (Xu et al. 2019a).

For a discontinuous exposure variable, due to the disjoint and nonconvex properties of such types of data, it would be problematic to fit it with a non-linear function. The dose-specific effects cannot be defined for non-integer doses, because these non-integer data points are inexistent (e.g. 1.5 of a birth). We may still establish a non-linear curve for a discontinuous variable with an outcome as if the discontinuous variable is continuous, but then this should be defined as "quasi-nonlinearity" and this should be mentioned and correctly explained in the context of such a DRMA. A more reasonable approach however is to fit the discontinuous variable by linear or piecewise linear model against the outcome. By doing so, we can explain the relationship as the changes of the effects for each unit increase (e.g. each birth increase) or decrease of the exposure (in each of the segments).

What types of study designs are to be synthesized?

Epidemiological theory categorizes studies into descriptive and analytic. Analytic studies could be observational or experimental and the observational cross-sectional study is generally used to describe the correlations between two (or more) variables (Doi and Williams 2013). The latter does not address whether A causes B or B causes A. Unlike the cross-sectional study, the other analytic studies aim to investigate the potential causal relationship between independent variables and the dependent variables. When conducting DRMA, it is recommended to pool cross-sectional studies separately in order to avoid reverse causality. However, this does not mean that pooling cohort or case-control studies is immune from reverse causality due to various forms of biases (e.g. confounders).

What types of non-linear approximating function to be fitted?

The commonly used non-linear functions include the restricted cubic splines (78.25%), the fractional polynomial (16.18%), and the conventional polynomial (< 5%) (Xu et al. 2019b). There is currently no consensus for which one of these is more appropriate or less biased for non-linear trend approximation in DRMA but it has been suggested that summarized curves generated from conventional polynomials may be misleading. Cubic splines (when compared to fractional polynomials) more adequately encompass sudden and important changes in relative risks and this is consistent with the frequency with which they are used in the literature (Durrleman and Simon 1989). A restricted cubic spline is defined as smoothly joined piecewise polynomial (divided by knots) with at most third-order polynomials fitted within each piece, and the left and (or) right tail of the curve are restricted to linearity. Inserting n knots (empirically 3−7 knots between the minimum and maximum values) would generate $n-1$ regression covariates with the first representing the linear spline and the second to $n-1$ representing the piecewise cubic splines.

When fitting these non-linear trends, testing should be done and commonly a Wald test (Gould 1996) is used. The use of the Wald test to test for the presence of an exposure-outcome association in the case of the restricted cubic spline function is to simultaneously test that the coefficients representing the cubic splines (2 to *n-1*) are zero. To test for non-linearity we test that each of the cubic spline coefficient (except the first) is zero. For example, inserting 3 knots would generate 2 cubic splines. We could test the null hypothesis that the coefficients of both cubic splines are simultaneously equal to zero and if rejected this is evidence for an association. We could also test the null hypothesis that the second spline coefficient is zero and if rejected then this is evidence for non-linearity.

What kind of synthesis approaches are to be employed?

There are three approaches that have been used to synthesize the dose-response evidence, including the traditional meta-regression (*TMR*), the generalized least squares for trend (*GLST*), and robust-error meta-regression (*REMR*). The *TMR* methods establishes the dose-response relationship by the mean dose of exposure of each study against the outcome, which does not take into account the within study correlation of effects such that the estimation is relatively crude, which is not recommended.

For the *GLST* model, the generalized least squares estimation, covariance information is imputed from the data and the regression coefficients are pooled by a "one-stage" or "two-stage" regression approach. The *REMR* model is a "one-stage" approach that treats each included study as a cluster, then the clustered robust variance is used to deal with the unknown correlations of effects within each cluster and the regression coefficient is estimated by weighted least squares estimation across the whole population. The *GLST* approach forces the curve to pass through the origin while the regression intercept is allowed in the *REMR* approach as the maximum weight is assigned to the reference which minimize the regression intercept deviations from the origin. Empirical evidence (and our simulation) suggests these two methods can reach similar trend estimation and the advantage of the *REMR* method is it does not require imputation of covariance information from the data.

References

Bekkering GE, Harris RJ, Thomas S et al (2008) How much of the data published in observational studies of the association between diet and prostate or bladder cancer is usable for meta-analysis? Am J Epidemiol 167(9):1017–1026

Cohen J (1988) Statistical power analysis for the behavioral sciences, 2nd edn. Hillsdale, NJ Erlbaum

Crippa A, Orsini N (2016) Dose-response meta-analysis of differences in means. BMC Med Res Methodol 2(16):91

Dobson AJ, Barnett AG (eds) (2008) An introduction to generalized linear models—third edition. Chapman and Hall/CRC Press, Boca Raton

Doi SA, Barendregt JJ, Khan S et al (2015) Advances in the meta-analysis of heterogeneous clinical trials I: the inverse variance heterogeneity model. Contemp Clin Trials 45(Pt A):130–138

Doi SAR, Williams GM (2013) Methods of clinical epidemiology. Springer, Germany

Durrleman S, Simon R (1989) Flexible regression models with cubic splines. Stat Med 8(5):551–561

Gould, WW (1996) crc43: Wald test of nonlinear hypotheses after model estimation. Stata Technical Bulletin 29:2–4. Reprinted in Stata Technical Bulletin Reprints, vol. 5, pp. 15–18. College Station. Stata Press, TX

Greenland S, Longnecker MP (1992) Methods for trend estimation from summarized dose-response data, with applications to meta-analysis. Am J Epidemiol 135(11):1301–1309

Hedges LV (1981) Distribution theory for glass's estimator of effect size and related estimators. J Edu Stat 6(2):107–128

Liu Q, Cook NR, Bergström A et al (2009) A two-stage hierarchical regression model for meta-analysis of epidemiologic nonlinear dose–response data. Comput Stat Data An 53:4157–4167

Orsini N, Bellocco R, Greenland S (2006) Generalized least squares for trend estimation of summarized dose-response data. Stata J 6(1):40–57

Orsini N, Li R, Wolk A, Khudyakov P, Spiegelman D (2012) Meta-analysis for linear and nonlinear dose-response relations: examples, an evaluation of approximations, and software. Am J Epidemiol 175:66–73

Steenland K, Deddens JA (2004) A practical guide to dose-response analyses and risk assessment in occupational epidemiology. Epidemiology 15(1):63–70

Takahashi K, Tango T (2010) Assignment of grouped exposure levels for trend estimation in a regression analysis of summarized data. Stat Med 29(25):2605–2616

Xu C, Doi SA (2018) The robust-error meta-regression method for dose-response meta-analysis. Int J Evid Based Healthcare 16(3):138–144

Xu C, Liu Y, Jia PL et al (2019a) The methodological quality of dose-response meta-analyses needed substantial improvement: A cross-sectional survey and proposed recommendations. J Clin Epidemiol 107:1–11

Xu C, Thabane L, Liu TZ et al (2019b) Flexible piecewise linear model for investigating dose-response relationship in meta-analysis: methodology, examples, and comparison. J Evid Based Medicine 12(1):63–68

Statistical Tables

© Springer Nature Singapore Pte Ltd. 2020
S. Khan, *Meta-Analysis*, Statistics for Biology and Health,
https://doi.org/10.1007/978-981-15-5032-4

The Standard Normal Table

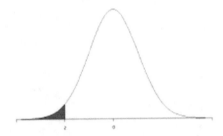

Standard Normal Probabilities for Negative Z-scores

z	0.00	0.01	0.02	0.03	0.04	0.05	0.06	0.07	0.08	0.09
-3.4	0.0003	0.0003	0.0003	0.0003	0.0003	0.0003	0.0003	0.0003	0.0003	0.0002
-3.3	0.0005	0.0005	0.0005	0.0004	0.0004	0.0004	0.0004	0.0004	0.0004	0.0003
-3.2	0.0007	0.0007	0.0006	0.0006	0.0006	0.0006	0.0006	0.0005	0.0005	0.0005
-3.1	0.0010	0.0009	0.0009	0.0009	0.0008	0.0008	0.0008	0.0008	0.0007	0.0007
-3.0	0.0013	0.0013	0.0013	0.0012	0.0012	0.0011	0.0011	0.0011	0.0010	0.0010
-2.9	0.0019	0.0018	0.0018	0.0017	0.0016	0.0016	0.0015	0.0015	0.0014	0.0014
-2.8	0.0026	0.0025	0.0024	0.0023	0.0023	0.0022	0.0021	0.0021	0.0020	0.0019
-2.7	0.0035	0.0034	0.0033	0.0032	0.0031	0.0030	0.0029	0.0028	0.0027	0.0026
-2.6	0.0047	0.0045	0.0044	0.0043	0.0041	0.0040	0.0039	0.0038	0.0037	0.0036
-2.5	0.0062	0.0060	0.0059	0.0057	0.0055	0.0054	0.0052	0.0051	0.0049	0.0048
-2.4	0.0082	0.0080	0.0078	0.0075	0.0073	0.0071	0.0069	0.0068	0.0066	0.0064
-2.3	0.0107	0.0104	0.0102	0.0099	0.0096	0.0094	0.0091	0.0089	0.0087	0.0084
-2.2	0.0139	0.0136	0.0132	0.0129	0.0125	0.0122	0.0119	0.0116	0.0113	0.0110
-2.1	0.0179	0.0174	0.0170	0.0166	0.0162	0.0158	0.0154	0.0150	0.0146	0.0143
-2.0	0.0228	0.0222	0.0217	0.0212	0.0207	0.0202	0.0197	0.0192	0.0188	0.0183
-1.9	0.0287	0.0281	0.0274	0.0268	0.0262	0.0256	0.0250	0.0244	0.0239	0.0233
-1.8	0.0359	0.0351	0.0344	0.0336	0.0329	0.0322	0.0314	0.0307	0.0301	0.0294
-1.7	0.0446	0.0436	0.0427	0.0418	0.0409	0.0401	0.0392	0.0384	0.0375	0.0367
-1.6	0.0548	0.0537	0.0526	0.0516	0.0505	0.0495	0.0485	0.0475	0.0465	0.0455
-1.5	0.0668	0.0655	0.0643	0.0630	0.0618	0.0606	0.0594	0.0582	0.0571	0.0559
-1.4	0.0808	0.0793	0.0778	0.0764	0.0749	0.0735	0.0721	0.0708	0.0694	0.0681
-1.3	0.0968	0.0951	0.0934	0.0918	0.0901	0.0885	0.0869	0.0853	0.0838	0.0823
-1.2	0.1151	0.1131	0.1112	0.1093	0.1075	0.1056	0.1038	0.1020	0.1003	0.0985
-1.1	0.1357	0.1335	0.1314	0.1292	0.1271	0.1251	0.1230	0.1210	0.1190	0.1170
-1.0	0.1587	0.1562	0.1539	0.1515	0.1492	0.1469	0.1446	0.1423	0.1401	0.1379
-0.9	0.1841	0.1814	0.1788	0.1762	0.1736	0.1711	0.1685	0.1660	0.1635	0.1611
-0.8	0.2119	0.2090	0.2061	0.2033	0.2005	0.1977	0.1949	0.1922	0.1894	0.1867
-0.7	0.2420	0.2389	0.2358	0.2327	0.2296	0.2266	0.2236	0.2206	0.2177	0.2148
-0.6	0.2743	0.2709	0.2676	0.2643	0.2611	0.2578	0.2546	0.2514	0.2483	0.2451
-0.5	0.3085	0.3050	0.3015	0.2981	0.2946	0.2912	0.2877	0.2843	0.2810	0.2776
-0.4	0.3446	0.3409	0.3372	0.3336	0.3300	0.3264	0.3228	0.3192	0.3156	0.3121
-0.3	0.3821	0.3783	0.3745	0.3707	0.3669	0.3632	0.3594	0.3557	0.3520	0.3483
-0.2	0.4207	0.4168	0.4129	0.4090	0.4052	0.4013	0.3974	0.3936	0.3897	0.3859
-0.1	0.4602	0.4562	0.4522	0.4483	0.4443	0.4404	0.4364	0.4325	0.4286	0.4247
0.0	0.5000	0.4960	0.4920	0.4880	0.4840	0.4801	0.4761	0.4721	0.4681	0.4641

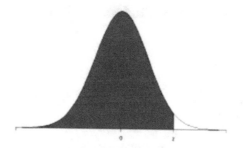

Standard Normal Probabilities for Positive Z-scores

z	0.00	0.01	0.02	0.03	0.04	0.05	0.06	0.07	0.08	0.09
0.0	0.5000	0.5040	0.5080	0.5120	0.5160	0.5199	0.5239	0.5279	0.5319	0.5359
0.1	0.5398	0.5438	0.5478	0.5517	0.5557	0.5596	0.5636	0.5675	0.5714	0.5753
0.2	0.5793	0.5832	0.5871	0.5910	0.5948	0.5987	0.6026	0.6064	0.6103	0.6141
0.3	0.6179	0.6217	0.6255	0.6293	0.6331	0.6368	0.6406	0.6443	0.6480	0.6517
0.4	0.6554	0.6591	0.6628	0.6664	0.6700	0.6736	0.6772	0.6808	0.6844	0.6879
0.5	0.6915	0.6950	0.6985	0.7019	0.7054	0.7088	0.7123	0.7157	0.7190	0.7224
0.6	0.7257	0.7291	0.7324	0.7357	0.7389	0.7422	0.7454	0.7486	0.7517	0.7549
0.7	0.7580	0.7611	0.7642	0.7673	0.7704	0.7734	0.7764	0.7794	0.7823	0.7852
0.8	0.7881	0.7910	0.7939	0.7967	0.7995	0.8023	0.8051	0.8078	0.8106	0.8133
0.9	0.8159	0.8186	0.8212	0.8238	0.8264	0.8289	0.8315	0.8340	0.8365	0.8389
1.0	0.8413	0.8438	0.8461	0.8485	0.8508	0.8531	0.8554	0.8577	0.8599	0.8621
1.1	0.8643	0.8665	0.8686	0.8708	0.8729	0.8749	0.8770	0.8790	0.8810	0.8830
1.2	0.8849	0.8869	0.8888	0.8907	0.8925	0.8944	0.8962	0.8980	0.8997	0.9015
1.3	0.9032	0.9049	0.9066	0.9082	0.9099	0.9115	0.9131	0.9147	0.9162	0.9177
1.4	0.9192	0.9207	0.9222	0.9236	0.9251	0.9265	0.9279	0.9292	0.9306	0.9319
1.5	0.9332	0.9345	0.9357	0.9370	0.9382	0.9394	0.9406	0.9418	0.9429	0.9441
1.6	0.9452	0.9463	0.9474	0.9484	0.9495	0.9505	0.9515	0.9525	0.9535	0.9645
1.7	0.9554	0.9564	0.9573	0.9582	0.9591	0.9599	0.9608	0.9616	0.9625	0.9633
1.8	0.9641	0.9649	0.9656	0.9664	0.9671	0.9678	0.9686	0.9693	0.9699	0.9706
1.9	0.9713	0.9719	0.9726	0.9732	0.9738	0.9744	0.9750	0.9756	0.9761	0.9767
2.0	0.9772	0.9778	0.9783	0.9788	0.9793	0.9798	0.9803	0.9808	0.9812	0.9817
2.1	0.9821	0.9826	0.9830	0.9834	0.9838	0.9842	0.9846	0.9850	0.9854	0.9857
2.2	0.9861	0.9864	0.9868	0.9871	0.9875	0.9878	0.9881	0.9884	0.9887	0.9890
2.3	0.9893	0.9896	0.9898	0.9901	0.9904	0.9906	0.9909	0.9911	0.9913	0.9916
2.4	0.9918	0.9920	0.9922	0.9925	0.9927	0.9929	0.9931	0.9932	0.9934	0.9936
2.5	0.9938	0.9940	0.9941	0.9943	0.9945	0.9946	0.9948	0.9949	0.9951	0.9952
2.6	0.9953	0.9955	0.9956	0.9957	0.9959	0.9960	0.9961	0.9962	0.9963	0.9964
2.7	0.9965	0.9966	0.9967	0.9968	0.9969	0.9970	0.9971	0.9972	0.9973	0.9974
2.8	0.9974	0.9975	0.9976	0.9977	0.9977	0.9978	0.9979	0.9979	0.9980	0.9981
2.9	0.9981	0.9982	0.9982	0.9983	0.9984	0.9984	0.9985	0.9985	0.9986	0.9986
3.0	0.9987	0.9987	0.9987	0.9988	0.9988	0.9989	0.9989	0.9989	0.9990	0.9990
3.1	0.9990	0.9991	0.9991	0.9991	0.9992	0.9992	0.9992	0.9992	0.9993	0.9993
3.2	0.9993	0.9993	0.9994	0.9994	0.9994	0.9994	0.9994	0.9995	0.9995	0.9995
3.3	0.9995	0.9995	0.9995	0.9996	0.9996	0.9996	0.9996	0.9996	0.9996	0.9997
3.4	0.9997	0.9997	0.9997	0.9997	0.9997	0.9997	0.9997	0.9997	0.9997	0.9998

The Student t Table

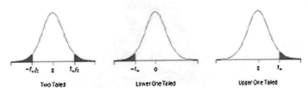

Two Tailed

Lower One Tailed

Upper One Tailed

t-distribution Critical Values

Two-tail probability	0.20	0.1	0.05	0.02	0.01
One-tail probability	0.10	0.05	0.025	0.01	0.005
df					
1	3.078	6.314	12.706	31.821	63.657
2	1.886	2.920	4.303	6.965	9.925
3	1.638	2.353	3.182	4.541	5.841
4	1.533	2.132	2.776	3.747	4.604
5	1.476	2.015	2.571	3.365	4.032
6	1.440	1.943	2.447	3.143	3.707
7	1.415	1.895	2.365	2.998	3.499
8	1.397	1.860	2.306	2.896	3.355
9	1.383	1.833	2.262	2.821	3.250
10	1.372	1.812	2.228	2.764	3.169
11	1.363	1.796	2.201	2.718	3.106
12	1.356	1.782	2.179	2.681	3.055
13	1.350	1.771	2.160	2.650	3.012
14	1.345	1.761	2.145	2.624	2.977
15	1.341	1.753	2.131	2.602	2.947
16	1.337	1.746	2.120	2.583	2.921
17	1.333	1.740	2.110	2.567	2.898
18	1.330	1.734	2.101	2.552	2.878
19	1.328	1.729	2.093	2.539	2.861
20	1.325	1.725	2.086	2.528	2.845
21	1.323	1.721	2.080	2.518	2.831
22	1.321	1.717	2.074	2.508	2.819
23	1.319	1.714	2.069	2.500	2.807
24	1.318	1.711	2.064	2.492	2.797
25	1.316	1.708	2.060	2.485	2.787
26	1.315	1.706	2.056	2.479	2.779
27	1.314	1.703	2.052	2.473	2.771
28	1.313	1.701	2.048	2.467	2.763
29	1.311	1.699	2.045	2.462	2.756
30	1.310	1.697	2.042	2.457	2.750
35	1.306	1.690	2.030	2.438	2.724
40	1.303	1.684	2.021	2.423	2.704
50	1.299	1.676	2.009	2.403	2.678
100	1.290	1.660	1.984	2.364	2.626
500	1.283	1.648	1.965	2.334	2.586
1000	1.282	1.646	1.962	2.330	2.581
∞	1.282	1.645	1.960	2.327	2.576
Confidence levels	80%	90%	95%	98%	99%

The Chi-squared Table

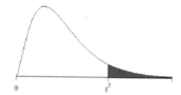

χ^2 Distribution Critical Values

df	Tail probability p						
	0.10	0.05	0.025	0.01	0.005	0.0025	0.001
1	2.71	3.84	5.02	6.63	7.88	9.14	10.83
2	4.61	5.99	7.38	9.21	10.60	11.98	13.82
3	6.25	7.81	9.35	11.34	12.84	14.32	16.27
4	7.78	9.49	11.14	13.28	14.86	16.42	18.47
5	9.24	11.07	12.83	15.09	16.75	18.39	20.52
6	10.64	12.59	14.45	16.81	18.55	20.25	22.46
7	12.02	14.07	16.01	18.48	20.28	22.04	24.32
8	13.36	15.51	17.53	20.09	21.95	23.77	26.12
9	14.68	16.92	19.02	21.67	23.59	25.46	27.88
10	15.99	18.31	20.48	23.21	25.19	27.11	29.59
11	17.28	19.68	21.92	24.72	26.76	28.73	31.26
12	18.55	21.03	23.34	26.22	28.30	30.32	32.91
13	19.81	22.36	24.74	27.69	29.82	31.88	34.53
14	21.06	23.68	26.12	29.14	31.32	33.43	36.12
15	22.31	25.00	27.49	30.58	32.80	34.95	37.70
16	23.54	26.30	28.85	32.00	34.27	36.46	39.25
17	24.77	27.59	30.19	33.41	35.72	37.95	40.79
18	25.99	28.87	31.53	34.81	37.16	39.42	42.31
19	27.20	30.14	32.85	36.19	38.58	40.88	43.82
20	28.41	31.41	34.17	37.57	40.00	42.34	45.31
21	29.62	32.67	35.48	38.93	41.40	43.78	46.80
22	30.81	33.92	36.78	40.29	42.80	45.20	48.27
23	32.01	35.17	38.08	41.64	44.18	46.62	49.73
24	33.20	36.42	39.36	42.98	45.56	48.03	51.18
25	34.38	37.65	40.65	44.31	46.93	49.44	52.62
26	35.56	38.89	41.92	45.64	48.29	50.83	54.05
27	36.74	40.11	43.19	46.96	49.64	52.22	55.48
28	37.92	41.34	44.46	48.28	50.99	53.59	56.89
29	39.09	42.56	45.72	49.59	52.34	54.97	58.30
30	40.26	43.77	46.98	50.89	53.67	56.33	59.70
40	51.81	55.76	59.34	63.69	66.77	69.70	73.40
50	63.17	67.50	71.42	76.15	79.49	82.66	86.66
60	74.40	79.08	83.30	88.38	91.95	95.34	99.61
80	96.58	101.88	106.63	112.33	116.32	120.10	124.84
100	118.50	124.34	129.56	135.81	140.17	144.29	149.45

Index

© Springer Nature Singapore Pte Ltd. 2020
S. Khan, *Meta-Analysis*, Statistics for Biology and Health,
https://doi.org/10.1007/978-981-15-5032-4

Printed in the United States
by Baker & Taylor Publisher Services